AF333006

1995
YEAR BOOK OF
OTOLARYNGOLOGY—
HEAD AND NECK SURGERY®

Statement of Purpose

The YEAR BOOK Service

The YEAR BOOK series was devised in 1901 by practicing health professionals who observed that the literature of medicine and related disciplines had become so voluminous that no one individual could read and place in perspective every potential advance in a major specialty. In the final decade of the 20th century, this recognition is more acutely true than it was in 1901.

More than merely a series of books, YEAR BOOK volumes are the tangible results of a unique service designed to accomplish the following:

- to *survey* a wide range of journals of proven value

- to *select* from those journals papers representing significant advances and statements of important clinical principles

- to provide *abstracts* of those articles that are readable, convenient summaries of their key points

- to provide *commentary* about those articles to place them in perspective

These publications grow out of a unique process that calls on the talents of outstanding authorities in clinical and fundamental disciplines, trained literature specialists, and professional writers, all supported by the resources of Mosby, the world's preeminent publisher for the health professions.

The Literature Base

Mosby subscribes to nearly 1,000 journals published worldwide, covering the full range of the health professions. On an annual basis, the publisher examines usage patterns and polls its expert authorities to add new journals to the literature base and to delete journals that are no longer useful as potential YEAR BOOK sources.

The Literature Survey

The publisher's team of literature specialists, all of whom are trained and experienced health professionals, examines every original, peer-reviewed article in each journal issue. More than 250,000 articles per year are scanned systematically, including title, text, illustrations, tables, and references. Each scan is compared, article by article, to the search strategies that the publisher has developed in consultation with the 270 outside experts who form the pool of YEAR BOOK editors. A given article may be reviewed by any number of editors, from one to a dozen or more, regardless of the discipline for which the paper was originally published. In turn, each editor who receives the article reviews it to determine whether or not the article should be included in the YEAR BOOK. This decision is based on the article's inherent quality, its probable usefulness to readers of that YEAR BOOK, and the editor's goal of representing a balanced picture of a given field in each volume of the YEAR BOOK.

In addition, the editor indicates when to include figures and tables from the article to help the YEAR BOOK reader better understand the information.

Of the quarter million articles scanned each year, only 5% are selected for detailed analysis within the YEAR BOOK series, thereby assuring readers of the high value of every selection.

The Abstract

The publisher's abstracting staff is headed by a physician-writer and includes individuals with training in the life sciences, medicine, and other areas, plus extensive experience in writing for the health professions and related industries. Each selected article is assigned to a specific writer on this abstracting staff. The abstracter, guided in many cases by notations supplied by the expert editor, writes a structured, condensed summary designed so that the reader can rapidly acquire the essential information contained in the article.

The Commentary

The YEAR BOOK editorial boards, sometimes assisted by guest commentators, write comments that place each article in perspective for the reader. This provides the reader with the equivalent of a personal consultation with a leading international authority—an opportunity to better understand the value of the article and to benefit from the authority's thought processes in assessing the article.

Additional Editorial Features

The editorial boards of each YEAR BOOK organize the abstracts and comments to provide a logical and satisfying sequence of information. To enhance the organization, editors also provide introductions to sections or individual chapters, comments linking a number of abstracts, citations to additional literature, and other features.

The published YEAR BOOK contains enhanced bibliographic citations for each selected article, including extended listings of multiple authors and identification of author affiliations. Each YEAR BOOK contains a Table of Contents specific to that year's volume. From year to year, the Table of Contents for a given YEAR BOOK will vary depending on developments within the field.

Every YEAR BOOK contains a list of the journals from which papers have been selected. This list represents a subset of the nearly 1,000 journals surveyed by the publisher and occasionally reflects a particularly pertinent article from a journal that is not surveyed on a routine basis.

Finally, each volume contains a comprehensive subject index and an index to authors of each selected paper.

The 1995 Year Book Series

Year Book of Allergy and Clinical Immunology: Drs. Rosenwasser, Borish, Gelfand, Leung, Nelson, and Szefler

Year Book of Anesthesiology and Pain Management: Drs. Tinker, Abram, Chestnut, Roizen, Rothenberg, and Wood

Year Book of Cardiology®: Drs. Schlant, Collins, Engle, Gersh, Kaplan, and Waldo

Year Book of Chiropractic: Dr. Lawrence

Year Book of Critical Care Medicine®: Drs. Parrillo, Balk, Calvin, Franklin, and Shapiro

Year Book of Dentistry®: Drs. Meskin, Berry, Currier, Kennedy, Leinfelder, Roser, and Zakariasen

Year Book of Dermatologic Surgery®: Drs. Swanson, Glogau, and Salasche

Year Book of Dermatology®: Drs. Sober and Fitzpatrick

Year Book of Diagnostic Radiology®: Drs. Federle, Clark, Gross, Latchaw, Madewell, Maynard, and Young

Year Book of Digestive Diseases®: Drs. Greenberger and Moody

Year Book of Drug Therapy®: Drs. Lasagna and Weintraub

Year Book of Emergency Medicine®: Drs. Wagner, Dronen, Davidson, King, Niemann, and Roberts

Year Book of Endocrinology®: Drs. Bagdade, Braverman, Horton, Kannan, Landsberg, Molitch, Morley, Nathan, Odell, Poehlman, Rogol, and Ryan

Year Book of Family Practice®: Drs. Berg, Bowman, Davidson, Dexter, Dietrich, and Scherger

Year Book of Geriatrics and Gerontology®: Drs. Beck, Burton, Goldstein, Reuben, Small, and Whitehouse

Year Book of Hand Surgery®: Drs. Amadio and Hentz

Year Book of Hematology®: Drs. Spivak, Bell, Ness, Quesenberry, Wiernik, and Blume

Year Book of Infectious Diseases®: Drs. Keusch, Barza, Bennish, Gelfand, Klempner, Snydman, and Skolnik

Year Book of Infertility and Reproductive Endocrinology®: Drs. Mishell, Lobo, and Sokol

Year Book of Medicine®: Drs. Bone, Cline, Epstein, Greenberger, Malawista, Mandell, O'Rourke, and Utiger

Year Book of Neonatal and Perinatal Medicine®: Drs. Fanaroff and Klaus

Year Book of Nephrology®: Drs. Coe, Favus, Henderson, Kashgarian, Luke, and Curtis

Year Book of Neurology and Neurosurgery®: Drs. Bradley and Wilkins

Year Book of Neuroradiology: Drs. Osborn, Eskridge, Grossman, Hudgens, and Ross

Year Book of Nuclear Medicine®: Drs. Gottschalk, Blaufox, McAfee, Wacker, and Zubal

Year Book of Obstetrics and Gynecology®: Drs. Mishell, Kirschbaum, and Morrow

Year Book of Occupational and Environmental Medicine®: Drs. Emmett, Frank, Gochfeld, and Hessl

Year Book of Oncology®: Drs. Simone, Bosl, Glatstein, Ozols, and Steele

Year Book of Ophthalmology®: Drs. Cohen, Adams, Augsburger, Benson, Eagle, Flanagan, Grossman, Laibson, Nelson, Rapuano, Reinecke, Sergott, Tasman, Tipperman, and Wilson

Year Book of Orthopedics®: Drs. Sledge, Cofield, Dobyns, Griffin, Poss, Springfield, Swiontkowski, Weisel, and Wilson

Year Book of Otolaryngology-Head and Neck Surgery®: Drs. Paparella and Holt

Year Book of Pain: Drs. Gebhart, Haddox, Jacox, Janjan, Marcus, Rudy, and Shapiro

Year Book of Pathology and Laboratory Medicine®: Drs. Mills, Bruns, Gaffey, and Stoler

Year Book of Pediatrics®: Dr. Stockman

Year Book of Plastic, Reconstructive, and Aesthetic Surgery: Drs. Miller, Cohen, McKinney, Robson, Ruberg, and Whitaker

Year Book of Podiatric Medicine and Surgery®: Dr. Kominsky

Year Book of Psychiatry and Applied Mental Health®: Drs. Talbott, Breier, Frances, Meltzer, Schowalter, Tasman, and Yudofsky

Year Book of Pulmonary Disease®: Drs. Bone and Petty

Year Book of Rheumatology®: Drs. Sergent, LeRoy, Meenan, Panush, and Reichlin

Year Book of Sports Medicine®: Drs. Shephard, Drinkwater, Eichner, Torg, Col. Anderson, and Mr. George

Year Book of Surgery®: Drs. Copeland, Bland, Deitch, Eberlein, Howard, Luce, Seeger, Souba, and Sugarbaker

Year Book of Thoracic and Cardiovascular Surgery®: Drs. Ginsberg, Lofland, and Wechsler

Year Book of Transplantation®: Drs. Sollinger, Eckhoff, Hullett, Knechtle, Longo, Mentzer, and Pirsch

Year Book of Ultrasound®: Drs. Merritt, Babcock, Carroll, Fagin, Finberg, and Fleischer

Year Book of Urology®: Drs. DeKernion and Howards

Year Book of Vascular Surgery®: Dr. Porter

1995

The Year Book of OTOLARYNGOLOGY— HEAD AND NECK SURGERY®

Otology

Editor

Michael M. Paparella, M.D.

Clinical Professor and Chairman Emeritus, Department of Otolaryngology, University of Minnesota; Director of Otopathology Laboratory and President, Minnesota Ear, Head, and Neck Clinic; Secretary, International Hearing Foundation

Head and Neck Surgery

Editor

G. Richard Holt, M.D., F.A.C.S.

Clinical Professor of Otolaryngology–Head and Neck Surgery, The University of Texas Health Science Center at San Antonio; Adjunct Institute Scientist, Southwest Research Institute, San Antonio

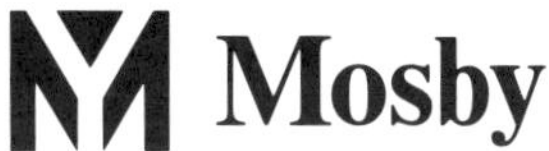

St. Louis Baltimore Boston Carlsbad Chicago Naples New York Philadelphia Portland
London Madrid Mexico City Singapore Sydney Tokyo Toronto Wiesbaden

Vice President and Publisher, Continuity Publishing: Kenneth H. Killion
Director, Editorial Development: Gretchen C. Murphy
Developmental Editor: Miranda Jackson
Acquisitions Editor: Jennifer Roche
Illustrations and Permissions Coordinator: Maureen Livengood
Manager, Continuity–EDP: Maria Nevinger
Project Manager, Editing: Tamara L. Smith
Assistant Project Supervisor: Sandra Rogers
Freelance Staff Supervisor: Barbara M. Kelly
Director, Editorial Services: Edith M. Podrazik, R.N.
Senior Information Specialist: Terri Santo, R.N.
Information Specialist: Nancy R. Dunne, R.N.
Senior Medical Writer: David A. Cramer, M.D.
Vice President, Professional Sales and Marketing: George M. Parker
Marketing Senior Manager: Eileen Lynch
Marketing Coordinator: Lynn Stevenson

1995 EDITION
Copyright © July 1995 by Mosby–Year Book, Inc.

Printed in the United States of America
Composition by Reed Technology and Information Services, Inc.
Printing/binding by Maple-Vail

Mosby–Year Book, Inc.
11830 Westline Industrial Drive
St. Louis, MO 63146
Editorial Office:
Mosby–Year Book, Inc.
200 North LaSalle Street
Chicago, IL 60601
International Standard Serial Number: 1041-892X
International Standard Book Number: 0-8151-0539-8

Table of Contents

Mosby Document Express xi
Journals Represented xiii

Otology, *edited by* MICHAEL M. PAPARELLA, M.D.

    Introduction 3

  1. VESTIBULAR FUNCTION 5

  2. HEARING AND TESTS OF HEARING 25

  3. INTERACTION OF THE MIDDLE EAR AND INNER EAR 41

  4. OTOSCLEROSIS 65

  5. FACIAL NERVE AND TUMORS 73

  6. EXTERNAL EAR, MIDDLE EAR, AND MASTOID. 95

Head and Neck Surgery, *edited by* G. RICHARD HOLT, M.D., F.A.C.S.

    Introduction 129

  7. ADVANCES IN HEAD AND NECK SURGERY RESEARCH 131

  8. RHINOLOGY AND PARANASAL SINUSES 163

  9. TRAUMA AND RECONSTRUCTIVE SURGERY 181

10. FACIAL PLASTIC SURGERY 199

11. LARYNX AND AIRWAY 217

12. HEAD AND NECK ONCOLOGY 231

13. COMPREHENSIVE OTOLARYNGOLOGY. 257

14. ENVIRONMENTAL HEALTH AND EPIDEMIOLOGY 275

    Subject Index 289

    Author Index 345

Mosby Document Express

Copies of the full text of the original source documents of articles abstracted or referenced in this publication are available by calling Mosby Document Express, toll-free, at 1 (800) 55-MOSBY.

With Mosby Document Express, you have convenient, 24-hour-a-day access to literally every article on which this publication is based. In fact, through Mosby Document Express, virtually any medical or scientific article can be located and delivered by FAX, overnight delivery service, international airmail, electronic transmission of bitmapped images (via Internet), or regular mail. The average cost of a complete, delivered copy of an article, including up to $4 in copyright clearance charges and first-class mail delivery, is $12.

For inquiries and pricing information, please call the toll-free number shown above. To expedite you order for material appearing in this publication, please be prepared with the code shown next to the bibliographic citation for each abstract.

Journals Represented

Mosby subscribes to and surveys nearly 1,000 U.S. and foreign medical and allied health journals. From these journals, the Editors select the articles to be abstracted. Journals represented in this YEAR BOOK are listed below.

Acta Oto-Laryngologica
Aesthetic Plastic Surgery
American Journal of Epidemiology
American Journal of Neuroradiology
American Journal of Otolaryngology
American Journal of Otology
American Journal of Respiratory and Critical Care Medicine
American Journal of Surgery
American Surgeon
Anesthesia and Analgesia
Annals of Allergy
Annals of Otology, Rhinology and Laryngology
Annals of the Royal College of Surgeons of England
Archives of Otolaryngology–Head and Neck Surgery
Bone Marrow Transplantation
British Journal of General Practice
British Journal of Plastic Surgery
British Medical Journal
Cancer
Cleft Palate-Craniofacial Journal
Clinical Pediatrics
ENT Journal
Head and Neck
International Journal of Cancer
International Journal of Pediatric Otorhinolaryngology
International Journal of Radiation, Oncology, Biology, and Physics
Journal of Allergy and Clinical Immunology
Journal of Applied Physiology: Respiratory, Environmental, and
    Exercise Physiology
Journal of Cranio-Maxillo-Facial Surgery
Journal of Craniofacial Surgery
Journal of Infectious Diseases
Journal of Laryngology and Otology
Journal of Long-Term Effects of Medical Implants
Journal of Neurosurgery
Journal of Nuclear Medicine
Journal of Oral and Maxillofacial Surgery
Journal of Otolaryngology
Journal of Sports Medicine and Physical Fitness
Journal of Trauma
Journal of the American Medical Association
Journal of the National Cancer Institute
Laryngoscope
Microsurgery
Neurology
New Zealand Medical Journal
ORL (Journal for Oto-Rhino-Laryngology)
Ophthalmic Plastic and Reconstructive Surgery
Otolaryngology–Head and Neck Surgery
Pediatric Infectious Disease Journal

Plastic and Reconstructive Surgery
Postgraduate Medicine
Respiratory Medicine
Scandinavian Journal of Plastic and Reconstructive Surgery and Hand Surgery
Southern Medical Journal
Surgery
Thorax
Western Journal of Medicine
World Journal of Surgery

STANDARD ABBREVIATIONS

The following terms are abbreviated in this edition: acquired immunodeficiency syndrome (AIDS), cardiopulmonary resuscitation (CPR), central nervous system (CNS), cerebrospinal fluid (CSF), computed tomography (CT), deoxyribonucleic acid (DNA), electrocardiography (ECG), health maintenance organization (HMO), human immunodeficiency virus (HIV), intensive care unit (ICU), intramuscular (IM), intravenous (IV), magnetic resonance (MR) imaging (MRI), and ribonucleic acid (RNA).

OTOLOGY

MICHAEL M. PAPARELLA, M.D.

Introduction

Biopsy vs. Modern Technology

Technology has brought us important new equipment and tools, such as MRI and CT scans, that help us diagnose and treat neurotologic and otologic diseases. At the same time, one should not lose sight of the importance of the patient's history, which will be exemplified in this introduction, or the importance of diagnosis of actual tissues in lieu of sophisticated radiologic assessment.

In the diagnosis and treatment of vestibular peripheral diseases, especially Meniere's disease, the patient's history remains paramount. Cost-effective diagnostic equipment that has been proved efficacious to date includes auditory brain stem–response (ABR) audiometry, which is less costly than MRI, to rule out a vestibular schwannoma; electronystagmography (ENG), of which the caloric test is most important in assessing vestibular hypofunction; and electrocochleography (ECoG), which adds important information regarding endolymphatic hydrops, the pathologic correlate of Meniere's disease. Other diagnostic tests, such as posturography and sinusoidal testing, which require expensive equipment and add cost to the diagnostic process, have been used and continue to be used by some practitioners. I have found these latter tests to be less relevant than ENG and ECoG in diagnosing and following up these dynamic, fluctuating diseases of the inner ear. Important diagnostic tools are the history, which I believe accounts for approximately 90% of the diagnosis of Meniere's disease in a patient, and audiometry; they remain the most important aspects of the diagnostic process.

Nobody would argue that MRI and CT have not been extremely helpful in enhancing the diagnosis of a variety of diseases in and around the temporal bone. Development and progress continue with regard to this technology, leading to improvements and enhancements in the diagnostic methods and equipment that are routinely used, such as MRI with gadolinium and CT with enhancement. Additional technologic development has led to spin-echo MR and MR angiography. These sophisticated neuroradiologic diagnostic tools, although costly, are helpful in diagnosis. Nevertheless, there is still a role for routine radiographs, which can provide a great deal of screening information. However sophisticated these neuroradiologic diagnostic tools may be, one should remember that radiology can neither be equated with nor supplant the diagnosis of pathologic tissue; too often, my colleagues and I have had a neuroradiologic interpretation of a CT scan suggesting debris or possible liquid in the middle ear cleft, only to find, at the time of surgical therapy, that a cholesteatoma is identified. The converse can also occur: The CT scan may diagnose a cholesteatoma, but at the time of surgery, granulation tissue or other pathologic conditions are identified. In this sense, in spite of sophisticated radiologic testing, every patient receiving ear surgery is, in effect, also having exploratory surgery to help identify anatomical pathologic conditions that are too often a variance with neuroradiologic findings.

Perhaps the following case will demonstrate this problem: An otolaryngologist in another state recently referred to us a patient who had a large (3-cm) "glomus jugulare" tumor diagnosed by MRI. This patient had a complete and comprehensive workup in every regard, including CT with enhancement, angiography, and embolization. According to modern-day tenets, this patient was offered an infratemporal approach with parotidectomy, rerouting of the facial nerve, and removal of deep aspects of the temporal bone. In short, the patient underwent a procedure requiring many hours in the operating room vs. an endaural exploratory procedure with removal of the lateral temporal bone and diagnosis and removal of pathologic tissue, which would have provided less chance of total removal of the tumor but, if required, could have allowed follow up by radiation therapy. This patient, seen in consultation with and treated by a competent neurosurgeon, chose to undergo total removal with the more radical approach. Even though all studies pointed to glomus jugulare with erosion of the skull base, the ultimate pathologic finding was plasmacytoma. In retrospect, this patient would have been better served by having a tissue diagnosis and by undergoing a less radical procedure followed by irradiative therapy.

There are many examples that could be cited in addition to that provided above, but it still remains true that a biopsy and diagnosis of pathologic tissue, whenever possible, will be critical to the management of patients with neurotologic disease.

Michael M. Paparella, M.D.

1 Vestibular Function

The Enlarged Vestibular Aqueduct Syndrome (EVA Syndrome)
Belenky WM, Madgy DN, Leider JS, Becker CJ, Hotaling AJ (Children's Hosp of Michigan, Detroit)
ENT J 72:746–751, 1993
130-95-1–1

Introduction.—The association of an enlarged vestibular aqueduct, in conjunction with other congenital otologic abnormalities, and sensorineural hearing loss has been recognized. A new association, the enlarged vestibular aqueduct (EVA) syndrome, consisting of an enlarged vestibular aqueduct, sensorineural hearing loss, and round window abnormalities, was described.

Patients.—Between 1988 and 1990, 3 males and 5 females, aged 1 to 5 years, with sensorineural hearing loss, were found to have unilateral or bilateral enlarged vestibular aqueducts on CT. In 6 evaluable patients, sensorineural hearing loss was mild-to-profound in a typical downsloping pattern.

Clinical Course.—During a prospective follow-up of 1 to 54 months, serial audiograms showed that 10 ears remained stable with no fluctuation or progression of hearing loss. Two ears had a fluctuating hearing level, 1 showed progressive loss, and another had sudden precipitous loss of hearing after mild head trauma. All 4 ears were explored, and round window abnormalities were documented in all 4 with a perilymphatic fistula in 1 ear. The round window abnormalities included enlarged diameters, anteriolateral placement with little anterior overhang, bipartite round window, absence of otic capsule development in the inferior posterior aspect of the window, absence of an apparent round window membrane, and a completely anomalous failure of development of the otic capsule in the round window area. In all 4 ears, obliteration of the round window was performed using free mucosal and fascial grafts after scarification of the mucosa. Postoperative follow-up revealed stabilization of hearing in 3 ears evaluated at 6 months to 1 year.

Implications.—All children with sensorineural hearing loss should undergo extensive evaluation to determine etiology of the loss, including CT scan of the temporal bone. The presence of an enlarged aqueduct should prompt consideration of the presence of a round window abnormality and the potential for predisposition to perilymph fistula.

▶ These authors describe a relationship between an enlarged vestibular aqueduct, sensorineural hearing loss, and the possibility of a perilymphatic fistula. An enlarged vestibular aqueduct can be a part of a variety of abnormalities of the inner ear; chief among these, most likely, is Mondini's dysplasia. If the vestibular aqueduct is enlarged, this (in and of itself) should not participate in the pathogenesis of a perilymphatic fistula, which relates to perilymph, not endolymph; the latter is processed via the vestibular aqueduct. This relationship is of interest. The authors are to be complimented for making this connection, but to identify this as a syndrome would, I think, be erroneous. These findings are nevertheless worth noting. Indeed, if there were a syndrome relating hearing loss and perilymphatic fistula, one would look to a patent modiolus or a patent cochlear aqueduct rather than an enlarged vestibular aqueduct.—M.M. Paparella, M.D.

Air Caloric Test With Continuous Thermal Change

Itaya T, Kitahara M (Shiga Univ of Med Science, Seta, Otsu, Japan)
Acta Otolaryngol S510:43–47, 1994   130-95-1–2

Objective.—The caloric test has several disadvantages, including nausea and vomiting, even with weak stimulation and occurrence of vestibular recruitment. A new caloric test was described for vestibular testing with an air caloric stimulator.

Technique.—An air caloric stimulator is connected to a computer, which regulates the air temperature (Fig 1–1). The nozzle of the stimulator is fixed in the ear 20 mm from the tragus, and the airflow is 6 L/min. Initially, air is passed into the external air meatus for 90 seconds at 37°C, and the air temperature is gradually decreased until nystagmus occurs. Nystagmus is observed under a Frenzel lens.

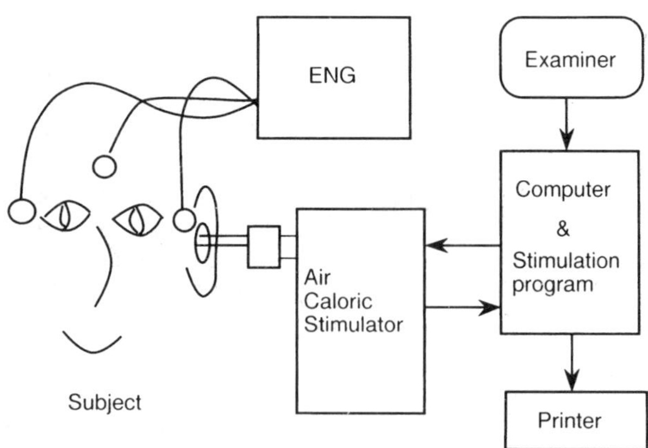

Fig 1–1.—Diagram of the vestibular testing system. Air temperature was controlled with a computer, and the temperature and time at which nystagmus occurred and the time when nystagmus stopped were recorded. The subject's eye movements were recorded by electronystagmography (ENG) during the test. (Courtesy of Itaya T, Kitahara M: *Acta Otolaryngol* S510:43–47, 1994.)

Results.—In a pilot study, the air caloric test with continuous thermal change was performed at 6 different rates of decrease: .01, .03, .05, .1, .15, and .2°C/seconds. The temperatures at which nystagmus occurred were 34.2°C, 33.1°C, 31.4°C, 28.5°C, 26.4°C, and 23.1°C, respectively. There was a linear relationship between the rate of decrease in air temperature and the temperature at which nystagmus occurred. The rate of .05°C/sec gave the smallest standard deviation for temperature threshold in normal subjects. When applied to 30 normal individuals, the temperature at which nystagmus occurred was 31.44°C, the duration of nystagmus was 77.3 seconds, and the maximum speed of the slow component of nystagmus was 2.2°C/sec. The mean interaural differences in temperature and in time when nystagmus occurred were −1.8 ±5.76, and the range of 2 SDs was less than 13%. This deviation had the narrowest normal limits when compared with other ordinary caloric tests by the coefficient of variation. There was no discomfort observed when the temperature decrease was .05°C/sec.

Conclusion.—The new air caloric test using thermal change may replace earlier caloric tests to obtain the nystagmus threshold. The temperature and time when nystagmus occurs are useful parameters to evaluate vestibular function.

▶ The air caloric test described by Itaya and Kitahara is interesting and should be tried by others. It makes sense, and perhaps it works. We would also like to try it. We have used air caloric tests for many years and have helped design the initial commercially available device. Air caloric stimulation can be used not only for Meniere's disease and other vestibular problems, but also for all forms of disease, even if there are pathologic conditions in the middle ear, such as a perforation of the tympanic membrane.—M.M. Paparella, M.D.

Vestibular Autorotation and Electronystagmography Testing in Patients With Dizziness

Murphy TP (Atlanta, Ga)
Am J Otol 15:502–505, 1994   130-95-1–3

Background.—Evaluation of the patient who has dizziness should include a thorough history, physical, and audiogram. However, when a patient's history does not provide a definitive etiology for dizziness, vestibular testing, such as electronystagmography (ENG), posturography, and evaluation of the vestibulo-ocular reflexes (VOR) may also be required. Vestibulo-ocular testing may be performed with sinusoidal harmonic acceleration, pseudorandom testing, high-frequency rotational chair testing, and vestibular autorotation testing (VAT). The efficacy of ENG and VAT in the initial evaluation of the patient with dizzinesss was studied, and reports were presented with regard to which symptoms or diagnoses might be best suited to each method of testing.

Method.—One hundred twenty patients with vestibular dysfunction were evaluated with ENG and VAT. Eighteen patients were unable to complete the VAT, largely because of difficulties with the vertical head-shake; they were excluded from the study. The 102 patients who completed both ENG and VAT were compared.

Results.—Forty-eight of 102 patients had abnormal ENG and VAT; of these, 17 had Meniere's disease. Twenty-two of the 102 patients had an abnormal ENG and a normal VAT; 9 of these patients had Meniere's disease, and 2 had acoustic neuromas. Twenty of the 102 patients had an abnormal VAT and a normal ENG. Of these, 4 had diagnoses that were clearly peripheral in origin; 3 had Meniere's disease, and 1 had a petrous apex cholesterol granuloma. Six patients had dizziness secondary to trauma, and the diagnosis of dizziness was made in 8 because nothing more definite could be assigned. In 12 of the 102 patients, both ENG and VAT were normal. Of these 3 patients with dizziness of peripheral origin, 2 had Meniere's disease and 1 had benign positional vertigo.

Conclusion.—Both ENG and VAT were found to provide valuable but different insights into dizziness. Electronystagmography has the highest yield and allows for the identification of dizziness thought to be of peripheral origin, but it may not give information regarding the brain's compensation for this dysfunction. Vestibular autorotation testing provides a broader, nonspecific test that examines the vestibulo-ocular reflexes, including the labyrinthine, brain stem, and oculomotor system. It also provides information regarding the body's ability to compensate for dizziness, but it does not permit identification of the site or side of the injury. The 2 tests may complement each other in examining difficult vestibular problems to assess the site of lesion and the extent of compensation for the dizziness.

▶ The VAT and ENG tests were assessed by Murphy, and his conclusions appear to be practical and useful. He notes that ENG is best for initial evaluation and that perhaps the most important aspect of ENG testing is its ability to determine the presence or absence of vestibular hypofunction by caloric stimulation. As indicated, patients who have had head trauma might be assessed with the VAT.—M.M. Paparella, M.D.

Study on Experimental Motion Sickness in Children
Takahashi M, Toriyabe I, Takei Y, Kanzaki J (Yamaguchi Univ School of Medicine, Japan; Keio Univ School of Medicine, Tokyo)
Acta Otolaryngol 114:231–237, 1994   130-95-1–4

Background.—Motion sickness may be induced by disorders of spatial orientation. Ataxia results from regulation based on erroneous orientation, and autonomic nervous symptoms are generated to alert a host against loss of spatial orientation. The relationship between autonomic

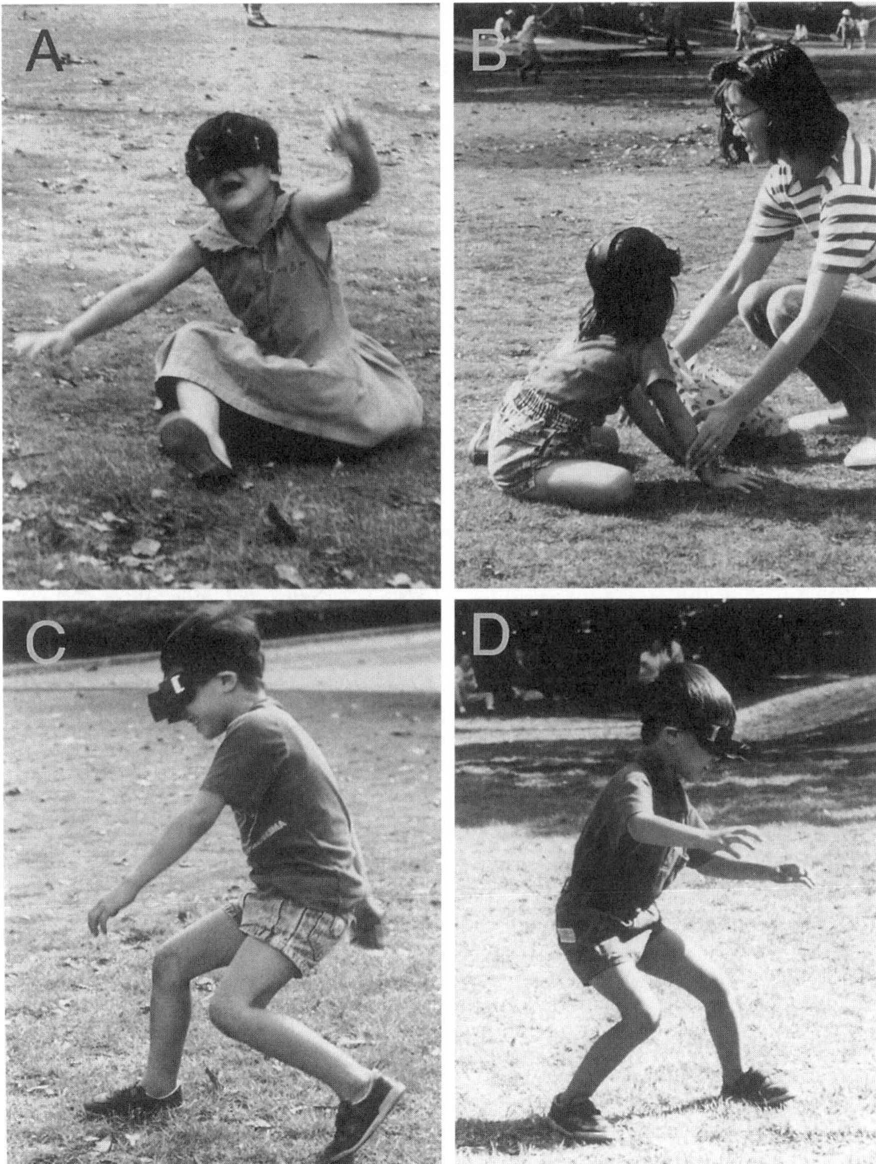

Fig 1–2.—Snapshots of subjects while wearing horizontally reversing prisms. Unpredictable falling of a 5-year-old girl (**A**), inability of a 4-year-old girl to stand up after falling (**B**), drunken gait in a 6-year-old boy (**C**), and frozen posture with a wide stance in a 4-year-old boy (**D**), (Courtesy of Takahashi M, Toriyabe I, Takei Y, et al: *Acta Otolaryngol* 114:231–237, 1994.)

nervous symptoms and instability may therefore change during growth in childhood.

Methods.—Ninety children, aged 4 to 15 years, were studied. Autonomic nervous symptoms and instability were evoked by having the children walk while wearing horizontally reversing goggles (Fig 1–2).

Findings.—Headache was the only autonomic nervous symptom evident in kindergarten children. In elementary school children, the frequency and severity of sickness increased gradually with age, whereas the frequency of headache decreased. The nausea syndrome commonly occurred in older elementary and junior high school students.

Conclusion.—The frequency and severity of sickness increased gradually during growth, whereas the severity of gait disorder became milder with increasing age. Thus, functions perceiving spatial orientation and action disorder are probably immature in young children. Once spatial orientation is impaired, instability becomes very severe, because no alarm function against disorientation stops insufficient control.

▶ The vestibular system is older, both embryologically and phylogenetically, than the cochlear labyrinthine system. It is amazing how many children and adults have motion sickness and how few studies are available that have addressed this common problem. The authors evaluate this problem in an innovative way, and it is hoped that others will attempt to explain the pathogenesis of motion sickness to us clinicians.—M.M. Paparella, M.D.

Vestibulopathy Induced by High Impact Aerobics. A New Syndrome: Discussion of 30 Cases
Weintraub MI (New York Medical College, Valhalla)
J Sports Med Phys Fitness 34:56–63, 1994   130-95-1–5

Introduction.—High-impact aerobic exercises are becoming an increasingly popular means of promoting cardiovascular fitness, but they may entail a risk of injury to the otoliths and cochlea, possibly producing vertigo, tinnitus, loss of balance, and impaired hearing.

Study Population.—The risk that repeated jarring will injure the inner ear structures was examined in 30 generally healthy women who had become symptomatic in conjunction with high-impact aerobic exercise. However, the participants had no specific lesions on CT or MRI that could explain the symptoms. In addition, they had not used ototoxic drugs or had ear infections. The subjects, who had a mean age of 35 years, included 12 instructors and 18 enthusiasts. The control group included 144 individuals who had exercised similarly but had not become symptomatic.

Findings.—Twenty-four of the 30 symptomatic individuals described vertigo, dizziness, and imbalance. Twenty reported tinnitus and muffling. Neurologic abnormalities were present in all but 4 of the 30 subjects.

Seventeen of 30 patients had positive findings during the Barany hanging-head maneuver, experiencing their specific symptoms. Sixty percent of subjects and 4% of controls were abnormally sensitive to barometric pressure and car travel. A typical 6,000-Hz hearing loss with "notching" was observed in 73% of the symptomatic group.

Implications.—High-intensity aerobic exercise is capable of injuring the cochlear-vestibular apparatus to an extent that may interfere with daily activities. Possible preventive measures include reducing exposure to noise, using better-insulated shoes, and performing stair or step exercises instead.

▶ This interesting study appeared in the *Journal of Sports Medicine and Physical Fitness*. Certainly aerobic exercise is a widespread craze, involving many males and females. This study suggests that there is involvement of the otolithic structures and, possibly, the organ of Corti during such exercise. A similar study should be undertaken in animal laboratories, which I think would provide a good corollary to this possibility occurring in humans.—M.M. Paparella, M.D.

Transdermal Scopolamine for the Reduction of Postoperative Nausea in Outpatient Ear Surgery: A Double-Blind, Randomized Study
Reinhart DJ, Klein KW, Schroff E (Univ of Utah, Ogden; Univ of Texas, Dallas)
Anesth Analg 79:281–284, 1994   130-95-1–6

Introduction.—Postoperative nausea, vomiting, and dizziness are common after outpatient middle ear surgery. In a double-blind, placebo-controlled study, it was determined whether these symptoms could be reduced by preoperative application of transdermal scopolamine, an agent that has successfully reduced postoperative nausea under various conditions.

Methods.—Eligible patients who were aged 18–65 years were scheduled for outpatient exploratory tympanotomy, mastoidectomy, or endolymphatic sac and oval and round window surgery. Two hours before surgery, 19 patients were randomly assigned to receive a transdermal patch containing scopolamine and 20, a placebo patch. The patches were placed behind the nonsurgical ear. An observer who was blind to patch composition recorded the incidence of nausea, vomiting, the length of stay in the postanesthesia care unit (PACU) and day surgery unit (DSU), and discharge time. Patients were given acetaminophen with codeine tablets to take every 4 hours as needed for pain relief. They also received a form to complete at home and were called 24 hours after discharge.

Results.—Thirty-two patients, 16 in each group, completed the study. The active treatment and placebo groups were similar in age, American Society of Anesthesiologists classification, baseline medical history, hours of patch placement before the end of surgery, type of procedure, and duration of surgery. They showed no significant differences in amount of time spent in the PACU or DSU, or the total postoperative time in the hospital. Nausea and vomiting during the hospital stay were similar for the scopolamine and placebo groups. After discharge, however, nausea was more common in the placebo group (62% of patients) than in the active patch group (31%). The active patch group also had a significantly lower incidence of vertigo after discharge (6.2% vs. 25%). Dry mouth was reported by 56% of the active patch group and 25% of the placebo patch group.

Conclusion.—Transdermal scopolamine reduces, but does not eliminate, the number of episodes of postoperative nausea, vomiting, and vertigo in outpatients undergoing middle ear surgery. The drug crosses the blood-brain barrier, blocking cholinergic stimulation of the emetic center from the gastrointestinal tract and the vestibular center.

▶ Our anesthesiologists routinely use transdermal scopolamine patches postoperatively, as was done in this study. Unfortunately, this medication and its system of delivery are not available because of a manufacturing deficiency at the present. This study, which appeared in an anesthesiology journal, is of interest and does suggest that there is some effect in reducing, but certainly not in eliminating, postoperative nausea and vomiting. The study does not control for diseases of the inner ear/vestibule or for relationships to other diseases that do not have a vestibular component.—M.M. Paparella, M.D.

Outcome of Sudden Deafness With and Without Vertigo
Nakashima T, Yanagita N (Nagoya Univ, Japan)
Laryngoscope 103:1145–1149, 1993   130-95-1-7

Objective.—Patients who experienced unilateral sudden deafness were reviewed to determine the clinical significance of vertigo and hearing loss. Several studies have reported that hearing recovery in sudden deafness is worse in patients with vertigo than in those without vertigo.

Patients and Methods.—Between 1972 and 1990, 1,313 patients were seen within 2 weeks after the onset of unilateral sudden deafness of unknown cause. The average age of the patients was 39.7 years. The shapes of their audiograms were classified as high-tone hearing loss, low-tone hearing loss, flat-type, profound loss, or other. Patients with high-tone hearing loss had an average loss between 4 and 8 kHz, and those with low-tone hearing loss had an average loss between .25 and .5 kHz. The proportion of cases with vertigo was calculated for each group.

Results.—Vertigo was present in 29.9% of the patients. The average age of the patients with vertigo was significantly lower than that of those without vertigo. Vertigo occurred most often in patients with profound deafness (74.2%), followed by patients with high-tone hearing loss (48.8%). The proportion of patients with these 2 types of audiograms was higher in patients aged 14 years or younger. Men and women did not differ significantly in audiogram distribution, although the percentage of profound loss was slightly higher in women. Even when initial hearing loss was the same, hearing recovery of high-tone frequencies was worse in patients with vertigo. Among patients with profound hearing loss, the initial and final hearing levels of those with vertigo were more impaired than the levels of patients without vertigo in all 6 frequencies.

Conclusion.—Anatomical factors may account for the close relationship between vertigo in sudden deafness and hearing loss in the high-tone frequencies. The cochlear basal turn in such cases is more proximal to the vestibular apparatus than the upper turn that receives low-frequency sounds. The increased incidence of profound sudden deafness in patients 14 years or younger may result from subclinical mumps.

▶ It is important to assess historical events in labyrinthine disease, including the problem of sudden deafness. This study is remarkable in that it has such a huge patient population—1,313 patients—accumulated during a period of only 18 years. The study suggests that recovery of hearing was worse in patients with vertigo than in those without vertigo. The authors attempt to provide a hypothetical explanation of pathogenesis.—M.M. Paparella, M.D.

Surgical Anatomy of the Endolymphatic Sac
Bagger-Sjöbäck D (Karolinska Inst, Stockholm)
Am J Otol 14:576–579, 1993   130-95-1–8

Background.—The majority of surgical procedures done to relieve vertigo belong to the destructive category. Endolymphatic sac-mastoid shunting is a relatively harmless and nondestructive procedure, but its success depends on the identification and penetration of the endolymphatic sac lumen.

Methods.—Ten human temporal bones were studied to define the fine structural anatomy and relationships of the endolymphatic duct and sac. The extratemporal extension of the endolymphatic sac was studied in 29 other specimens.

Findings.—The human emdolymphatic sac is formed by the union of the saccular duct and the utricular duct a distance away from the vestibule. The proximal endolymphatic duct tapers to its narrowest portion within the vestibular aqueduct and widens again to gradually transform into the proximal endolymphatic sac. The widest portion of the sac, the intermediate or rugose portion, is situated in the distal part of the vestibular aqueduct. In this portion, a majority of cases demonstrate a clear extraosseous extension of the sac but with varied appearance. Its single lumen may be replaced by confluent lumina with a parallel orientation,

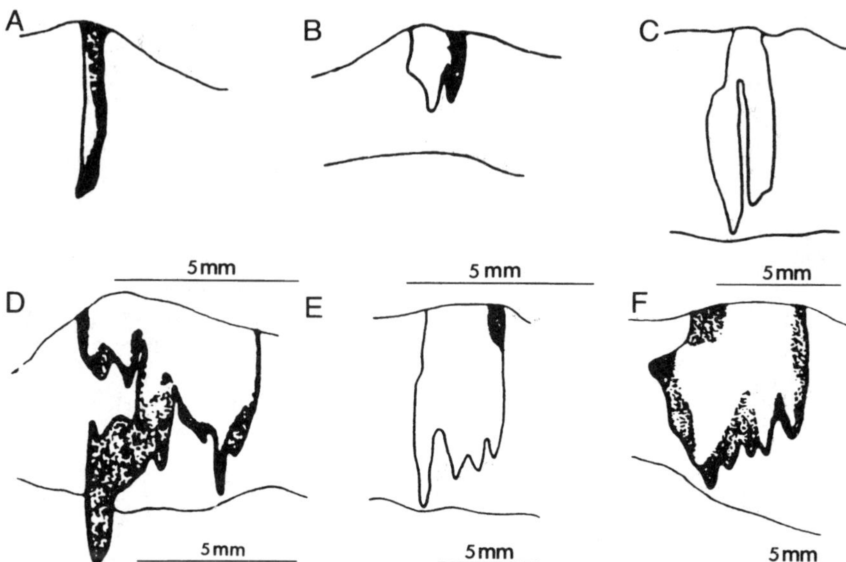

Fig 1–3.—Examples of graphic reconstruction of the extratemporal portion of the human endolymphatic sac. The *upper horizontal line* represents the opening of the vestibular aqueduct. The *lower horizontal line* represents the anterior margin of the sigmoid sinus. The *unfilled area* in the sacs represents a confluent lumen, and the *dotted areas* represent the portion of the sac that is made up of parallel epithelial tubules. Note the large variation in size. Although the sac in **A** has an area of approximately 2 mm^2, the largest specimen in **F** covers approximately 35 mm^2. (Courtesy of Bagger-Sjöbäck D: *Am J Otol* 14:576–579, 1993.)

thereby producing a single lumen, a single lumen divided at places by thin fibrous strands, a single lumen surrounded by small tubules, or a tubular appearance (Fig 1–3, A–F). The distal portion of the sac in the dura mater outside the temporal bone usually presents as a system of parallel tubules. In 2 cases, no extraosseous extension of the endolymphatic sac is evident, indicating that the entire sac must be confined to the lumen of the vestibular aqueduct. In the same individual, it is also common to have some differences in the 2 sides.

Implication.—There is a large interindividual variety in the size and shape of the human endolymphatic sac. Most studies report a success rate of 60% to 70% with endolymphatic sac surgery. It is possible that, in the remaining 30% to 40%, the surgeon has not actually approached the endolymphatic sac because of the considerable individual variation of the human endolymphatic sac.

▶ This is an excellent study of the surgical anatomy of the endolymphatic sac. The author indicates that it is essential to identify the lumen of the sac to obtain an efficacious result. This may not always be the case. By decompressing the dura, one may also allow for nanoliters of endolymph to diffuse to even a hypoplastic sac. Nevertheless, this is an important study that provides us with useful information regarding surgical anatomical factors.—M.M. Paparella, M.D.

Absorption Activity and Barrier Properties in the Endolymphatic Sac: Ultrastructural and Morphometric Analysis
Hoshikawa H, Furuta H, Mori N, Sakai S-I (Kagawa Med School, Japan)
Acta Otolaryngol 114:40–47, 1994   130-95-1–9

Introduction.—The endolymphatic sac plays a major role in maintaining homeostasis in the inner ear. It is believed that the endolymphatic sac absorbs macromolecules, but studies of its absorptive activity and barrier characteristics have been limited. Recently, a technique to inject materials directly into the endolymphatic sac lumen was developed.

Method.—Using the microelectrode insertion procedure, a constant volume of horseradish peroxidase (HRP) was injected directly into the endolymphatic sac lumen of the guinea pig (Fig 1-4). Ultrastructural and morphometric methods were used to analyze the reaction products at 1 to 10 hours after the tracer injection. For control purposes, a glass microelectrode filled with Tris buffer was inserted into the endolymphatic sac on the opposite side.

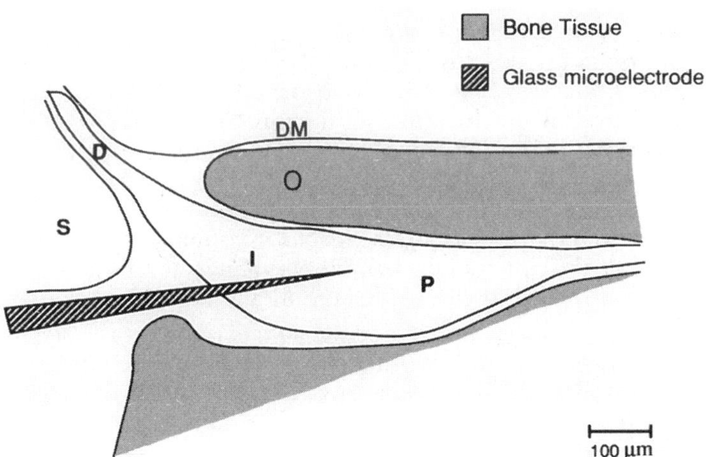

Fig 1–4.—Schematic view of the procedure for injection of horseradish peroxidase (HRP) into the endolymphatic sac (ES) lumen. First, the sigmoid sinus is detached medially from the medial surface of the temporal bone until the operculum is seen. Next, a microelectrode filled with HRP is inserted into the lumen of the intermediate portion of the ES, and a positive direct current is recorded. While monitoring this potential, the electrode is inserted 200–200 μm further, in the direction of the vestibular aqueduct. With this insertion procedure, the tip of the electrode is expected to locate near the portion between the intermediate and proximal portions. The HRP is injected into the ES lumen by electrophoresis without mechanical force. *Abbreviations: D* represents the distal portion of the ES; *DM*, dura mater; *I*, intermediate portion of the ES; *O*, operculum; *P*, proximal portion of the ES; *S*, sigmoid sinus. (Courtesy of Hoshikawa H, Furuta H, Mori N, et al: *Acta Otolaryngol* 114:40-47, 1994.)

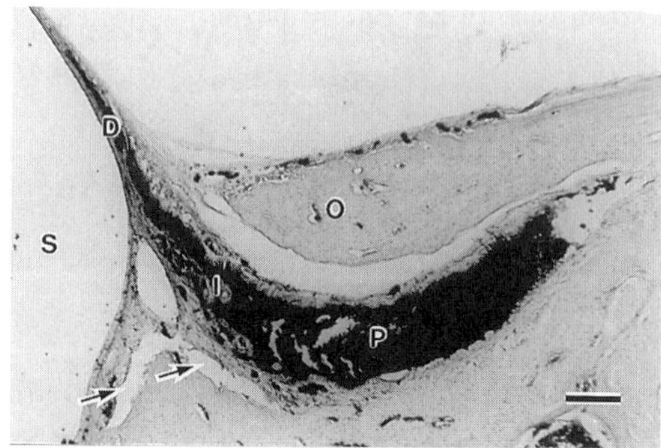

Fig 1–5.—Light micrograph of the endolymphatic sac (ES) of the guinea pig 15 minutes after the injection of horseradish peroxidase (HRP). The reaction spreads from the proximal portion of the distal portion of the ES. The sigmoid sinus and the intermediate portion of the ES are detached from the temporal bone (*arrows*). D represents the distal portion of the ES; *I*, intermediate portion of the ES; O, operculum; *P*, proximal portion of the ES; *S*, sigmoid sinus. Magnification, ×90. *Bar* = .1 mm. (Courtesy of Hoshikawa H, Furuta H, Mori N, et al: *Acta Otolaryngol* 114:40–47, 1994.)

Findings.—Fifteen minutes after the injection of HRP, the intraluminal HRP diffused steadily from the proximal to the distal portion of the sac (Fig 1–5); no staining was observed in the controls. In the proximal portion of the endolymphatic sac, the epithelial cells did not absorb the intraluminal HRP at any intervals after the tracer injection. In the intermediate portion, the epithelial cells were classified into 2 distinct types based on their absorption activity. The active-absorptive cells reached maximal uptake 8 hours after the tracer injection and then decreased. The nonactive cells scarcely absorbed the tracer, suggesting that these cells were not involved in the macromolecular absorption. In the distal portion of the endolymphatic sac, the absorption activity was significantly lower than that of the active-absorptive cells in the intermediate portion at 1 to 8 hours after HRP injection, but it was significantly higher at 10 hours after the injection. No intraluminal HRP permeated either beyond the junctional complexes between epithelial cells or through the cytoplasm of the epithelium in any portion of the endolymphatic sac.

Implications.—Both the intermediate portion of the endolymphatic sac and the distal portion may play an active role in the macromolecular absorption. It is possible that there is a tight barrier to the intraluminal macromolecules in the epithelial linings of the sac.

▶ This very good, basic study gives us more stereometric information concerning the absorptive capacity of the endolymphatic sac. It suggests that the intermediate portion and the distal portion may play an active role in macromolecular absorption. It also allows us to better understand the physiology of the normal endolymphatic sac and, therefore, to have, eventually, more insight into possible clinical management.—M.M. Paparella, M.D.

Particulate Matter Within the Membranous Labyrinth: Pathologic or Normal?

Kveton JF, Kashgarian M (Yale Univ, New Haven, Conn)
Am J Otol 15:173–176, 1994   130-95-1-10

Background.—Particulate matter identified in the membranous part of the posterior semicircular canal may be responsible for the development of positional vertigo. The presence of particles in the endolymphatic space was investigated in patients with no initial complaints of positional vertigo.

Methods and Findings.—Particulate matter in the endolymphatic space was found in 9 of 10 patients undergoing the translabyrinthine approach for acoustic neuroma removal. None of these patients had a primary complaint of positional vertigo, although 7 described occasional imbalance, 1 had a 2-year history of mild positional vertigo, 1 had recurrent vertigo, and 1 had an isolated episode of true vertigo years before tumor was diagnosed. The tumors ranged in size from 6 to 33 mm. In the specimen adequate for thorough assessment with transmission electron microscopy, granular particles of various electron-density characteristics of partially mineralized protein were identified in the lumen of the membranous labyrinth (Fig 1–6). Particles with a rhomboid configura-

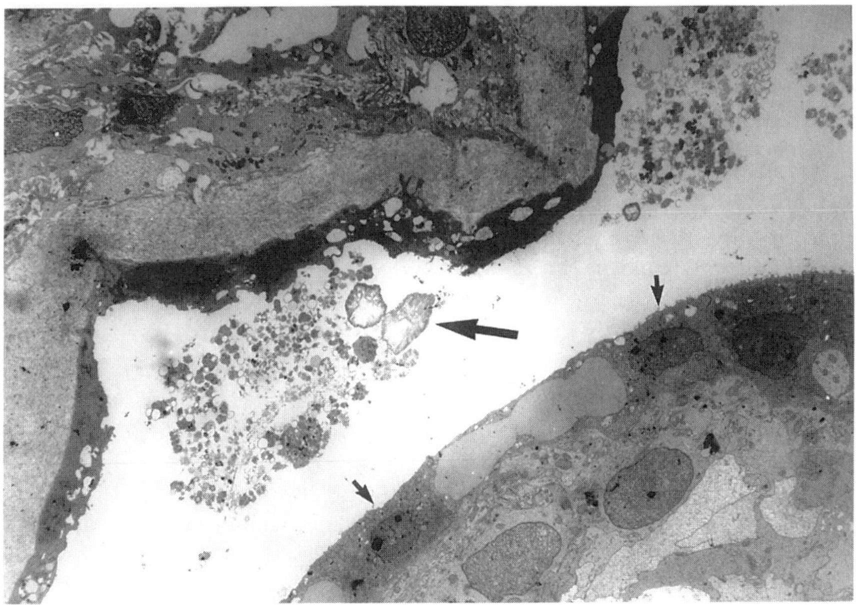

Fig 1–6.—Low-power transmission electron micrograph of the nonampullary portion of the membranous labyrinth of the posterior semicircular canal. Granular densities (*large arrow*) are evident within the lumen, and low cuboidal epithelium lines the lumen (*small arrows*). (Courtesy of Kveton JF, Kashgarian M: *Am J Otol* 15:173–176, 1994.)

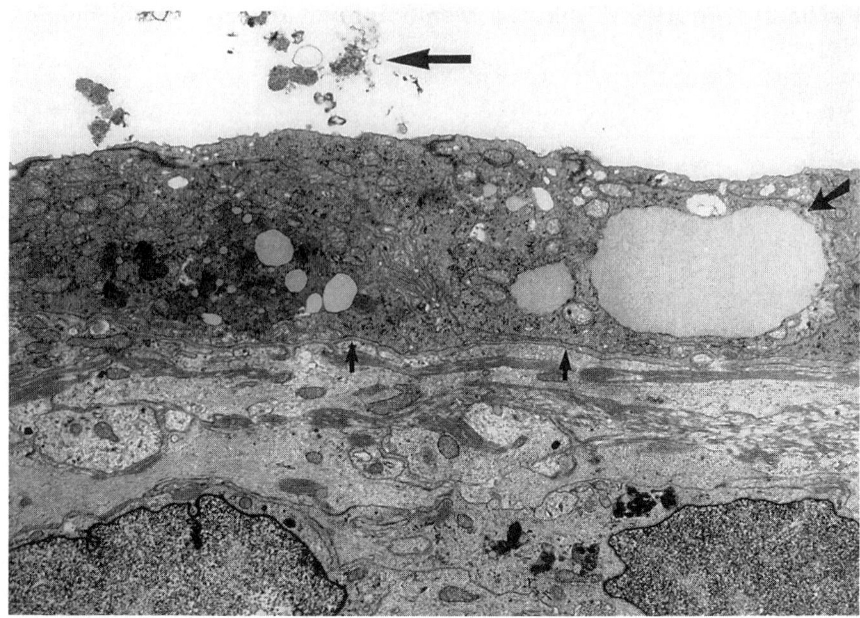

Fig 1–7.—Higher-power photomicrograph shows granular densities (*large arrow*). Irregular vacuoles are within the lumen epithelium (*medium arrow*). The basement membrane separates the epithelium from supporting cells (*small arrows*). (Courtesy of Kveton JF, Kashgarian M: *Am J Otol* 15:173–176, 1994.)

tion were thought to represent degenerating otoconia, fragments of apoptotic cells, or mineralized secreted protein extruded into the lumen (Fig 1-7). The labyrinthine epithelium consisted of a single layer of cuboidal cells with abundant mitochondria and microvilli similar to epithelial cells of the spiral prominence. Large irregular vacuoles containing lipid or moderately electron-dense material consistent with protein were noted in the cytoplasm (Fig 1-8).

Conclusion.—Electron microscopy demonstrated particles in the membranous labyrinth that seemed to be of mixed proteinaceous and mineral content. Further research is needed before the theory of endolymphatic particle migration can be confirmed as the cause of positional vertigo.

▶ These authors were able to fenestrate the posterior semicircular canal and identify particulate matter in the membranous labyrinth, which is quite an accomplishment. They achieved this in patients who underwent removal of acoustic tumors, most of whom did not have positional vertigo preoperatively. It would have been more effective to study this problem in the temporal bones of patients who had acoustic tumors; surgical intervention may create a possible contaminating factor. Although cupulolithiasis remains an attractive theory to explain benign postural vertigo, many questions never-

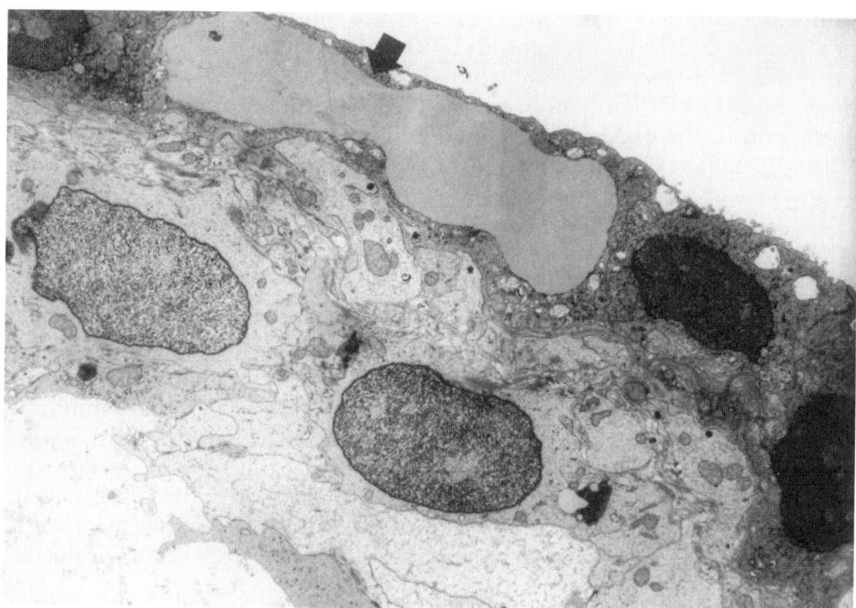

Fig 1–8.—High-power photomicrograph. A large irregular vacuole (*arrow*) containing either lipid or protein close to the lumen. The significance of this structure is unknown. (Courtesy of Kveton JF, Kashgarian M: *Am J Otol* 15:173–176, 1994.)

theless remain regarding the pathophysiology and pathogenesis of this all-too-common problem.—M.M. Paparella, M.D.

Immunological Approach to Ménière's Disease: Vestibular Immune Injury Following Immune Reaction of the Endolymphatic Sac

Tomiyama S, Nonaka M, Gotoh Y, Ikezono T, Yagi T (Nippon Med School, Tokyo)

ORL J Otorhinolaryngol Relat Spec 56:11–18, 1994   130-95-1-11

Introduction.—The endolymphatic sac is the only site in the inner ear that contains immunocompetent cells and secretory IgA, suggesting a role for the sac in the immunodefense of the inner ear. Dysfunction of the sac may be one cause of Meniere's disease. The pathophysiology of immune injury of the vestibule and its relation to the inner ear immune response after direct antigen challenge to the sac were studied.

Methods.—Experiments were done using female Hartley guinea pigs. The relation of caloric tests results and spontaneous nystagmus to the histologic changes of the sensory epithelium of the vestibular organ and perilymph antibody levels were investigated after direct antigen challenge to the sac. Keyhole limpet hemocyanin (KLH) in an associated form, diluted in phosphate-buffered saline (pH, 6.4), was used. The caloric reaction was examined on days 1, 7, 14, 21, 28, and 35, after KLH inoculation to the sac. The onset and duration of spontaneous nystagmus were observed at 8-hour intervals from days 0 to 7 and at 1-hour intervals from days 0 to 2. Perilymph, serum, and temporal bone were harvested at the end of the experiments for histologic study.

Results.—In a secondary KLH challenge to the sac, irritative nystagmus was followed by paralytic nystagmus and a suppression of caloric reaction. Good correlation was observed between these findings and the degree of degeneration of the sensory epithelium of the vestibular organ and the levels of perilymph antibody. Vestibular function was not disturbed by phosphate-buffered saline inoculation, primary KLH challenge to the sac, or by a secondary KLH challenge to the intradural space.

Conclusion.—The physiologic changes of the vestibular organ appear to be derived from the secondary immune reaction of the endolymphatic sac. These results were confirmed by histologic investigation and assessment of perilymph anti-KLH antibody levels. In this animal model, evidence suggested that the immune response to soluble foreign proteins in the sac leads to a disorder of vestibular function resembling Meniere's disease. This suggests that the immune response of the sac may hold the key to the pathogenesis of this disorder.

▶ This study by Tomiyama and colleagues makes the intriguing suggestion that the immune response of the sac may possibly be an important key to the pathogenesis of Meniere's disease. I would agree. It is my opinion, on the basis of observations in both laboratory and clinic, that the endolymphatic sac and duct play a role in physical obstruction leading to endolymphatic malabsorption, and that there can also be a chemical factor including not only factors of relationships of osmotic pressure but, also, immune factors, as suggested by this study.—M.M. Paparella, M.D.

Diuretic and Diet Effect on Menière's Disease Evaluated by the 1985 Committee on Hearing and Equilibrium Guidelines
Santos PM, Hall RA, Snyder JM, Hughes LF, Dobie RA (Southern Illinois Univ, Springfield; Palm Springs, Calif; Univ of Washington, Seattle; et al)
Otolaryngol Head Neck Surg 109:680–689, 1993   130-95-1–12

Objective.—Fifty-four patients with Meniere's disease who were treated with diuretics and a low-salt diet were studied retrospectively, using the most recent recommendations of the 1985 Committee on Hearing and Equilibrium (CHE) of the American Academy of Otolaryngology–Head and Neck Surgery for vertigo and hearing changes. In addition, treatment results were evaluated using other methods to determine the usefulness of the 1985 CHE guidelines.

Methods.—The first method of vertigo evaluation, which used the 1985 CHE guidelines, specified the ratio of post-treatment vertigo frequency and pretreatment vertigo frequency. The second method calculated the difference of pretreatment vertigo frequency from post-treatment vertigo frequency. The third method compared raw data at different times before and during medical therapy. Hearing level assessment evaluated the pure-tone thresholds decibel (dB) hearing level and word discrimination scores. Different puretone averages were evaluated.

Results.—After 24 months of therapy, 79% of patients achieved complete or substantial control of vertigo, 19% achieved limited or insignificant control, and 2% became worse based on the 1985 CHE guidelines. Hearing improved in 35% of patients, remained unchanged in 29%, became worse in 22%, and could not be classified by CHE guidelines in 14%. Comparison of individual thresholds before medical therapy and at 22 and 74 months after the start of medical therapy showed stabilization of low- and mid-threshold frequencies. The average rate of hearing loss approximated 0 dB/year with 74 months of follow-up. There was also a significant threshold loss at 4 and 8 kHz from pretreatment to 74 months post treatment, and the rate of hearing loss at these higher frequencies was approximately 1.5 dB/year.

Conclusion.—Diuretics and low-salt diet may decrease the natural progression of sensorineural hearing loss in patients with Meniere's disease. The 1985 CHE guidelines lack the sensitivity to evaluate hearing changes. Because the CHE guidelines specify that vertigo is to be evaluated by a ratio, there is loss of information and loss of statistical power. Comparison of the differences of vertigo also have the same drawbacks. In contrast, analysis of raw data of episodes per month preserves the most information, is sensitive, and should be recommended for evaluation of vertigo and hearing changes.

▶ This study is of interest. Most of us recommend diuretics and a low-salt diet, on an empirical basis, in our attempt to manage patients who have Meniere's disease. It is too simplistic, however, to assume that this method would "cure" or resolve the problem in the majority of cases. The authors found that the treatment is efficacious from the design of this study. My recollection is that Perlman and Lindsay did a careful study many years ago in hospitalized patients who were receiving diuretics, and they found no significance objectively in terms of substantial elimination of the symptoms of Meniere's disease. Further studies should be done.

Certainly, most of us will continue to recommend diuretics, but in combination with many other medications that also play an empirical role and are not curative. As I tell every one of my patients with Meniere's disease, "There is no cure for Meniere's disease, but there is lots of hope and lots of help and many ways of treating the condition," placing emphasis on conservative measures.—M.M. Paparella, M.D.

Endolymphatic Sac Ballooning Surgery for Meniere's Disease

Huang T-S, Lin C-C (Chang Gung Med College, Taipei, Taiwan, Republic of China)
Ann Otol Rhinol Laryngol 103:389–394, 1994   130-95-1–13

Background.—Endolymphatic sac ballooning surgery (ESBS) enhances endolymphatic sac volume. The procedure incorporates the "T-strut" technique, and insertion and fanfolding of a Silastic sheet. The ESBS may prevent or retard osteoneogenosis and provide long-term control of the symptoms of Meniere's disease. The results obtained with ESBS in 112 patients were described.

Surgical Procedure.—After induction of general anesthesia, complete mastoidectomy was accomplished. The bony plate overlying the dura of the posterior fossa between the posterior semicircular canal and the lateral sinus was removed. The endolymphatic sac was delineated anteriorly and inferiorly to Donaldson's line as a whitish, dense thickening of the dura. The superior endolymphatic sac margin was incised, and its lumen was well defined, layer by layer, with a whirlybird. A .005-in thick ribbon of Silastic sheet was inserted into the sac lumen and then fanfolded within the lumen to enlarge and balloon the sac medially and laterally. The ribbon tail was left outside the sac (Fig 1–9). The entire mastoid

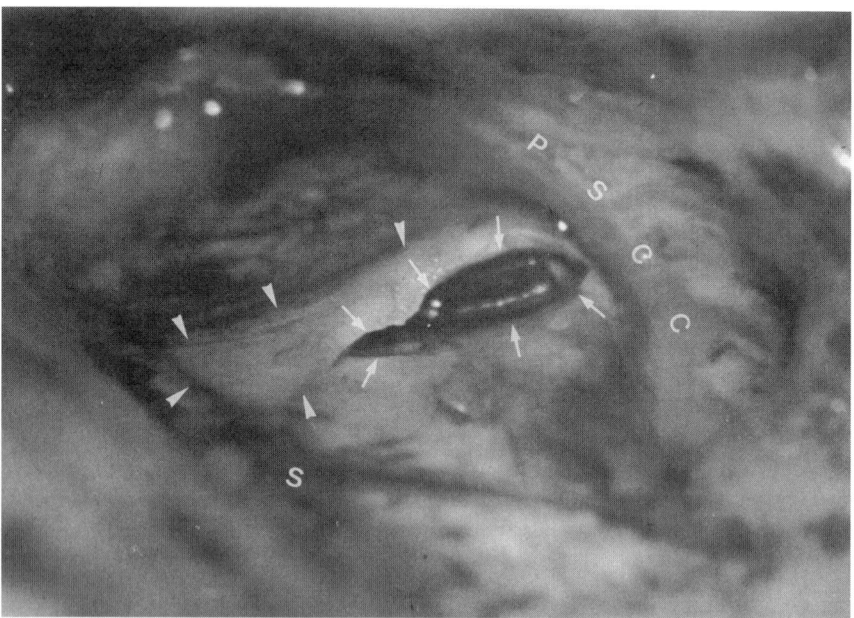

Fig 1–9.—Endolymphatic sac ballooning technique used in the left ear. *Arrowheads* indicate the endolymphatic sac; *arrows,* the endolymphatic sac lumen enlarged by fan-folded Silastic sheet; *PSCC,* the posterior semicircular canal; and S, sigmoid sinus. (Courtesy of Huang T-S, Lin C-C: *Ann Otol Rhinol Laryngol* 103:389–394, 1994.)

cavity was packed with Gelfoam to control bleeding into the middle ear cavity. The wound was closed in layers, and a mastoid dressing applied.

Results.—The results achieved with ESBS in patients with incapacitating Meniere's disease symptom complex have been superior to those achieved with primary endolymphatic sac surgery with either nonballooning sac techniques or ESBS revision operations using nonexpansion techniques. The ESBS completely or substantially controlled vertigo in 91.7% of 109 patients who had classic Meniere's disease or endolymphatic hydrops, and it improved or stablized hearing in 91.7%.

Conclusion.—Endolymphatic sac ballooning surgery preserves sac integrity, expands the lumen, and may prevent surgically induced damage. The procedure may be more effective than other endolymphatic sac surgical procedures in the drainage of hydropic endolymph.

▶ Dr. Huang has had a very broad experience in successfully treating Meniere's disease with endolymphatic sac surgery. This technique of ballooning surgery is intriguing because it accomplishes many of the objectives of endolymphatic sac enhancement, namely to decompress, increase the lumen for absorption of nanoliters of endolymph, create a corollary blood supply, and perhaps enhance immune properties. In any case, this interesting technique seems reasonable and most likely is efficacious, as the study indicates. The technique I continue to use certainly incorporates the concept as described by Huang and Lin.—M.M. Paparella, M.D.

Surgery for Vertigo in the Nonserviceable Hearing Ear: Transmastoid Labyrinthectomy or Translabyrinthine Vestibular Nerve Section
Langman AW, Lindeman RC (Virginia Mason Clinic, Seattle)
Laryngoscope 103:1321–1325, 1993   130-95-1–14

Introduction.—Episodic vertigo that cannot be managed medically can be treated with several surgical procedures. When it is caused by an ear with hearing impairment, 2 typical approaches are used: a transmastoid labyrinthectomy (TL) or a translabyrinthine vestibular nerve section (TLVNS). Because TLVNS removes all preganglionic vestibular tissue, it may better prevent recurrent or persistent vertigo, but it also sacrifices all hearing in the affected ear. In a retrospective review, the relative superiority of either TL or TLVNS in relieving vertigo was determined.

Methods.—The records of patients who had at least 1-year of follow-up after having either a TL (43 patients) or a TLVNS (15 patients) were reviewed. Preoperatively, the patients were classified into 4 diagnostic categories: Meniere's disease, chronic otitis media, poststapedectomy, and vertigo with sensorineural hearing loss. Postoperative equilibrium was the outcome measure.

Results.—The average follow-up was 3.3 years and ranged from 1 to 13 years. Preoperatively, all patients had significant hearing loss, and

2 Hearing and Tests of Hearing

The Validity of Tuning Fork Tests in Diagnosing Hearing Loss
Miltenburg DM (Univ of Manitoba Health Sciences Centre, Winnipeg)
J Otolaryngol 23:254–259, 1994   130-95-2–1

Introduction.—Although the tuning fork test (TFT) remains a traditional part of the otologic examination, its present usefulness is uncertain. A study was designed to test the sensitivity and bias of the Weber, Rinne, and Bing TFTs; to describe how mixed hearing loss behaves on a TFT; to determine whether masking improves the validity of the Rinne test; to explore how TFTs are influenced by the frequency of the hearing loss; and to compare the otologic diagnosis with TFT results.

Methods.—The study participants were all patients at least 9 years of age who were referred to a general hospital for audiologic assessment between December 1, 1991, and March 31, 1992. Controls were those who were found to have normal hearing on audiologic assessment. The TFT was performed within 24 hours of audiometric evaluation and without knowledge of the patient's diagnosis and audiometry results. Seven TFTs were randomly administered to each of the 68 patients: Weber, Rinne unmasked and masked for each ear, and the Bing for each ear. Signal Detection Theory was used to compare results of TFTs with pure-tone air- and bone-conduction audiometry.

Results.—The Weber test tended to report hearing loss when hearing was normal and was correct only half the time. The Rinne test had a high overall sensitivity, whereas the Bing test was insensitive. Sensitivity of the Rinne test remained high whether hearing loss was severe or moderate and regardless of the frequency of the hearing loss. The masked Rinne test was different from the unmasked Rinne test in only 8 of 68 patients. Sensitivity of the 3 TFTs was not appreciably changed with the type of hearing loss (sensorineural, conductive, or mixed).

Conclusion.—Because TFTs are subjective, response bias must be accounted for in assessing their validity as diagnostic tools. The Rinne test, with a 256-Hz fork, is a sensitive and unbiased test that was not affected by hearing loss frequency and was equally sensitive to different types of hearing loss. The Rinne test is nonspecific, however, and cannot distinguish between conductive and mixed hearing loss. Both the Weber and Bing tests are insensitive and have no role as independent tests.

▶ The question of TFTs arises once again. The author makes some interesting observations. I would agree with them in the main but would differ slightly. I find that TFTs are helpful for both Weber and Rinne testing, whether we are dealing with a conductive loss, large or small, or a mixed loss. With time and experience, it usually is possible, using the tuning fork, to corroborate the audiogram and to identify small vs. large conductive losses using these well-established tests. When doing the Rinne test, I always use an electric masker on the opposite side to eliminate crossover hearing from the opposite side. I believe TFTs should be a common part of routine assessment of patients in the otologic clinic.—M.M. Paparella, M.D.

Laboratory Diagnosis of Immune Inner Ear Disease
Hughes GB, Moscicki R, Barna BP, San Martin JE (Cleveland Clinic Found, Ohio; Massachusetts Gen Hosp, Boston; Massachusetts Eye and Ear Infirmary, Boston)
Am J Otol 15:198–202, 1994   130-95-2–2

Introduction.—Immune inner ear disease is a newly recognized and distinct clinical entity that typically results in rapidly progressive sensorineural hearing loss. Middle-aged women are affected most often. The disorder usually is bilateral and may be limited to the inner ear, but it may also be part of a systemic immune complex disorder involving specific target organs for reasons that are as yet poorly understood.

Laboratory Tests.—Antigen-specific tests are available with which to identify specific cellular or humoral immune reactivity with inner ear tissues. Both the lymphocyte transformation test (LTT) and the migration inhibition tests are used. These tests assume that a population of circulating lymphocytes is present that recognizes and responds to inner ear antigens. The LTT is illustrated in Figure 2–1. Antigen-specific tests of humoral immunity include the indirect immunofluorescence and enzyme-linked immunoassay procedures and the Western blot immunoassay.

Pathogenesis.—The nature of the antigens involved in immune inner ear disease remains uncertain, but there is evidence that type II collagen may be involved. It is a major structural protein of the inner ear.

▶ Hughes and co-workers have a large experience in the laboratory testing and diagnosing of immune disease of the inner ear. I think the 2 tests, lymphocyte transformation and Western blot immune tests, are of interest for diagnostic purposes. I must say that we frequently search for autoimmune disease of the inner ear and seldom find it, but we will continue to search.—M.M. Paparella, M.D.

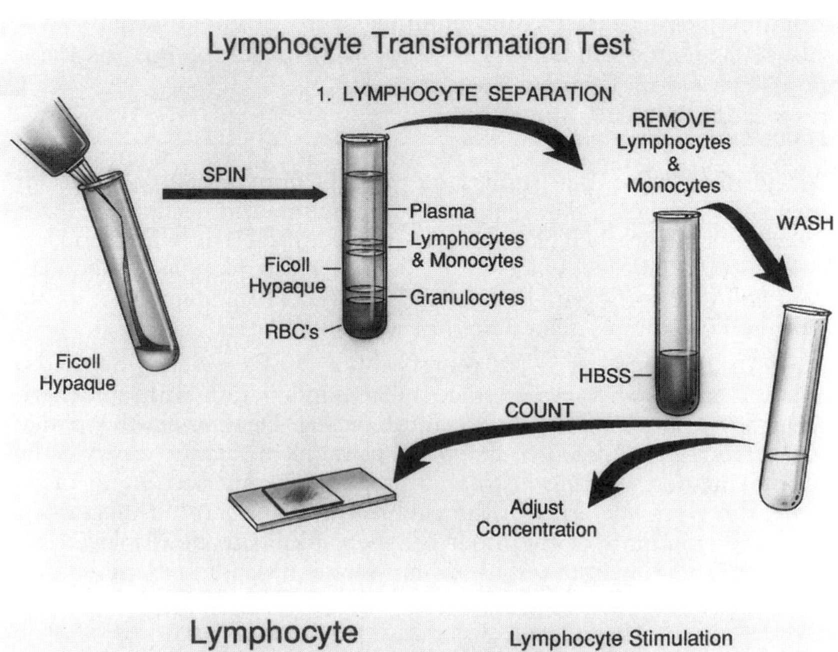

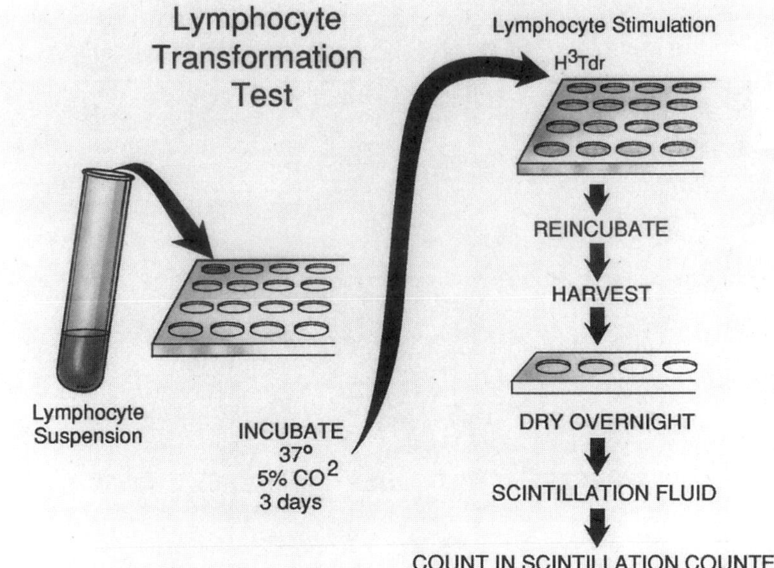

Fig 2–1.—**Top,** in the lymphocyte transformation test, whole fresh blood is obtained from the patient when symptoms are active and immunosuppressive medication is not given. **Bottom,** mononuclear leukocytes are separated by centrifugation. Cells are mixed with inner ear proteins in microtiter plates with exposure to tritiated thymidine. Results are interpreted by comparing activity in cells exposed to medium alone with cells exposed to antigen. (Courtesy of Hughes GB, Moscicki R, Barna BP, et al: *Am J Otol* 15:198–202, 1994.)

Otopathology in a Case of Multichannel Cochlear Implantation

Nadol JB Jr, Ketten DR, Burgess BJ (Harvard Med School, Boston; Massachusetts Eye and Ear Infirmary, Boston)
Laryngoscope 104:299–303, 1994   130-95-2-3

Background.—Previous studies of patients undergoing cochlear implantation have shown that temporal bone trauma can occur to supporting elements of the cochlea as a consequence of electrode insertion, tissue reaction to the presence of implanted electrodes, and secondary degeneration of spiral ganglion cells. The effects of implantation on the spiral ganglion cell population are not well understood.

Methods and Findings.—The temporal bones of a patient who died of unrelated causes 10 weeks after cochlear implantation with a Richards Ineraid device were studied histopathologically. Deafness in this patient resulted from a prolonged course of IV gentamicin treatment 5 years before implantation. During histologic preparation and sectioning of the sample, the electrode array of the cochlear implant was left in situ. The supporting structures of the inner ear were found to be displaced and disrupted, especially in the 6- to 15-mm range measured from the round window (Fig 2–2). The basilar membrane, spiral ligament, stria vascularis, and Reissner's membrane were disrupted in this area (Fig 2–3). In

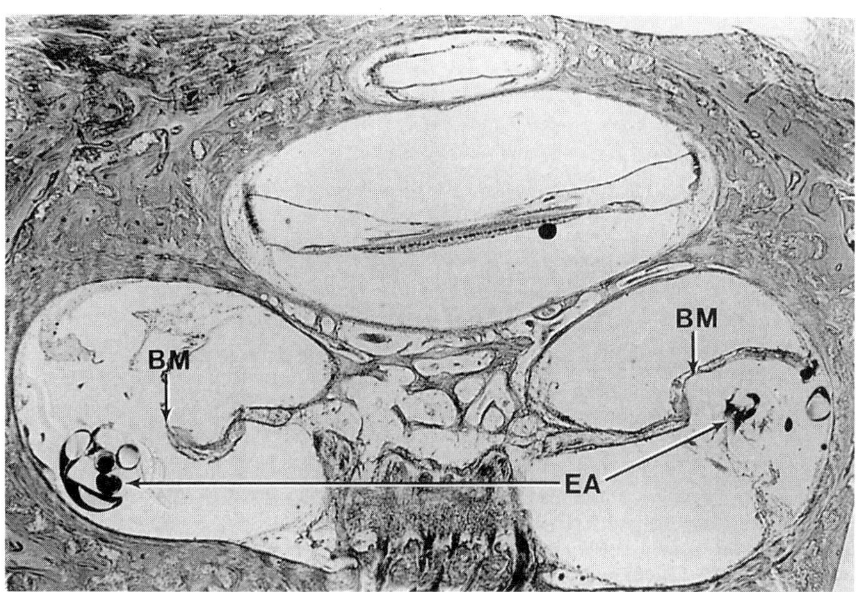

Fig 2–2.—Unstained 35-μm axial section of the ear with the implant. The electrode array (*EA*) was sectioned in situ. Disruption of the basilar membrane (*BM*) is evident on the left, approximately 11 mm from the round window membrane, and displacement of the basilar membrane is evident on the right, approximately 18 mm from the round window membrane (original magnification, ×28). (Courtesy of Nadol JB Jr, Ketten DR, Burgess BJ: *Laryngoscope* 104:299–303, 1994.)

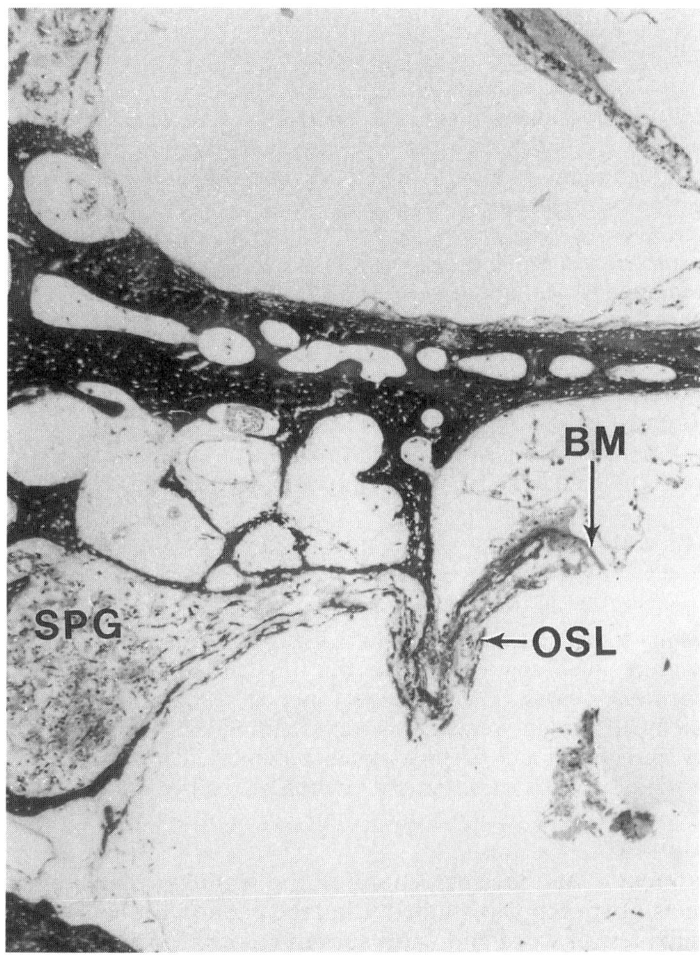

Fig 2–3.—Remounted 5-μm section of the 11- to 12-mm region of the implanted cochlea. Fracture and displacement of the osseus spiral lamina (*OSL*) and basilar membrane (*BM*) are evident. Spiral ganglion cells (*SPG*) and their dendritic processes are seen in Rosenthal's canal. (Toluidine blue stain; original magnification, ×75.) (Courtesy of Nadol JB Jr, Ketten DR, Burgess BJ: *Laryngoscope* 104:299–303, 1994.)

the 16- to 24-mm range, the supporting elements of the organ of Corti showed no disruption; however, they were significantly displaced toward the scala vestibuli, with the electrode array placed in the normal location of the scala media. The mean densities of spiral ganglion cells did not differ on the implanted and unimplanted sides.

Conclusion.—The findings in this patient provide evidence that, despite significant disruption of supporting elements of the inner ear, which occurs commonly during cochlear implantation, there seems to be little effect on the residual spiral ganglion cell count. These results only reflect short-term effects.

▶ Nadol and colleagues make an interesting observation of otopathology but also, in my opinion, a correct conclusion. They state that trauma to the supporting elements of the organ of Corti, particularly the pillar cells, has little effect on the residual counts of spiral ganglion cells, "at least in the short term." Studies by Schuknecht and others would suggest that, in the long term, degeneration of ganglial cells indeed occurs subsequent to such structural damage.—M.M. Paparella, M.D.

Performance of Prelingually or Postlingually Deafened Adults Who Were Using a Single or Multichannel Cochlear Implant

Hinderink JB, Snik AFM, Mens LHM, Brokx JPL, van den Broek P (Univ Hosp Nijmegen, The Netherlands; Inst for the Deaf, St Michielsgestel, The Netherlands)
ENT J 73:180–183, 1994   130-95-2-4

Objective.—A number of studies have shown that postlingually deafened adults who use multichannel cochlear implants perform better than those with a single-channel device, but few studies have assessed prelingually deafened adults. Accordingly, speech recognition ability 2 years after cochlear implant placement was examined in 4 pairs of prelingual patients and in 4 pairs of postlingual patients, all of whom were profoundly deaf in both ears. Patients matched for the onset and duration of deafness received either a multichannel cochlear implant or a single-channel device.

Assessment.—Auditory perception of the segmental and suprasegmental aspects of speech was studied using the Monosyllable-Trochee-Spondee (MTS) test of word and word pattern recognition. Patients were also asked to identify recorded environmental sounds, and they took the Continuous Discourse Tracking (CDT) test to assess the ability to repeat words correctly as they are read to each subject.

Results.—Prelingually deafened patients performed comparably with single-channel and multichannel implants, although in 3 of 4 instances the multichannel user scored at least 25% higher than the single-channel user in recognizing environmental sounds. Prelingually deaf users of a single-channel implant most often did better than multichannel implant users on the suprasegmental part of the MTS test. In postlingual patients, the multichannel implant gave better results. In postlingually deaf patients, use of a multichannel implant provided better results on the segmental part of the MTS test. The CDT test results indicated that, for postlingual patients, the multichannel implant produced much better performance.

Conclusion.—Postlingually deaf patients do better with a multichannel cochlear implant than with a single-channel implant. For prelingually deaf patients, however, the analogue stimulation mode of the single-channel implant may provide better performance than the digitally coded mode used by multichannel implants.

▶ The authors did not find multichanneled systems to be superior in prelingually deafened adults, as compared with the single-channeled implant. As they appropriately conclude, further studies are indicated. If a single-channeled implant will be as efficacious as or, we hope, less costly than a multichanneled implant, this would have broader applications and might be better adopted by gatekeepers in the large HMOs developing nationwide.—M.M. Paparella, M.D.

Sudden Hearing Loss as the Initial Monosymptom of Multiple Sclerosis

Drulović B, Ribarić-Jankes K, Kostić VS, Šternić N (Univ Clinical Ctr, Belgrade, Serbia)
Neurology 43:2703–2705, 1993   130-95-2–5

Introduction.—Hearing loss occurs in some patients with multiple sclerosis (MS), but it has not been reported as an early symptom before. However, in 2 patients who were definitively given a diagnosis of MS, unilateral sudden hearing loss was the first manifestation of the disease.

Case 1.—A woman, 20, was seen with sudden hearing loss and tinnitus in her right ear. She had no other signs or symptoms. Audiometry confirmed severe sensorineural hearing loss in the right ear and normal hearing in the left ear. The right ear had a normal tympanogram, an absent stapedial reflex, a normal electronystagmogram (ENG), and abnormal brain stem auditory evoked potentials (BAEPs). Magnetic resonance imaging studies revealed cerebral lesions and demyelination on the right side of the pontomedullary junction. Although she recovered her hearing in 14 days, the right BAEPs remained abnormal. Within 2 months she experienced a temporary numbness in her legs, which recurred 14 months later along with Lhermitte's sign.

Case 2.—A woman, 33, had sudden hearing loss and tinnitus in her left ear, as well as subjective mild dysequilibrium. Her neurologic examination was normal. Unilaterally, she had audiometrically confirmed hearing loss, normal tympanometry, absent stapedial reflex, abnormal BAEPs, and a normal ENG. The MRI identified several cerebral demyelinating lesions and 1 small left pontine lesion. The BAEPs remained abnormal after her hearing returned. She experienced more symptoms during the following year and was subsequently given a diagnosis of MS.

Discussion.—The absent stapedial reflex in both patients suggests that a retrocochlear demyelinating lesion may cause unilateral hearing loss in patients with MS. The BAEP responses with absent peak II in the first patient suggests a cochlear lesion; the absent peaks III–V in the second patient suggest a lesion in the upper pontine or midbrain.

▶ This study, which appeared in the journal *Neurology*, describes 2 patients who had sudden deafness. One cannot rule out the possibility that, although there might be central findings on MRI, there could also be a concurrently occurring peripheral event, such as labyrinthine deafness caused by viral endolymphatic labyrinthitis. We have the opportunity to work closely with a director of a large clinic for patients with MS. Such patients usually are referred because they have peripheral otologic problems, which can occur with any systemic illness. Nevertheless, others should look for this finding and, if possible, corroborate it. The pathogenesis of the 2 cases in this study remains enigmatic.—M.M. Paparella, M.D.

Otosyphilis: Diagnostic and Therapeutic Update
Linstrom CJ, Gleich LL (New York Med College, Valhalla; New York Eye and Ear Infirmary)
J Otolaryngol 22:401–408, 1993   130-95-2-6

Introduction.—Patients with otosyphilis often experience fluctuating hearing loss, tinnitus, and vertigo. The diagnosis is confirmed by serologic screening. Treatment with penicillin and steroids is effective in some patients. A trial of penicillin and corticosteroids was undertaken to determine the profile of patients with otosyphilis most likely to respond to treatment.

Methods.—Eighteen patients with sensorineural hearing loss, hearing fluctuation, tinnitus, or dysequilibrium and positive syphilis serology were tested to exclude any other known etiology and to detect allergy. Lumbar puncture was performed to determine HIV status. The patients were treated with penicillin (or tetracycline if allergic to penicillin) and prednisone. Hearing loss was monitored audiometrically during and after treatment; dysequilibrium was monitored with an electronystagmography battery.

Results.—The CSF obtained by lumbar puncture was abnormal in 7 patients: 5 had elevated protein, 1 had elevated glucose and protein, and 2 had HIV positivity. Significant treatment response was achieved in 4 of 16 patients (25%) with hearing loss, 10 of 14 patients (71.4%) with tinnitus, and 6 of 9 patients (86%) with vertigo. Of those with improved hearing, 50% had improved speech reception threshold scores and 75% had improved discrimination. Of the 5 patients with elevated CSF protein, 1 had improvements in hearing, tinnitus, and vertigo, and another had decreased tinnitus but no hearing improvement. Of the 2 HIV-positive patients, 1 had decreased tinnitus but no hearing improvement, and the other had decreased vertigo. Patients with fluctuating symptoms and less than 5 years of hearing loss and who were younger than age 60 were more likely to respond to treatment.

Discussion.—Elderly patients with steady or progressing symptoms lasting longer than 5 years will probably not respond to antibiotic and steroid treatment. However, a patient of any age with fluctuating symptoms should be treated. Patients with no fluctuation should be treated if they have disabling tinnitus or vertigo or if they have tinnitus or vertigo but no hearing loss. Patients with recent syphilis infection are more likely to respond to treatment.

▶ This is a good update study that alerts us to the continuing presence of syphilis as a disease that can mimic Meniere's disease and other labyrinthine difficulties. The authors have an excellent experience, explain the problem well, and describe a therapeutic protocol that would be helpful for these patients.—M.M. Paparella, M.D.

Clinical Features of Idiopathic Bilateral Sensorineural Hearing Loss
Yagi M, Harada T, Yamasoba T, Kikuchi S (Saitama Med Ctr, Japan; Univ of Tokyo; Kameda Gen Hosp, Chiba, Japan)
ORL J Otorhinolaryngol Relat Spec 56:5–10, 1994   130-95-2–7

Introduction.—The Research Committee of the Ministry of Health and Welfare in Japan has determined the diagositic criteria of idiopathic bilateral sensorineural hearing loss (IBSH): quickly progressive bilateral hearing loss of an unknown etiology. The clinical features of IBSH were studied with long-term observation.

Methods.—Both physiologic hearing deterioration and pathologic progression were evaluated with audiometry for at least 3 years in 20 patients, aged 8 to 27 years. Known etiologies were excluded with audiometry, serologic tests, and radiologic studies.

Results.—Most patients had mild or moderate hearing loss, which deteriorated to profound hearing loss. Audiograms had gradually descending or flat patterns. Thirteen experienced bilateral progression of hearing loss; 7 had unilateral progression of hearing loss. Although the initial audiograms were asymmetrical in 15 patients, progression of either type produced symmetrical final audiograms in 15 patients. The speed of progression varied widely and was not age-dependent, but the speed of progression tended to slow when the hearing loss became profound. Patients with fixed hearing experienced rapid or slow pathologic progression only or both rapid and slow phases of progression. Temporary improvement of hearing loss occurred in a minority of the patients with steroid therapy.

Discussion.—It is suggested that a physiologic progression of hearing loss of more than 15 dB per year in 2 adjacent frequencies be added to the pathologic progression diagnostic criteria defining IBSH. Hearing loss often progressed from higher to lower frequencies. This pattern also occurs in patients with hereditary hearing loss, suggesting that IBSH may have a genetic etiology. However, the response to steroid treatment may indicate an immunogenic factor. Continued research is required to identify the pathogenesis of IBSH.

▶ First of all, not all bilateral sensorineural hearing loss is idiopathic; there is a cause, or there may be multiple causes. When extrinsic factors such as trauma, infection, and the like are eliminated, this, by definition, leaves intrinsic factors, which means genetic problems that can lead to progressive sensorineural loss during a lifetime. The more we can avoid using the word "idiopathic," the better chance we have of identifying the etiologic bases of these disorders. Patient history continues to be the most important part of the workup, along with, of course, audiometric and appropriate other studies.—M.M. Paparella, M.D.

Hearing Loss After Neurosurgery: The Influence of Low Cerebrospinal Fluid Pressure
Walsted A, Nielsen OA, Borum P (Gentofte Univ Hosp, Denmark; Glostrup Hosp, Denmark)
J Laryngol Otol 108:637–641, 1994   130-95-2–8

Background.—In patients undergoing neurosurgery, decreases in volume and pressure in the CSF may affect hearing. The extent and cause of any hearing loss after neurosurgery were systematically evaluated in a prospective study.

Patients and Methods.—Thirty-two patients, aged 19 to 72 years, who underwent neurosurgery and 32 control patients, aged 19 to 73 years, who had surgical procedures without puncture or drainage of the subdural space were evaluated. Patients were asked about existing audiologic symptoms, and all underwent preoperative assessments, including otoscopy, pure tone audiometry, speech audiometry, and tympanometry. All patients underwent 2 postoperative tests, with the first scheduled between days 1 and 3 and the second between days 4 and 7. Any new subjective symptoms, including hearing loss, fullness, tinnitus, and dizziness or nausea, were reported at this time.

Results.—Seventeen patients undergoing neurosurgery had a significant hearing loss during the first postoperative week. The threshold shift toward worse hearing was more common at frequencies of 125, 250, and 500 Hz, but was also noted at 4 and 8 kHz. In the entire neurosurgery group, 49 significant threshold changes showing worse hearing at the first postoperative audiometry were noted, compared with only 6 in the control patients. Among the neurosurgery group, 2 patients reported subjective postoperative symptoms of nausea, 3 had dizziness, 3 felt fullness in the ears, 8 reported decreased hearing, and 9 reported a new symptom of tinnitus. Only 1 patient in the control group reported subjective symptoms, which comprised a sensation of occlusion in the ears, confirmed by audiometry and tympanometry. The latter patient was among those in the control group who had a significant threshold decrease.

Conclusion.—In patients undergoing neurosurgery, the mechanism of hearing loss results from a decrease in pressure and/or volume of the CSF, which is reflected within the perilymphatic fluid and is similar to a transitory endolymphatic hydrops. Further studies that can help clarify the pathophysiologic mechanisms leading to hearing loss after CSF leakage are suggested.

▶ This interesting study should be replicated by others. I am not aware of a similar study in which surgery, namely having puncture or drainage of the subdural space, is followed by significant hearing loss in the immediate postoperative period. If this result is true, this will tell us something about the relationship between CSF and perilymph and their interaction via the modiolus and cochlear aqueduct. This would be relevant in assessing other forms of hearing loss. Incidentally, permanent hearing loss usually does not occur after neurosurgery.—M.M. Paparella, M.D.

Ultrastructural Findings in the Cochlea of AIDS Cases
Pappas DG, Sekhar HKC, Lim J, Hillman DE (New York Univ Med Ctr, NY)
Am J Otol 15:456–465, 1994   130-95-2–9

Objective.—Whether specific pathologic changes or pathogens are found in the cochlea in individuals dying of AIDS was studied.

Cases.—Temporal bones were available from 8 adults with confirmed HIV-1 infection that had progressed to AIDS. The patients, 31 to 62 years of age, had died of AIDS-related complications or disease. All had received potentially ototoxic drugs.

Observations.—Inner sulcus cells and Deiters' cells were swollen and appeared watery and broken. Organisms were found in the endolymphatic space and in blood vessel lumens. Extracellularly, HIV-like particles were found embedded in the tectorial membrane and, in one case, appeared to be trapped within lacunae (Fig 2–4). Virus-like particles also were seen over the limbus epithelium within lacunae and embedded in the filamentous attachment of the tectorial membrane. Dense amorphous masses were seen shrouding bundles of collagen fibers and contacting fibrocytes; some had highly ordered striations extending from their borders. The hair cells had pathologic alterations in their cytoplasm. Viral-like particles were present within connective tissue cells, endothelial cells, and the epithelium of the organ of Corti. Globular-dense particulate bodies of varying size accompanied viral cisterns within infected cells.

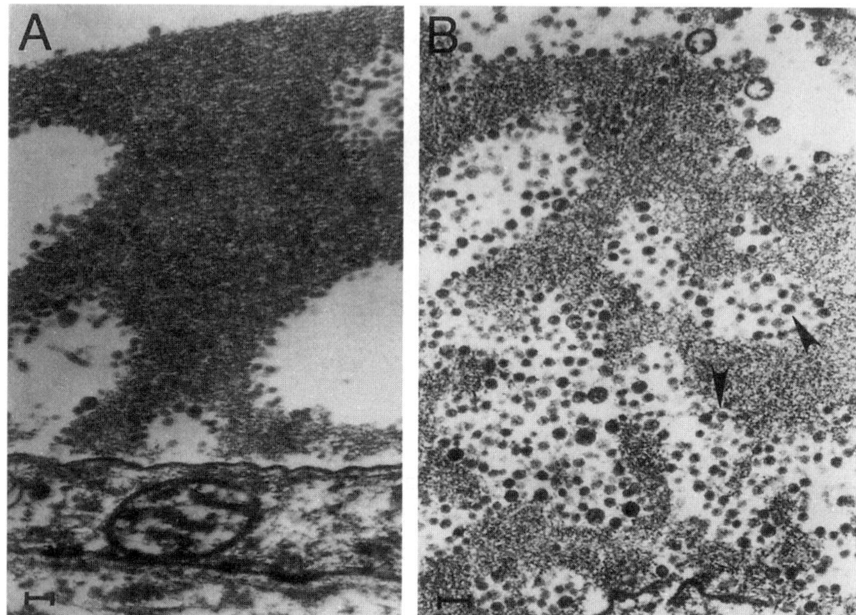

Fig 2–4.—Electron micrographs of the extracellular and intracellular viral-like particles with a comparison micrograph of HIV-1 cell culture. **A,** low-power view of the tectorial membrane overlying attachment to the limbus, showing the dense filament substructure of the tectorial membrane. **B,** high-power view showing viral-like particles (*arrowheads*) lining the under surface and lodged in lacunae. These viral-like particles ranged in diameter from 90 to 120 μm. Conical cores are seen in a few parti-

(continued)

Conclusion.—It appears that HIV-1 grows within the endolymph. Infected temporal bones might prove very useful for studying the morphogenesis of HIV-1 disease.

▶ Pappas and colleagues have brought to our attention an epidemic problem, namely AIDS, and how it can affect the cochlea. Extracellular virus-like particles were identified in 3 patients on the tectorial membrane. This excellent paper would be enhanced if we had an opportunity to study pathologic conditions in the temporal bone of patients in addition to the useful method of study that was used.—M.M. Paparella, M.D.

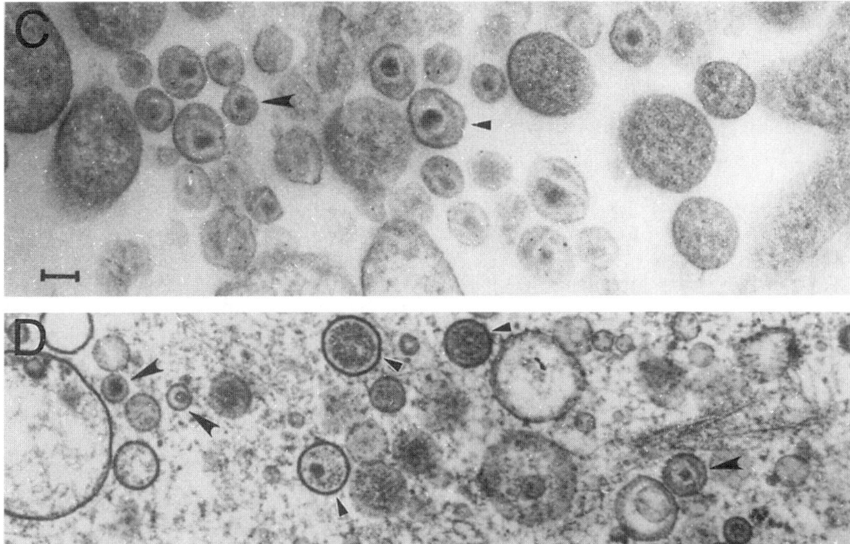

Fig 2–4 (cont).

cles that are sectioned longitudinally. **C,** micrograph of lymphocyte cell culture infected with HIV-1 (*arrowheads*). Note that the viral envelope contains various shaped cores and varying amounts of particulate material. **D,** cochlear connective tissue cell from an AIDS case. Compare the viral-like particles indicated by larger arrowheads to HIV-1 particles in **C.** Note *small arrowheads* indicating enlarged envelopes forming cisterns containing particulate material. The small cisterns have a dense core almost filling the cistern space and a few cisternal particles aligned around the core. *Bar* represents 100 nm. (Courtesy of Pappas DG, Sekhar HKC, Lim J, et al: *Am J Otol* 15:456–465, 1994.)

Hypnosis as an Aid for Tinnitus Patients

Kaye JM, Marlowe FI, Ramchandani D, Berman S, Schindler B, Loscalzo G (Medical College of Pennsylvania, Philadelphia)
ENT J 73:309–315, 1994   130-95-2–10

Introduction.––Hypnosis has been effectively used to relieve such symptoms as pain, nausea, and vomiting, and it has allowed some patients with chronic disorders to function better. Hypnotherapy also has proved useful in patients with tinnitus, but objective measurements were not obtained.

Objective.—Hypnosis was compared with stress management in 14 patients with intractable tinnitus (mean age, 60 years). All were evaluated by a psychiatrist.

Methods.—A psychologist saw the patients for 1 hour, 3 times per week. Hypnosis was induced by visualization methods and by the home use of self-hypnosis cassette tapes. Hypnotic suggestions were individualized. Stress management involved identifying sources of stress, instructing patients in ways of coping, and practicing coping strategies in actual stressful situations. In addition to a tinnitus questionnaire-rating scale, patients were evaluated using the NIMH Diagnostic Interview Schedule, the SCL 90R, and the Beck Depression Index.

Results.—Sleep indices did not change significantly after treatment. Beck depression scores decreased after hypnotherapy. Stress management was associated with reductions in the Global Severity Index, Positive Symptom Total, and Anxiety Dimension components of the SCL-90R.

Conclusion.—Behavioral techniques appear to have potential value in patients with intractable tinnitus.

▶ Tinnitus continues to be a common problem in every otolaryngologist's practice. The usual methods of managing tinnitus, namely with identification of the problem, reassurance of the patient, and instructions regarding behavioral listening, usually suffice. As we all know, some patients have such severe problems that they threaten suicide. These patients are best managed by a psychologist who can use methods such as hypnosis, described very nicely in this study. Other techniques of psychological counseling, biofeedback, and the like can also be usefully used.—M.M. Paparella, M.D.

Prevalence of Hearing Loss Among People Aged 65 Years and Over: Screening and Hearing Aid Provision
Wilson PS, Fleming DM, Donaldson I (Selly Oak Hosp, Birmingham, England)
Br J Gen Pract 43:406–409, 1993   130-95-2–11

Introduction.—Audiometric screening can identify patients who would benefit from using a hearing aid. These patients often do not realize that they have hearing loss. However, patients usually receive hearing aids after they realize they have a significant loss and seek treatment. Studies of the prevalence of hearing loss in the elderly have reported widely varying findings. The prevalence of hearing impairment in individuals aged 65 years and older was studied, using audiometric screening to identify patients who would benefit from hearing aids. These patients were offered hearing aids.

Methods.—All patients aged 65 years and a 20% random sample of patients older than 65 years seen in a large general practice were invited to have a hearing assessment. The 322 patients were assessed by history, physical examination, tuning fork tests, and audiometry. Patients who had a hearing loss of at least 35 decibels were offered a hearing aid. The relative risk for significant hearing loss with a history of occupational noise exposure was calculated. Patients with audiometric evidence of asymmetric sensorineural hearing loss were referred for acoustic neuroma screening.

Results.—Thirty-four of the 322 patients already had hearing aids. An additional 142 patients had significant hearing loss and were offered hearing aids; 69 (49%) accepted them. A history of occupational noise exposure was not a significant risk factor, and only 5 patients with a history of noise exposure showed the audiometric pattern characteristic of hearing loss from exposure to noise. Twenty-four patients had indications of asymmetric sensorineural hearing loss; none had acoustic neuroma.

Discussion.—The prevalence of hearing impairment in these patients was 54%. None of the patients had serious pathologic conditions requiring major intervention. Screening the hearing of elderly patients in a practice-based general service is more feasible and efficient than screening in patients in a hospital-based specialist service.

▶ This study was done in Birmingham with a computerized record system. It nicely confirms statistically the prevalence of hearing loss among older citizens as well as the reluctance or difficulty for those individuals to acquire amplification via a hearing aid. It is my understanding that approximately one fifth of patients, mostly among the elderly, who could benefit from a hearing aid actually do so, which means that many *could* benefit but do not. We hope that, over time, this problem will be improved.—M.M. Paparella, M.D.

3 Interaction of the Middle Ear and Inner Ear

Efficacy of Surgical Treatments for Squamous Cell Carcinoma of the Temporal Bone: A Literature Review
Prasad S, Janecka IP (Univ of Pittsburgh School of Med, Pa)
Otolaryngol Head Neck Surg 110:270–280, 1994   130-95-3–1

Introduction.—Squamous cell carcinoma of the temporal bone is rare. Several treatments have been used to manage it. Data on survival as it is related to the depth of invasion, the optimal treatment for each disease manifestation, and the effect of invasion of surrounding tissues on prognosis were analyzed.

Methods.—Twenty-six articles containing information on 144 patients were reviewed. The extent of disease involvement, treatments, outcome, and survival were analyzed.

Results.—All but one of the studies were case series that did not use controls; the remaining study was a nonrandomized historical cohort comparison. When the disease was confined to the external canal, survival was similar regardless of whether the lesion was treated by mastoidectomy, lateral temporal bone resection (TBR), or subtotal TBR. When disease extended into the middle ear, survival was slightly enhanced if the disease was treated with a subtotal TBR compared with lateral TBR or mastoidectomy. The value of preoperative or postoperative radiation therapy is generally unclear, although it appears to improve survival in patients treated with mastoidectomy. Involvement of the dura, internal carotid artery, or the temporal lobe severely reduced survival. Surgical treatment and radiation did not appear to increase survival in these patients, but incomplete data and lack of comparisons precluded definitive analysis.

Discussion.—Mastoidectomy or lateral or subtotal TBR are similarly effective treatments when the carcinoma is confined to the external canal. However, subtotal TBR and radiation provide the best treatment results when disease has extended into the middle ear. The role of surgical resection of the surrounding tissue when the tumor has shown aggressive invasion is unclear. These findings should be clarified or confirmed by randomized clinical trials.

▶ This study is of interest from a critical point of view, and it also demonstrates that squamous cell carcinoma of the temporal bone can occupy several components of the temporal bone to include the middle ear cleft, the dura, and the labyrinth as well as the petrous apex. Thus, cancer can involve various aspects of the temporal bone simultaneously. It is also possible for a tumor of the temporal bone in one site, such as the middle ear, to invade another site, such as the inner ear, and vice versa; also, there are tumors that arise primarily in the petrous apex that can secondarily involve and invade the middle ear cleft.—M.M. Paparella, M.D.

The Otological Manifestations of Wegener's Granulomatosis

Fenton JE, O'Sullivan TJ (South Infirmary/Victoria Hosps Complex, Cork, Ireland)

J Laryngol Otol 108:144–146, 1994　　　　　　　　　　　　　130-95-3–2

Introduction.—Three women aged 31, 27, and 32 years were seen with Wegener's granulomatosis, a rare disease that primarily affects the respiratory and renal systems. The common presenting features were otalgia and otorrhea and a myringitis with middle ear involvement. Two women had a history of right-sided and left-sided facial pain. The erythrocyte sedimentation rate (ESR) was noted in each patient before and after treatment.

Case Report.—Woman, 27, with a 5-week history of right-sided facial pain additionally complained of left-sided otorrhea and bloodstained nasal discharge. After an examination, acute otitis media of the left ear, a right middle ear effusion, and an enlarged right inferior turbinate were revealed. An audiogram revealed a conductive hearing loss on the left side. Radiographs were suggestive of a maxillary sinusitis and, therefore, the woman was treated with IV antibiotics. Initially, her ESR was 108 mm/hr. Generous amounts of pus were aspirated from the sinus after a left antral lavage procedure. Because she did not improve, a right radical antrostomy was performed. Although tuberculosis was suggested, Wegener's granulomatosis was diagnosed. Cyclophosphamide and prednisolone were prescribed and the patient made an excellent recovery. Two months after treatment started, her ESR was 11 mm/hr and her hearing was normal.

Discussion.—In all 3 patients, the facial or postauricular pain was very severe and the ESR was elevated, indicating a basis for middle ear disease activity. If not treated early, and if renal involvement sets in, this disease can be fatal. These patients had a correct diagnosis and were treated early, leading to a marked improvement in their morbidity and survival. Treatment with cyclophosphamide and prednisolone can lead to 95% remission of the disease.

▶ This article describes, in 3 patients who have Wegener's granulomatosis, development of otitis media and/or sensorineural hearing loss and vertigo, which indicates that, here again, both the middle ear cleft and the labyrinth can be involved, either individually or together.—M.M. Paparella, M.D.

Extensive Otosclerosis and Endolymphatic Hydrops: Histopathologic Study of Temporal Bones

Li W, Schachern PA, Paparella MM (Univ of Minnesota, Minneapolis; Minnesota Ear, Head, and Neck Clinic, Minneapolis; Int Hearing Found, Minneapolis, Minn)

Am J Otolaryngol 15:158–161, 1994   130-95-3–3

Background.—Otosclerosis and Meniere's syndrome have long been known to coexist. Otosclerosis generally has a single focus. Multiple invasions are rare and have been reported in only a few studies of temporal bone. One patient provided investigators an opportunity to study another temporal bone with otosclerosis and concomitant Meniere's disease.

Case Report.—Woman, 64, was seen with a 40-year history of severe hearing loss in both ears and severe, acute vertigo with nausea and vomiting. The histo-

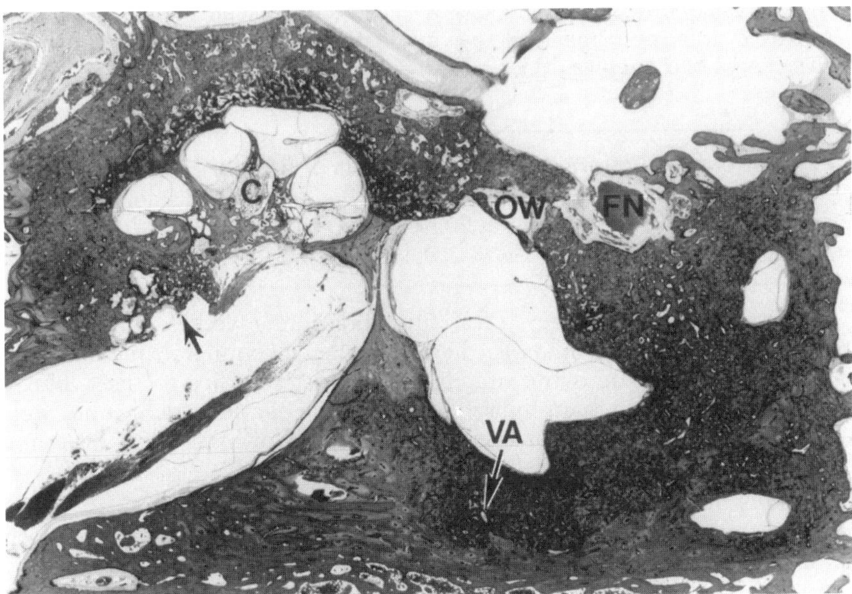

Fig 3–1.—Extensive otosclerosis surrounding the oval window (OW), bony cochlear labyrinth, vestibular aqueduct (VA; *arrow*), semicircular canals, facial nerve canal (FN), and involving the anterior wall (*arrow*) of the internal auditory canal in the right ear. *Abbreviation:* C, cochlea. Original magnification, ×9. (Courtesy of Li W, Schachern PA, Paparella MM: *Am J Otolaryngol* 15:158–161, 1994.)

logic findings in her temporal bones were comparable. Although the external and middle ear were normal, there was extensive otosclerosis involving the oval window, round window, bony cochlear labyrinth, vestibule, vestibule aqueduct, semicircular canals, anterior wall of the internal auditory canal, and facial nerve canal (Fig 3–1). Fibrosis was noted in the scala tympani. The basilar membrane in the middle turn of the left cochlea was distorted. New bone formation was noted in the scala tympani of the middle and basal turns in the right cochlea. Otosclerosis completely involved and distorted the cochlear capsule. Severe endolymphatic hydrops occurred in all cochlear turns. Mildly atrophic changes in the organ of Corti were found in the left ear. In the right ear, these changes were severe. Severe atrophy was noted in all turns of the stria vascularis. Both footplates at the anterior and posterior margins showed otosclerotic involvement of the stapes.

Conclusion.—The most common focus for otosclerosis is the front of the oval window, followed by the round window. Stapedectomy/sacculotomy is one treatment option for improving hearing and controlling vertigo in patients with otosclerosis and Meniere's syndrome.

▶ This patient had extensive or "malignant" otosclerosis, occurring initially, to be followed by endolymphatic hydrops or extensive Meniere's disease that caused vertigo and sensorineural deafness secondarily. Therefore, we have a disease of the inner ear (otosclerosis) that can cause symptoms in the middle ear, such as conductive hearing loss, which in turn can cause another disease (Meniere's disease) in the inner ear by obstructing the vestibular aqueduct and sac.—M.M. Paparella, M.D.

Vestibular and Audiometric Consequences of Blast Injury to the Ear
Sahupak A, Doweck I, Nachtigal D, Spitzer O, Gordon CR (Israeli Naval Hyperbaric Inst, Haifa, Israel; Central Emek Hosp, Afula, Israel)
Arch Otolaryngol Head Neck Surg 119:1362–1367, 1993   130-95-3–4

Objective.—Five members of a patrol boat crew were examined after they experienced blast injury to the ear by the close-range explosion of a TNT device. The ear is the organ that is most sensitive to blast injury, and the effects of such an injury on the middle ear and cochlea are well documented. The vestibular and auditory effects of blast injury have not been fully described.

Patients and Methods.—The 5 patients ranged in age from 19 to 30 years. Two had minor bruises and lacerations from the blast. Auditory symptoms included tinnitis, hearing loss, and vertigo. Only one patient reported no symptoms. Eardrum perforations were present in all cases. During the week after the blast, the men were examined with audiometry studies, electronystagmography (ENG), and the rotatory-chair smooth harmonic acceleration (SHA) test. Otoscopic examinations were performed at 2-week intervals. All patients had normal audiograms 2 to 5 months before the blast.

Results.—Eight tympanic membranes were perforated, all in the pars tensa. Seven perforations were central and 1 was marginal; none occupied more than 20% of the tympanic membrane area. The initial audiologic examination found only 4 ears to have a conductive hearing loss component greater than 20 dB. There was no correlation between magnitude of conductive hearing loss and size and location of the perforations. Three ears had sensorineural hearing impairment. Three patients were given a diagnosis of peripheral vestibulopathies, but all were free of vestibular signs and symptoms at the first follow-up examination. Tinnitus had disappeared by the second follow-up in 3 of 4 affected patients. All 7 central tympanic membrane perforations healed spontaneously within 1 month of the injury. The marginal perforation had to be closed by myringoplasty 6 months later. Follow up ENG and SHA tests showed permanent damage to the vestibular end organ, as indicated by the finding of canal paresis, in 2 patients.

Conclusion.—Tympanic membrane perforation is the most common finding after blast injury. Patients exposed to blasts should be monitored for vestibular damage, because long-term deficits may affect an individual's balance in situations that might prove life-threatening.

▶ It is well known that blast injuries to the ear can cause cochlear deafness via acoustic trauma. This also reaffirms that injuries caused by blasts can cause vestibular difficulties as well. We know that such injuries can occasionally cause problems in the middle ear cleft when the blast is strong enough.—M.M. Paparella, M.D.

An Unusual Otolaryngologic Manifestation of Lightning Strike

Todd DH, Meyers A (Colorado Univ Health Sciences Ctr, Denver)
Otolaryngol Head Neck Surg 110:126–130, 1994   130-95-3–5

Background.—In the United States, lightning strikes are responsible for 300 to 600 deaths annually. Related injuries can sometimes be of concern to the otolaryngologist, such as burns to the auricle and external auditory canal, tympanic membrane rupture, middle ear injury, and sensorineural hearing loss. A case of lightning strike in which the patient experienced prolonged dysphagia as well as the expected otologic manifestations was reported.

Case Report.—Woman, 64, was struck by lightning while horseback riding. She fell from the horse and was found pulseless and apneic. Immediate cardiac resuscitation restored the pulse after 45 seconds, and the patient was intubated and admitted to the hospital. On initial evaluation, the patient was intubated and was comatose with first-degree burns to the forehead and right thigh and buttock. She regained consciousness the next day and was extubated. Cognition was normal, except for delayed thought processing and retrograde amnesia. She reported hearing loss and a sense of imbalance. Otolaryngologic evaluation showed bilateral near-total perforations of the tympanic membranes with intact annulus and ossicles bilaterally. The patient's audiogram revealed moderate mixed hearing loss with significant conductive component. She coughed when attempting to swallow liquids. The nasopharynx, oropharynx, hypopharynx, and larynx were normal, and the mucosa was intact without burns. Speech therapy revealed minimal-to-mild left lingual and velar weakness, although speech was normal. A tailored barium swallow was obtained, showing normal oral phase, absent pharyngeal phase with flaccid paralysis, and delayed esophageal motility without reflux. Marked aspiration from the oropharynx and piriform sinuses with intact cough reflex was noted.

Because of the dysphagia and risk of aspiration, all oral feeding was discontinued, and the patient was maintained with a nasointestinal feeding tube and transferred home. Three months later her dysphagia had improved. A barium swallow revealed slight persistent vallecular filling and minimal pharyngeal transit delay. The patient was eating normally, and her hearing had improved. An audiogram showed improving mixed hearing loss with significant conductive component. Otologic evaluation also showed improving tympanic membrane perforations bilaterally. Tympanoplasty will be considered if the perforations fail to heal. The patient has no tinnitus or vertigo and can ambulate with the help of a walker.

Conclusion.—The most common otolaryngologic injury reported in lightning strike accidents is tympanic membrane rupture. The lightning strike-induced dysphagia is uncommon and is thought to be associated with an isolated CNS defect, isolated pharyngeal anesthesia, or motor dysfunction. Because the patient had intact gag reflexes and soft palate elevation, the central defect appears to be the most likely explanation in this case.

Lightning Injury of the Tympanic Membrane

Redleaf MI, McCabe BF (Univ of Iowa Hosps and Clinics, Iowa City)
Ann Otol Rhinol Laryngol 102:867–869, 1993   130-95-3–6

Introduction.—Lightning strikes have caused a variety of injuries to the ear, including large tympanic membrane perforations, sensorineural hearing loss, and disequilibrium. Although soft tissues are injured, bony structures are left intact. Direct electrical conduction is the mechanism of injury to the ear when lightning damage occurs.

Patients.—Three patients, a 27-year-old male farmer, a 46-year-old male jogger, and an 8-year-old girl, were all found to have burns on the neck and face area after being struck by lightning. External auditory canals were normal. Tympanic membranes of the farmer consisted of the annulus only. An audiogram showed that he had bilateral conductive hearing loss. The right tympanic membrane had healed completely 9 months later, but the patient subsequently required anterior myringoplasty because of scar tissue under the left anterior tympanic membrane. In the remaining 2 patients, the right tympanic membrane had a large perforation. Both the jogger and the young girl had conductive hearing loss in the right ear and underwent successful myringoplasty. The jogger has never recovered vestibular function, however, and the girl needed a ventilation tube for persistent effusion.

Discussion.—The tympanic membrane appears to disintegrate during lightning injury but usually heals spontaneously. There is no bony damage, suggesting a direct flow of electrical energy through the patient. Histologic evidence also indicates a subcutaneous energy transfer along the external auditory canal. Disintegration of the tympanic membrane probably results from electrical burn to its small central vessels. The edges of the membrane remain intact, allowing regeneration. Therefore, a lightning strike causes a direct electrical transmission of electrical charge from an entry point through the soft tissues of the head, ears, and blood vessels.

▶ The preceding 2 articles (Abstracts 130-95-3–5 and 130-95-3–6) both describe the possible effects of lightning on the temporal bone. In the first article, associated audiologic and otologic problems were accompanied by prolonged dysphagia. In the second article, 3 cases of injury by lightning occurred; the injuries were considered to be direct conduction of electricity from the scalp to the soft tissues of the tympanic membrane, and they caused injury to the central area of the tympanic membrane. Associated injuries are documented in these 2 articles. The usual treatment will be based on the anatomical pathologic conditions that result.—M.M. Paparella, M.D.

Malignant External Otitis in Nondiabetic Patients
Shpitzer T, Stern Y, Cohen O, Levy R, Segal K, Feinmesser R (Beilinson Med Ctr, Petah-Rtiqva, Israel)
Ann Otol Rhinol Laryngol 102:870–872, 1993   130-95-3–7

Introduction.—Malignant external otitis (MEO) has been described primarily in elderly diabetic patients, but some patients without diabetes have this severe bacterial infection. Nine patients without diabetes who had MEO were reviewed to better characterize the infection in this small but significant population.

Patients and Methods.—Thirty patients with a diagnosis of MEO were treated at the study institution from 1987 to 1991. Diagnosis was based on the presence of severe, painful inflammation of the external auditory canal, failure of antibiotic therapy or an abnormal radionuclide bone scan, and isolation of *Pseudomonas aeruginosa* from the exudate. All patients were treated with oral ofloxacin, removal of the granulation tissue, and instillation of neomycin sulfate or gentamicin sulfate, or both. Patients without a history of diabetes mellitus were evaluated during follow-up for results of the oral glucose tolerance test, glycolated hemoglobin values, and fructosamine levels.

Results.—The 6 men and 3 women with MEO and no history of diabetes had a mean age of 71 years. All lived on the Mediterranean coast, an area of high humidity during the summer, and they first experienced symptoms during the summer months. All patients had otalgia, and 6 had necrotic tissue or abcess formation, or both. The mean duration of symptoms before diagnosis was 32 days. In all 8 patients who had a ^{99m}Tc scan, the findings were abnormal; *P. aeruginosa* was isolated from the external auditory canal in all 9 patients. Ofloxacin (200 mg twice daily) was administered for 14 to 28 days. Symptoms subjectively improved after 5 days of treatment and objectively improved after 7 to 12 days. During follow-up of at least 6 months after recovery, all patients had normal glycolated hemoglobin and fructosamine levels, and 7 had normal glucose tolerance.

Conclusion.—The age of these patients with MEO and the absence of a history of diabetes suggests that age-related, small-vessel disease may be involved in the development of MEO. None of the patients had a history of ear disease, and most did not show impaired glucose tolerance. The diagnosis of MEO should be considered in otherwise healthy patients with *P. aeruginosa* infection of the external auditory meatus and other characteristic signs of the condition.

▶ This important article reminds us that MEO can occur in patients who do not have diabetes. Nine of 32 patients studied did not have diabetes. External otitis may initiate in the external auditory canal, but it can cause great damage to the middle ear and inner ear, as well as to the associated intracranial structures, including the cranial nerves.—M.M. Paparella, M.D.

Malignant Hyperthermia in the Otology Patient: The UCLA Experience

Wackym PA, Blackwell KE (Univ of California, Los Angeles)
Am J Otol 15:371–375, 1994   130-95-3–8

Background.—The incidence of malignant hyperthermia (MH) during otologic surgery is unknown. Among 280 MH crises reported during anesthesia for head and neck surgery, 6.8% occurred during anesthesia for general otologic procedures such as myringoplasty, tympanoplasty, or mastoidectomy. A protocol has been established for anesthetic and surgical management of MH-susceptible patients. Experience using the protocol during otologic surgery in MH-susceptible patients was described.

Methods.—Seven patients who had previously experienced MH or had a strong family history of MH were anesthetized with nitrous oxide, barbiturates, opiates, tranquilizers, and nondepolarizing muscle relaxants. Prophylactic dantrolene was not administered. Cardiac performance, end-tidal PCO_2, and rectal temperature were monitored. Vastus lateralis muscle biopsy and caffeine/halothane contracture studies were performed.

Results.—Bilateral myringotomy with tympanostomy tube insertion was performed in 5 patients; tympanoplasty in 1; and tympanomastoidectomy in 1. Six muscle biopsy specimens responded positively to the caffeine/halothane contracture test. Preoperative, intraoperative, and postoperative temperature and cardiac monitoring and tactile muscle tone assessment did not indicate impending MH crisis. None of the patients had any clinical signs of MH develop.

Conclusion.—This protocol enhances the safety of otologic surgery in patients susceptible to MH crisis. Patients at risk for having MH crisis develop can undergo otologic surgical procedures safely with appropriately selected anesthesia.

MR Imaging and MR Angiography in the Evaluation of Pulsatile Tinnitus
Dietz RR, Davis WL, Harnsberger HR, Jacobs JM, Blatter DD (Univ of Utah Med Ctr; LDS Hosp, Salt Lake City, Utah)
AJNR 15:879–889, 1994   130-95-3–9

Background.—Pulsatile tinnitus is associated with a spectrum of lesions, which makes assessment by imaging a challenge. The differential diagnosis includes congenital and acquired vascular lesions as well as skull base tumors. One experience with MR and MR angiographic (MRA) imaging in patients with pulsatile tinnitus was reported.

Methods.—Forty-nine patients were evaluated from February 1991 through December 1992. The patients were 31 females and 17 males, aged 12 to 80 years. Spin-echo MR and MRA were done in all. In 10 cases, CT images were available for review. Conventional angiography was also done in 17 patients.

Findings.—Twenty-eight patients had vascular lesions or paraganglioma on imaging. Forty-six percent of these lesions were seen best on MRA, and 36% were seen only on MRA. The most common lesion identified was dural arteriovenous fistula (AVF), seen in 9 patients. Associated MR and MRA findings were increased number and size of extracranial vessels, visualization of transosseous collateral vessels, abnormal flow in the dural sinus or other venous channels, stenosis or occlusion of the transverse sinus, and abnormal signal from the calvarium overlying the site of the fistula. Extracranial direct AVF was observed in 3 patients. Because of the large vascular channels and high flow associated with these lesions, they were readily identified on MR and MRA. The other lesions detected were paraglanglioma in 5 patients, jugular bulb variants in 3, aberrant internal carotid artery in 1, internal carotid artery stenosis in 1, tortuous internal carotid artery in 1, carotid dissection with pseudoaneurysms in 1, stenosis of the transverse sinus in 2, and ateriovenous malformation in 2.

Conclusion.—The spectrum of lesions associated with pulsatile tinnitus can be imaged effectively with MR and MRA. The latter contributes significant information to that provided by spin-echo MR and is useful or necessary in determining the cause of pulsatile tinnitus in most patients. Angiography should still be performed in patients with troublesome pulsatile tinnitus who have normal MR and MRA findings.

▶ New technology has evolved in MR and MRA in conjunction with spin-echo imaging, enhancing the ability of MR to diagnose lesions that cause pulsatile tinnitus. Such lesions can involve the middle ear cleft, with secondary labyrinthine involvement, or vice versa.—M.M. Paparella, M.D.

Management of Petrous Bone Fractures in Children: Analysis of 127 Cases

Glarner H, Meuli M, Hof E, Gallati V, Nadal D, Fisch U, Stauffer UG (Univ Children's Hosp, Zurich, Switzerland; Univ Hosp Zurich, Switzerland)
J Trauma 36:198–201, 1994

130-95-3–10

Introduction.—Petrous bone fractures (PBFs) are relatively common in children with head trauma. Complications may be life threatening or lead to permanent hearing loss. The etiology of PBF, the frequency and type of complications associated with this injury, and means of treating and preventing meningitis were determined retrospectively.

Methods.—The charts of children younger than 16 years of age admitted to the study institution between 1980 and 1989 with PBF were reviewed for mechanism of injury, complications, and treatment. Palsy of the facial nerve was described as immediate when diagnosed on the day of the accident and late when occurring with a delay of 24 hours or more. An early meningitis occurred during the first 2 weeks after trauma, whereas a late meningitis appeared after months or years.

Results.—During the study period, 139 PBFs were found in 127 children, 77 boys and 50 girls with a median age of 7 years 10 months. There were 110 unilateral and 22 bilateral longitudinal fractures (LFs) and 7 unilateral transverse fractures (TFs). An LF does not involve the inner ear, whereas a TF passes through the inner ear and always leads to deafness. All but 6 of the children had been injured in traffic collisions (49.6%) or falls (45.7%). Conductive hearing loss was common but generally transient after LF. Sensorineural hearing loss occurred in 9 patients after LF, 1 of whom remained deaf despite surgical revision. Another patient with LF had irreversible bilateral deafness after late meningitis. Irreversible deafness occurred in 7 patients after TF. Unilateral peripheral facial nerve palsy was seen in 8.3% of the LF group and 28.6% of the TF group. Both cases of facial palsy after TF showed immediate onset. Liquorrhea was diagnosed in 19 patients (14.4%) after LF and in 4 patients (57.1%) after TF. Altogether, 11 patients (8.6%) required surgery for complications of PBF.

Conclusion.—Severe complications of PBF may result in further morbidity and irreversible defects and thus require aggressive diagnostic and therapeutic measures. Children with PBF should be monitored daily during hospitalization for evidence of cranial nerve palsy, liquorrhea, and meningitis. Routine audiometric examinations and antibiotic prophylaxis are also indicated. Subtotal petrosectomy after TF and vaccination against *Streptococcus pneumoniae* are recommended to lower the incidence of posttraumatic meningitis.

▶ These injuries involve not only the labyrinth but also other aspects of the temporal bone. This is an interesting series because it contains such a large number of patients. The study, presented in the *Journal of Trauma,* will help alert otolaryngologists to such findings subsequent to trauma.—M.M. Paparella, M.D.

Extracranial and Intracranial Complications of Suppurative Otitis Media: Report of 102 Cases
Kangsanarak J, Fooanant S, Ruckphaopunt K, Navacharoen N, Teotrakul S (Chiang Mai Univ, Thailand)
J Laryngol Otol 107:999–1004, 1993   130-95-3–11

Introduction.—The risk of complications of acute and chronic otitis media has decreased significantly since the advent of antibiotics. However, severe complications can still occur as the result of physician inexperience, changing bacterial virulence, and the individual patient's condition. This report from Thailand examines the prevalence of complications of acute and chronic otitis media.

Patients.—A total of 17,144 cases of suppurative otitis media were treated during an 8-year period. During this time, there were 102 patients with intracranial (IC) or extracranial (EC) complications. Prevalence was .24% for IC and .45% for EC complications. The common EC complications included facial paralysis, subperiosteal abscess, and labyrinthitis; the IC complications included meningitis and brain abscess. Multiple complications were seen in 44% of the IC group and 25% of the EC group.

Warning signs of IC complications included fever, headache, earache, vestibular symptoms, meningeal signs, and impaired consciousness. The organisms most commonly associated with both types of complications were *Proteus spp., Pseudomonas aeruginosa,* and *Staphylococcus spp.* In both complication groups, cholesteatoma and granulation or polyp in the middle ear or mastoid were important findings. Nineteen percent of the IC group died. The morbidity rate was 14.3% in the EC group and 27.9% in the IC group.

Conclusion.—Even with appropriate antibiotic therapy, patients with suppurative otitis media can have EC or IC complications. Early diagnosis relies on recognition of the clinical signs and symptoms, culture, and CT scan. Patients with complications should be referred to an experienced otologist, who will decide the priority of treatments (e.g., systemic antibiotics, neurosurgery, or treatment for ear lesions).

▶ I have had the occasion to visit Chiang Mai, a beautiful small city in upper Thailand. This very large series of 102 patients certainly reminds us that otitis media can secondarily cause serious complications in the IC space as well as the EC space.—M.M. Paparella, M.D.

A Contactless Electromagnetic Implantable Middle Ear Device for Sensorineural Hearing Loss

Maniglia AJ, Ko WH, Rosenbaum M, Zhu W-L, Werning J, Belser R, Drago P, Falk T, Frenz W (Case Western Reserve Univ, Cleveland, Ohio; Wilson Greatbatch Ltd, Clarence, NY)
ENT J 73:78–90, 1994   130-95-3–12

Introduction.—A contactless electromagnetic implantable hearing device has been developed after basic science experiments, improvement of precision micromechanics and electronic design, and development of different prototypes.

The Device.—The device consists of external and internal units (Fig 3–2). The external unit consists of an electret microphone, amplitude modulated radiofrequency amplifier, antenna (copper coil), and battery. The external unit is packaged in a $12 \times 12 \times 5$-mm plastic case to be concealed in a postauricular skin pocket. The electrical signal is picked up by the platinum iridium (PI) coil implanted over the squamous portion of the temporal bone. A titanium supporting shaft affixes the electronic case and driving coil. The PI wire is introduced in a glass-insulated feedthrough into a titanium, hermetically sealed, laser-welded case and is connected to a hybrid electronic circuit. The solid state, hybrid circuit transforms radio signals into auditory signals that activate a titanium-encased air core coil copper wire. This drive coil or vibrator generates a magnetic field that activates, in a contactless manner, the neodymium-iron-boron magnet encapsulated in titanium (14 mg of weight per magnet) and surgically and permanently fixed in the incus.

Experiments.—The device (Fig 3–3) was successfully implanted in cats. In acute experiments with the incus out, the minimal auditory brainstem response recorded was at the 105-dB sound pressure level (SPL) (conductive hearing loss). When the magnet was cemented to the stapes and

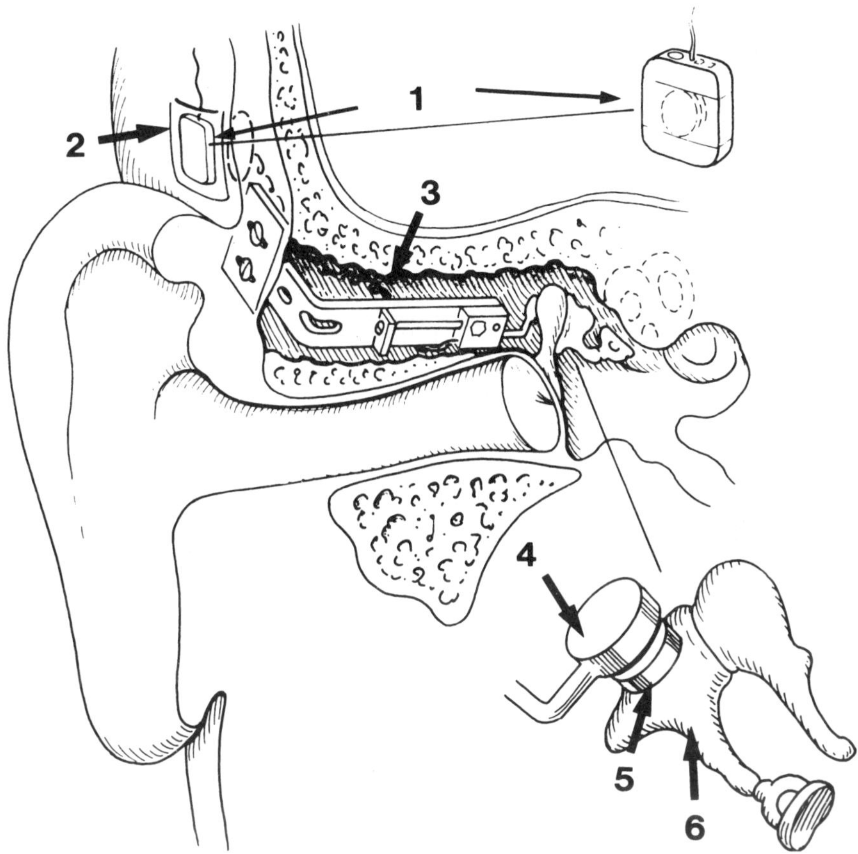

Fig 3–2.—Depiction of device implanted in the human mastoid antrum and attic. The external unit (1) is lodged in the skin pocket (2), supporting the shaft, electronics, and coil (3). The **inset** shows the coil (4) and magnet (5) on the incus (6). (Courtesy of Maniglia AJ, Ko WH, Rosenbaum M, et al: *ENT J* 73:78–90, 1994.)

the device affixed 1.0 mm away from the magnet, the threshold improved to a 55-dB SPL, for a gain of 50 dB.

Summary.—The contactless electromagnetic implantable middle ear device can be suitable for the treatment of moderate to severe sensorineural hearing loss. Chronic experiments in cats and rabbits are ongoing to test the components of the device. When favorable results are achieved, the device will be implanted in fewer than 10 volunteers, pending reviews and approvals. The lifetime of the coil, magnet, and implanted electronics and antenna could be unlimited, and the external unit can always be improved and upgraded as technology advances.

▶ Maniglia and co-workers continue to contribute to our understanding and knowledge of a device that, we hope, will someday come to fruition: a mid-

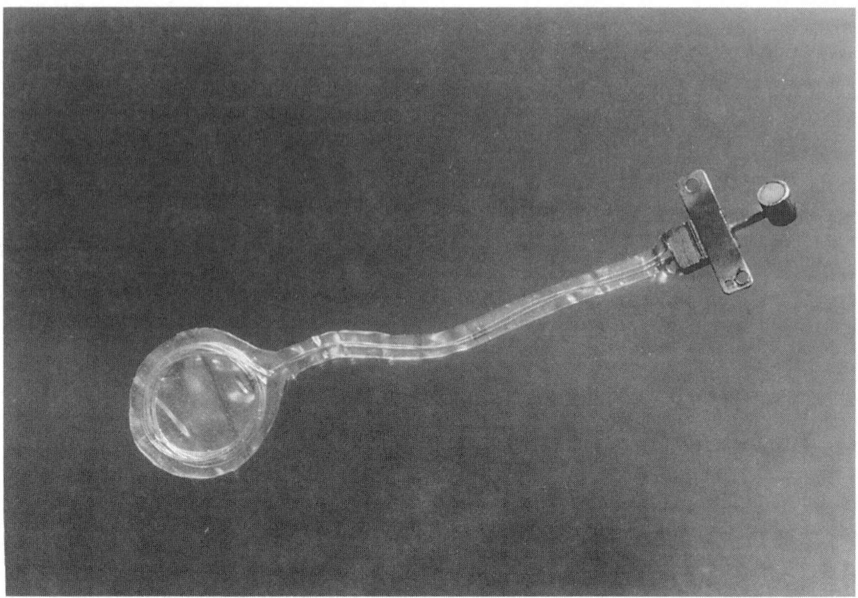

Fig 3–3.—Implantable device designed for the cat experiment. At the left, the platinum-iridium coil (antenna) is encapsulated in silicone. At the right is the titanium housing for the electronics and coil. (Courtesy of Maniglia AJ, Ko WH, Rosenbaum M, et al: *ENT J* 73:78–90, 1994.)

dle ear implant that will help many patients with sensorineural hearing loss. This will be a means of using the middle ear to enhance function in the inner ear. This update is interesting and provides us a glimpse of the future. It is anticipated that this device will not only enhance auditory perception but will also avoid feedback and other problems associated with hearing aids inserted in the external auditory canal.—M.M. Paparella, M.D.

Implantation of Electromagnetic Ossicular Replacement Device

Tos M, Salomon G, Bonding P (Gentofte Hosp, Hellerup, Denmark; Glostrup Hosp, Copenhagen)
ENT J 73:92–103, 1994   130-95-3–13

Introduction.—Six patients undergoing surgery for chronic otitis media underwent implantation of a semi-implantable hearing aid. The Heide system of the semi-implantable hearing device consists of a permanent middle ear implanted magnet, either partial ossicular replacement prostheses (PORPs) or total ossicular replacement prostheses (TORPs) driven by an electromagnet placed in the ear canal (Fig 3–4).

Techniques.—In 2 patients with a fixed malleus, disruption of the ossicular chain was performed with extrusion of the incus, resection of the malleus head, and interposition of a magnetic PORP between the stapes and the ear drum. In 2 patients with a posterosuperior perforation of

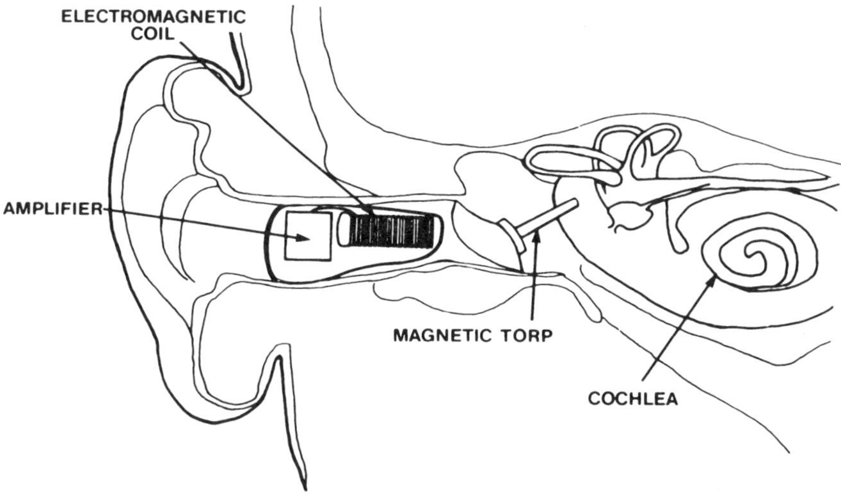

Fig 3–4.—Schematic drawing of the Heide system of the semi-implantable hearing device, in situ, in the external acoustic meatus. A TORP is located between the drum and the footplate. (From Heide J, Tatge G, Sander T, et al: Development of a semi-implantable hearing device, in Hoke M [ed]: *Advances in Audiology, Volume 4.* Middle Ear Implant. Implantable hearing aids. Basel, Switzerland, Karger, 1988. Courtesy of Tos M, Salomon G, Bonding P: *ENT J* 73:92–103, 1994.)

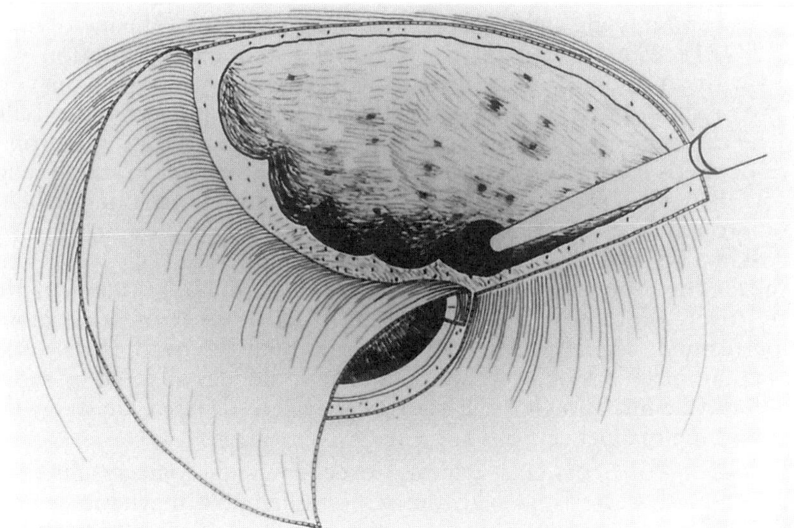

Fig 3–5.—Method of removal of the protrusion from the posterosuperior ear canal by elevation of the superiorly pedicled skin flap and gradual drilling of the bone. After drilling, the flap is replaced in its original position. (From Tos M: *Manual of Middle Ear Surgery.* Stuttgart, Germany, Thieme, 1993. Courtesy of Tos M, Salomon G, Bonding P: *ENT J* 73:92–103, 1994.)

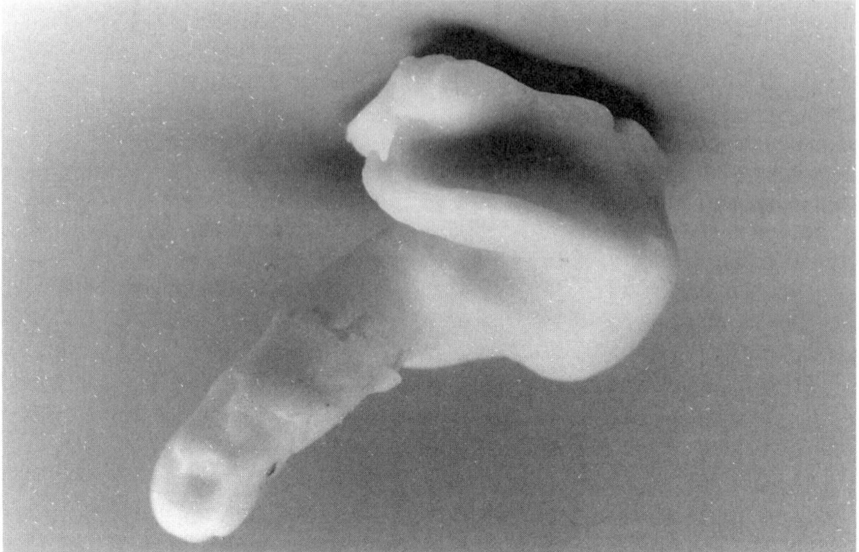

Fig 3–6.—Impression of the head of the prosthesis on the silicone mold, indicating a shortening of 1 to 2 mm of the impression mold to provide an optimal distance between the driver and the prosthesis. (Courtesy of Tos M, Salomon G, Bonding P: *ENT J* 73:92–103, 1994.)

pars tensa and missing stapedial arch and long process of the incus, magnetic TORPs were placed on the footplate, and the perforation was closed with an underlay fascia graft. Two patients with a previous conservative radical cavity underwent partial reconstruction of the middle ear. The eardrum was reconstructed with a fascia placed onto the prominence of the horizontal semicircular canal and the fallopian canal; magnetic TORPs were placed on the footplate. In 3 patients, anterior bulging or prominences of the ear canal were removed by elevating the ear canal skin flap and drilling off the bony prominence (Fig 3–5). After healing of the tympanoplasty and the ear canal, the adjustment of the future driver, which was designed on the basis of an impression mold, was performed. The impression of the drum with the head of the prosthesis could often be seen on the mold. The mold was adapted by shortening 1 to 2 mm, allowing the shortest possible distance between the driver and the magnet (Fig 3–6).

Outcome.—All 6 patients achieved excellent audiologic results. The transmission characteristics with the semi-implantable magnetic hearing aid varied between patients, but a functional gain of 40 to 70 dB was obtained for the entire frequency range of the audiogram. This gain was obtained by using a battery that lasted 6 to 7 hours.

▶ Tos and associates have now applied this device in 6 patients, and this too appears to be a promising approach, along with the former approach described by Maniglia. We await further developments with eagerness and anticipation.—M.M. Paparella, M.D.

Perilymphatic Fistula: The Value of Diagnostic Tests
Podoshin L, Fradis M, Ben-David J, Berger SI, Feiglin H (Bnai Zion Med Centre, Haifa, Israel; The Bruce Rappaport Faculty of Medicine, Haifa, Israel; Technion-Israel Inst of Technology, Haifa)
J Laryngol Otol 108:560–563, 1994   130-95-3–14

Background.—Perilymphatic fistula (PLF) remains a challenging problem in otologic practice. Controversy still surrounds the accuracy of its clinical diagnosis, and many studies have been done to achieve a better diagnosis of this entity. The value of diagnostic tests in identifying this condition was investigated, and the indications for an explanatory tympanotomy were verified.

Method.—Fifty-two patients (53 ears) who underwent explorative tympanotomy for suspected PLF were studied. The criteria for explorative tympanotomy included suggestive anamnesis such as trauma, including barotrauma, and severe physical efforts; fluctuating hearing loss without other symptoms of Meniere's disease; and sudden hearing loss with findings suggestive of relief in the electronystagmography (ENG) testing.

Results.—Of the 53 tympanotomies performed, PLF was found in 40 ears. In all patients with a clear anamnesis of trauma or physical effort a PLF was found. Six patients with an upper respiratory tract infection and strenuous cough also had a PLF, whereas in 3 with the same anamnesis a PLF was not found. No significant correlation was found regarding a complaint of vertigo and PLF, despite the fact that in the literature vertigo and nystagmus are regarded as an indicator of PLF. Neither was any audiologic pattern found characterizing PLF. A positive fistula test in ENG was found to be suggestive of PLF in 75% of patients, with the presence of a positive caloric test in 78%, and with the additional presence of positional nystagmus in 100%. Of 13 ears in which the ENG findings were negative, a PLF was found in only 3. The only positive finding was that 100% of patients in whom a fistula was identified had a positive fistula test and positional nystagmus. None of the patients in whom no fistula was found had a positive fistula test and positional nystagmus.

Conclusion.—No single test has yet been considered diagnostic for perilymphatic fistulas, and it has not been possible to be certain if the clinical entity exists without surgical exploration. The results suggest that the diagnosis of perilymphatic fistulas can be based on the clinical picture and a number of laboratory diagnostic tests. However, further research is required to identify a single test that allows for diagnosing this condition preoperatively.

▶ I am in concurrence with these authors' conclusion that there is not any one test that will diagnose PLF but, rather, that history plays the most important role and laboratory tests can be supportive or supplementary. I personally believe the history is most important, as is suggested by this study.—M.M. Paparella, M.D.

Absent Round Window Reflex: Possible Relation to Step-Wise Hearing Loss
Harvey SA, Millen SJ (Med College of Wisconsin, Milwaukee)
Am J Otol 15:237–242, 1994   130-95-3–15

Introduction.—A perilymphatic fistula was sought in 4 children with marked hearing impairment whose losses progressed in a stepwise manner after a period of relative stability. Instead of a fistula, these patients were found to have a normally mobile stapes but no round window reflex, and the secondary tympanic membrane appeared full or tense.

Case Report.—Woman, 18, had been hearing impaired since birth. The hearing loss had been stable for many years. At exploration of the left ear 10 years before, no round window reflex was obtained despite a normally mobile stapes footplate. Hearing in the right ear, the only one with useful hearing, decreased abruptly 6 months before referral. Hearing recovered after 1 week of steroid treatment. The patient received diazepam for mild motion-related unsteadiness. Hearing in the right ear again decreased 2 months later, in association with recruitment and imbalance. Neuro-otologic assessment, including a fistula test, was negative. Audiography disclosed a speech awareness threshold of 80 dB on the left with no discrimination, and a speech reception threshold of 90 dB on the right with 32% discrimination. High-resolution CT of the temporal bones was negative. On exploration of the right ear, the round window membrane appeared full and tense and no reflex was elicited. The stapes was mobile. Paracentesis of the round window membrane led to a rapid flow of perilymph. Hearing recovered to baseline within 4 weeks of surgery. The patient currently receives a diuretic.

Interpretation.—This clinical picture may reflect altered fluid dynamics within the inner ear. It is possible that a fistula developed earlier and healed spontaneously. These patients do not necessarily require surgical exploration.

▶ The round window reflex is an important step in considering phase-differential interactions of the middle ear and inner ear, and conduction of sound along the basilar membrane. There are a variety of causes that can influence the round window reflex, such as perilymphatic hypertension, a growth in the scala tympani adjacent to the round window membrane (such as otosclerosis), and other causes. It is useful to study this perplexing finding, and it continues to have clinical relevance; however, there are so many factors that can affect a round window reflex test.—M.M. Paparella, M.D.

Inner Ear Injury Caused by Air Intrusion to the Scala Vestibuli of the Cochlea

Kobayashi T, Sakurada T, Ohyama K, Takasaka T (Tohoku Univ, Sendai, Japan)
Acta Otolaryngol 113:725–730, 1993   130-95-3–16

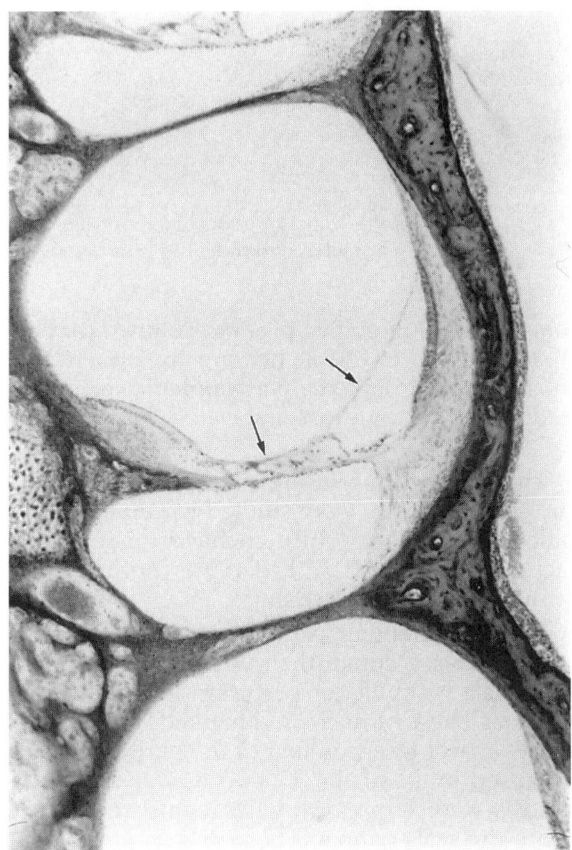

Fig 3–7.—A photomicrograph of the second cochlear turn perfused with air in the scala vestibuli for .5 minutes at a flow rate of 6 μL/min. Severe collapse of the endolymphatic space of the cochlear duct is prominent, and Reissner's membrane (*arrows*) is seen to drape over the organ of Corti. (Magnification, × 10.) (Courtesy of Kobayashi T, Sakurada T, Ohyama K, et al: *Acta Otolaryngol* 113:725–730, 1993.)

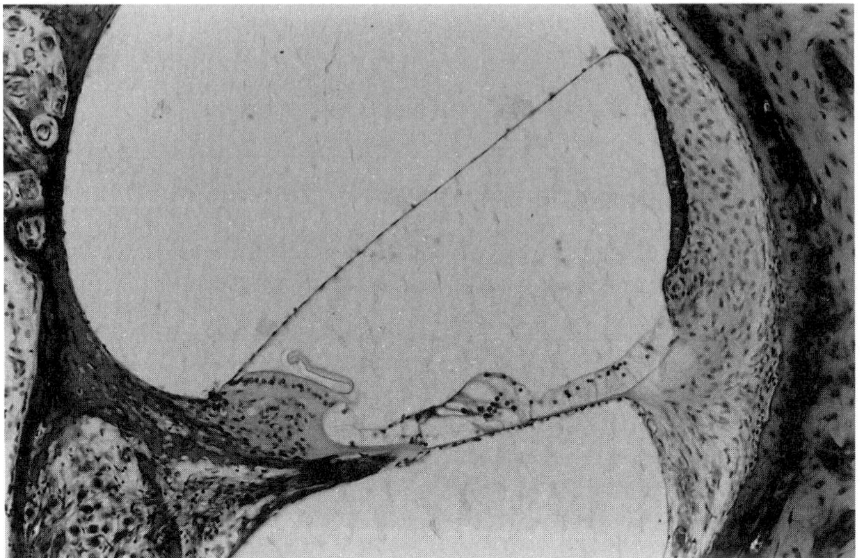

Fig 3–8.—A representative histopathology of the cochlea after air perfusion of the scala tympani for 60 minutes at a very high flow rate (200 μL/min). Little change was observed in the cochlear structures. (Magnification, $\times$13.) (Courtesy of Kobayashi T, Sakurada T, Ohyama K, et al: *Acta Otolaryngol* 113:725–730, 1993.)

Introduction.—Studies in guinea pigs have shown that air perfusion in the scala tympani leads to reversible hearing impairment. It has been suggested that intrusion of air into the perilymphatic space, or pneumolabyrinth, may lead to the hearing loss associated with perilymphatic fistula formation.

Methods.—The effects of perfusing air into the scala vestibuli, as compared with the scala tympani, were studied in guinea pigs by monitoring the endocochlear dc potential (EP), cochlear microphonics (CM), and compound action potential (CAP). Air was perfused using a syringe pump at flow rates of 3 to 60 μL/minute.

Results.—Cochlear potentials were depressed more markedly by perfusing air into the scala vestibuli than was previously noted in the scala tympani. In the scala vestibuli, air perfusion reduced the negative EP in response to anoxia. The CM decreased markedly at the start of air perfusion and did not recover after refilling of the perilymph. Reissner's membrane was collapsed in 12 of the 17 cochleas examined (Fig 3–7). The histologic changes were impressive when compared with the results of perfusing air into the scala tympani (Fig 3–8).

Implications.—A very small amount of air may suffice to damage the inner ear structures. If pneumolabyrinth has a role in the development of perilymphatic fistula, patients with an oval window fistula may have a worse outlook than those with a round window fistula. Air inflation of the middle ear would appear to be dangerous if an oval window fistula is present.

▶ It is possible that air entering the inner ear can be part of the pathogenesis of why perilymphatic fistulas cause sensorineural hearing loss. Another possibility is contamination from the nasopharynx via the eustachian tube through the round window membrane. In any case, these authors continue to study the role of air in the pathogenesis of PLF, and I think this is useful and continues to add to our understanding of the problem. It is likely that the fistula per se does not cause problems, but secondary effects, such as this one to the inner ear, may best explain the pathogenesis of this form of middle ear/inner ear interactive disease.—M.M. Paparella, M.D.

Intratympanic Gentamicin in Bilateral Meniere's Disease
Pyykkö I, Ishizaki H, Kaasinen S, Aalto H (Univ Hosp, Helsinki; Hamamatsu School of Medicine, Japan)
Otolaryngol Head Neck Surg 110:162–167, 1994   130-95-3–17

Background.—Some animal experiments have indicated that intratympanic gentamicin may be less ototoxic than systemic streptomycin, which is commonly used in bilateral Meniere's disease. Vestibular ablation with streptomycin is often followed by oscillopsia and gait problems. The use of unilateral intratympanic gentamicin on the recovery of postural stability in bilateral, intractable Meniere's disease was evaluated.

Methods.—Fourteen patients, 24 to 74 years of age (mean, 52 years), with a mean duration of disease of 19.4 years were studied. Six of them had undergone previous surgical treatment. Baseline complete electronystagmographic series were obtained. Postural stability was measured with eyes closed on a force platform connected to a computer. The system recorded the center point of forces on the platform, and the velocity was determined. Buffered gentamicin, 20 mg, was injected into a topically anesthetized spot on the lower quadrant of the tympanic membrane. Patients received 1 injection per day, for a total of 1 to 4 injections. Follow-up evaluations were done at 2 weeks and at 1, 3, 6, 12, and 24 months.

Results.—The pretreatment severity of attacks of vertigo had a significant inverse correlation, with gait problems and Tumarkin attacks being directly correlated with gait problems. The degree of hearing loss, gait disturbance, and severity of rotary vertigo were the significant factors affecting work capacity. The treatment abated the vertigo (rotary and Tumarkin) attacks in all but 3 patients. These 3 had substantially less severe vertigo after therapy. Four patients had persistent diminished work capacity. This residual disability was significantly associated with increased age and gait disturbance. Hearing was not significantly changed. Postural stability was worsened at the 2-week evaluation and gradually returned to baseline by 2 years. The labyrinths became calorically unresponsive to ice water in 8 patients, reduced response in 4, and normal in 2. This responsiveness correlated inversely with gait disturbance. Three patients had relapses of vertigo during the first year and were reinjected. One patient was reinjected when relapse occurred after 2.5 symptom-free years.

Discussion.—Other studies of intratympanic gentamicin have shown positive effects on vertigo, but severe hearing complications have resulted from more than 4 treatments. In these bilateral cases, only 1 or 2 treatments given 2 weeks apart benefited the patients in relieving vertigo. It is imperative that this treatment only be used when the causative ear can be identified. These patients all participated in a habituation program to help them cope with postural instability and recovery. Larger series of patients may help to delineate the ideal dosage and number of treatments as well as the relapse rate.

▶ We know that ototoxic drugs can cause problems of sensorineural deafness, if they are instilled into the middle ear. We also know that ototoxic drugs, if used in a controlled manner (such as gentamicin is used for Meniere's disease), can be efficacious in terms of treatment. This study describes this method of causing chemical ablation of the vestibular labyrinth with attempts to preserve auditory function using a mechanism of interaction between middle ear and inner ear.—M.M. Paparella, M.D.

Cochlear Polyamines: Markers of Otitis Media-Induced Cochlear Damage

Naguib MB, Hunter RE, Henley CM (Baylor College of Medicine, Houston; Military Med Academy, Cairo, Egypt)
Laryngoscope 104:1003–1007, 1994   130-95-3–18

Introduction.—There have been few reports of specific biochemical changes in response to otitis media-induced cochlear damage. In an experimental study, polyamine tissue levels in separate cochlear tissue of the guinea pig were characterized, and the effects of *Streptococcus pneumoniae* otitis media on polyamine metabolism in the inner ear were determined.

Methods.—Twenty albino guinea pigs weighing 200 g were separated into an experimental group and a control group, each with 10 animals. The ears of experimental animals were inoculated with a bacterial suspension containing *S. pneumoniae* and the ears of controls with sterile tryptic soy broth. The guinea pigs were divided for sacrifice on days 3, 7, 14, 21, and 28 postinfection, but analyzed collectively. High-performance liquid chromatography set to the femtoliter sensitivity level was used to identify and quantify the polyamines spermidine and spermine, as well as the diamine putrescine in the different tissues of the inner ears. The tissues examined were the lateral wall, the organ of Corti, and the cochlear nerve.

Results.—Cochlear tissue of the control guinea pigs exhibited the diamine putrescine and the polyamines spermidine and spermine. The relative amounts of putrescine, spermidine, and spermine were similar in the organ of Corti and the lateral wall. In the cochlear nerve, however, the level of spermidine was 3 times greater than that of putrescine and 20 times greater than that of spermine; the level of putrescine was 6 times greater than spermine. Total polyamine content was significantly higher in the organ of Corti and the cochlear nerve than in the lateral wall in control animals. The experimental group showed a trend for lower putrescine levels in the organ of Corti and the lateral wall. The mean levels of putrescine in the organ of Corti of *S. pneumoniae*-treated guinea pigs were 54.1% of those of control guinea pigs. Spermine significantly increased in the organ of Corti and the lateral wall of the experimental animals.

Conclusion.—Differences in polyamine profiles observed in the inner ear tissues of infected vs. noninfected guinea pigs suggest the presence of a specific biochemical response to injury. Polyamines may be involved in a repair process of the inner ear and are potential biochemical markers for inner ear damage associated with acute otitis media.

▶ These authors believe that polyamines may involve tissues of the inner ear secondarily to acute otitis media. A number of markers have been studied, and this investigation appears to be an interesting attempt to understand the pathogenesis of why, in certain patients and certainly in animals, otitis media can cause cochlear dysfunction. These studies should continue.—M.M. Paparella, M.D.

Suppression of Tinnitus by Cochlear Implantation
Ito J, Sakakihara J (Otsu Red Cross Hosp, Shiga, Japan; Kyoto Univ, Japan)
Am J Otolaryngol 15:145–148, 1994   130-95-3–19

Background.—Transcutaneous electrical stimulation provides relief to approximately 33% of patients with tinnitus; transpromontory electrical stimulation, to 60%. Many patients experience relief of tinnitus after multichannel cochlear implant surgery. Cochlear implant may be superior to transcutaneous or transpromontory electrical stimulation in relieving tinnitus because the implant stimulates the cochlear nerve directly. The change in tinnitus after cochlear implant surgery was evaluated.

Methods.—Tinnitus was documented and quantified in 18 hearing-impaired or totally deaf patients before cochlear implant surgery. Before surgery, the effectiveness of promontory stimulation in relieving tinnitus was tested. After implantation, the change in tinnitus was determined.

Results.—Before cochlear implantation, tinnitus was marked in 5 patients and slight in 13. Promontory stimulation relieved tinnitus in 72%

of patients: Tinnitus disappeared in 4, was suppressed in 9, and did not change in 5. Cochlear implantation effectively relieved tinnitus in 83% of patients: Tinnitus was abolished in 8, suppressed in 7, unchanged in 2, and aggravated in 1.

Conclusion.—Cochlear implantation suppresses tinnitus in many patients. The mechanism of this suppression remains unclear.

▶ The fundamental indication for cochlear implantation is to allow for audition and speech development, to the optimal degree possible. It may be that, as studies such as this one evolve, we may find an additional indication: the relief of tinnitus in individuals who are deaf. It is interesting that, under the design of this study, 72% of these patients had relief of tinnitus.—M.M. Paparella, M.D.

4 Otosclerosis

Effect of Drinking Water Fluoridation on Hearing of Patients With Otosclerosis in a Low Fluoride Area: A Follow-Up Study
Vartiainen E, Karjalainen S, Nuutinen J, Suntioinen S, Pellinen P (Univ of Kuopio, Finland)
Am J Otol 15:545–548, 1994　　　　　　　　　　　　　　130-95-4–1

Objective.—Because sodium fluoride (NaF) reportedly has a beneficial effect on hearing in otosclerotic ears, the effects of drinking fluoridated water were examined in 280 patients with conductive hearing loss of otosclerotic origin. A total of 344 ears underwent surgery.

Methods.—Stapedectomy was done using a Teflon piston prosthesis in 182 ears, and a posterior crus stapedectomy (or stapedioplasty) was used in 162 ears. Samples of stapes footplate were taken in 50 cases to estimate fluorine content. The posterior crus was sampled in 12 cases and the posterior meatal wall in 41. The patients were followed for a mean of 9.6 years.

Results.—The fluorine content of the stapes footplate and meatal wall was slightly higher in patients who drank fluoridated water than in those drinking fluoride-poor water, but the difference was not significant. No fluoride-related differences in air or bone conduction thresholds were apparent preoperatively or at last follow-up. Air conduction thresholds in unoperated ears were significantly worse in patients who drank low-fluoride water. The same was true for bone conduction thresholds at 2 and 4 kHz.

Conclusion.—A NaF intake of 2 to 3 mg daily benefits the hearing of unoperated patients with otosclerosis who live in a low-fluoride region, but does not significantly influence hearing in operated ears.

▶ Since the fluoridation of drinking water has become widespread throughout the United States, dental caries have apparently significantly reduced. One wonders, from an epidemiologic point of view, whether this might also reduce the incidence of otosclerosis. This study provides insight into this mechanism, and it would be interesting if such an epidemiologic study could be undertaken.—M.M. Paparella, M.D.

"

Far-Advanced Otosclerosis

Lippy WH, Battista RA, Schuring AG, Rizer FM (Northeastern Ohio College of Medicine, Warren, Ohio; EAR Consultants of Michigan, Royal Oak)
Am J Otol 15:225–228, 1994 130-95-4–2

Introduction.—Far-advanced otosclerosis (FAO) may be difficult to distinguish from a profound sensorineural hearing loss because many patients with FAO have no measurable air or bone conduction thresholds. Surgery can be worthwhile, however, when patients with FAO have cochlear reserve. A review of 59 patients (73 ears) examines outcome relative to severity of preoperative air and bone conduction thresholds.

Patients and Methods.—The patient group included 30 men and 29 women and had a mean age of 61 years. All underwent surgery performed by the senior author from 1961 to 1991. Group 1 (31 ears) had untestable preoperative air and bone conduction thresholds. Group 2 (14 ears) had air conduction thresholds greater than 85 dB and untestable bone conduction thresholds. Group 3 (11 ears) had untestable air conduction thresholds and fragmentary bone response only at 500 Hz. Group 4 (10 ears) had air conduction thresholds greater than 85 dB and fragmentary bone response only at 500 Hz. Included in group 5 were patients operated on after 1985 when improved audiometric equipment became available. Bone conduction testing could be provided to 80 dB versus the previous limit of 65 dB. All group 5 patients had air conduction thresholds greater than 90 dB and bone conduction thresholds greater than 65 dB. Surgical success was defined as improvement in at least 2 of 3 measures: the 3-frequency pure-tone average air conduction threshold, speech discrimination score, or improvement with use of an aid.

Results.—In 77% of ears there was improvement of 20 dB or more in air conduction thresholds. Discrimination scores improved 15% or greater in 54% of cases, and 75% showed improvement with use of a hearing aid. The success rate, based on improvements on at least 2 of 3 measures, was 67% overall. Individual groups achieved success rates ranging from 45% (group 3) to 100% (group 5). Footplate drilling was required in 37% of ears. The 14 patients with bilateral FAO had similar surgical outcomes (6 successes and 8 failures) in the initial and contralateral ear.

Conclusion.—Because successful results were obtained in all 5 groups, the severity of postoperative hearing loss does not determine surgical outcome in FAO. If the first ear fails, however, the second should not undergo surgery. Exploration is recommended only when there is evidence of cochlear reserve, as in the patient's ability to hear a 512-Hz tuning fork on the teeth, dentures, or gums.

▶ These authors selected patients with far-advanced otosclerosis for study. They find that stapedectomy is efficacious for this group, which matches my experience as well. The best results, in patients with far-advanced otosclerosis, are in those who have little or no measurable hearing on a routine audiogram. If there is any kind of a conductive hearing loss, these are the "miracle" results, such as those in a patient who was literally deaf being brought to a speech-reception threshold of 60 or 70 dB and being able to use a hearing aid. This is far more impressive and conservative than considering the cochlear implant for such otherwise "deaf" patients.—M.M. Paparella, M.D.

Long-Term Hearing Results Following Stapedotomy
Dornhoffer JL, Bailey HAT Jr, Graham SS (Ear and Nose Throat Clinic, Little Rock, Ark; Univ of Arkansas, Little Rock)
Am J Otol 15:674–678, 1994   130-95-4-3

Background.—Stapedectomy continues to be the treatment of choice for the conductive hearing loss caused by otosclerosis. However, there has been a recent trend away from total removal of the stapes footplate toward a technique that creates a small hole in the footplate, known as the small fenestra technique (SFT) or stapedotomy. This method has shown encouraging early postoperative results, but few long-term follow-up data are available. The long-term hearing results of patients undergoing this type of surgery for otosclerosis were investigated.

Method.—The medical records of 35 patients who had undergone SFT between 1979 and 1986 were reviewed. Data were also examined for 27 nonoperated contralateral ears. The follow-up ranged from 5 to 11 years. Audiograms that included air conduction, and bone conduction thresholds, speech discrimination scores, and speech reception thresholds were done for both ears preoperatively, 1 month postoperatively, and at variable long-term follow-ups.

Results.—The long-term hearing results of the SFT technique compared favorably with those achieved with total stapedectomy. However, a statistical analysis proved difficult because of the differing methods used to report the data. After good initial hearing gain, the air conduction thresholds saw a linear decrease over a time of .4 dB/year for the pure-tone average. An initial improvement was also seen in the pure-tone average for bone conduction that continued for 2 years after surgery, followed by deterioration at a rate of .49 dB/year in the long term. Although there was good initial closure of the air-bone gap at all measured frequencies, there was no significant increase in conductive hearing loss with time. Bone conduction for the speech frequencies was seen to deteriorate in the nonoperated ear at a rate significantly higher than that for the operated ear, probably as a result of Carhart's effect.

Conclusion.—Small fenestra stapes surgery appears to produce long-term hearing results that are favorable to those of total stapedectomy.

► These authors compared the long-term results of stapedotomy with those of stapedectomy and found the long-term results to be fairly comparable. The number of patients is relatively small for a study of this type; nevertheless, this finding is of interest. I suspect that the results have a great deal to do with the skill and technique used by the surgeons as much as with the method per se. I might add that patients who have a very small oval window (and I find this represents a significant percentage of patients in my practice who have otosclerosis) benefit more by having a complete stapedectomy, because making a stapedotomy in an already small footplate in a small oval window only encourages the possibility of fixation and regrowth of bone at a subsequent date.—M.M. Paparella, M.D.

The Role of KTP Laser in Revision Stapedectomy

McGee TM, Diaz-Ordaz EA, Kartush JM (Michigan Ear Inst, Farmington Hills; Naval Hosp, Portsmouth, Va)
Otolaryngol Head Neck Surg 109:839–843, 1993   130-95-4-4

Introduction.—The difficulty and risk associated with surgically dissecting scar tissue account for some of the poor results of conventional revision stapedectomy. However, laser technology allows the safe removal of scar tissue covering the oval window and accurate placement of the new prosthesis. The safety and efficacy of revision stapes surgery with the laser were compared with those of conventional revision stapedectomy.

Methods.—During a 7-year period, 77 patients underwent revision stapes surgery involving (1) removal of middle ear and oval window adhesions; and (2) oval window opening with laser followed by insertion of a new prosthesis. The patients were evaluated audiometrically before and 2 to 6 months after surgery.

Results.—The most common indications for revision stapes surgery were prosthesis displacement, followed by fibrous or bony closure of the oval window. None of the patients experienced either intraoperative or postoperative vertigo. Tinnitus did not increase in any patients. After revision stapedectomy, audiometric testing showed air-bone gap closure to within 10 dB in 80.5% of the patients, significantly improved hearing in 62.3%, and better speech discrimination in 7.8%, with no change in speech discrimination in 90.9%.

Discussion.—These audiometric improvements compare favorably with reports of other studies of revision stapes surgery leaving the oval window closed or using conventional techniques to open the oval window. A significant postoperative hearing loss, particularly loss of speech discrimination, and mechanical injury to the vestibule have been seen in patients undergoing conventional revision stapedectomy. Using the laser to remove scar tissue and to open the oval window improves safety and efficacy of revision stapes surgery.

▶ This article is selected in respect and in honor of Dr. McGee, who died recently. Dr. McGee was an excellent technician, did beautiful surgery, and, therefore, this article is of interest. He was my friend and senior resident, and I know we shall all miss him greatly. The effect of his contributions to our understanding of otology will continue for decades to come, as indicated by this article on the application of the KTP laser in revision stapedectomy.—M.M. Paparella, M.D.

Otosclerosis Regrowth

Robinson M (Brown Univ, Providence, RI)
Laryngoscope 103:1383–1384, 1993   130-95-4–5

Introduction.—Otosclerosis regrowth after stapedectomy is a rare delayed complication that results in conductive hearing loss. This problem, its incidence, and its etiology are briefly reviewed.

Etiology.—The osseous closure may result from reactivation of the otospongiotic lesion with initially high vascular new bone and subsequent sclerosis of the spongy lesion. Other cases might develop because of new bone formation with an increase in osteoblastic activity and diminished osteoclastic activity.

Differential Diagnosis.—Osseous closure of the oval window after stapedectomy must be distinguished from other causes of a delayed conductive-type hearing loss, including prosthesis displacement, incus necrosis, loosening of a wire prosthesis on the long process of the incus, malleus fixation, perilymphatic fistula, and tympanofibrosis. In patients with reclosure of the oval window, tuning fork tests will confirm the conductive component. Speech discrimination scores usually remain high. The prosthesis position and status of the oval window can be revealed by CT.

Discussion.—One review found an incidence of 3 regrowths per 1,000 stapedectomy cases. More than half (53%) underwent successful revision. In juvenile otosclerosis, footplate drilling was required in 27.8% of patients who underwent early surgical treatment; after age 18, 45.2% required drilling. Drilling of the otosclerotic footplate indicates advanced or aggressive disease. Overall, most bony reclosures have occurred in stapedectomies that have required the use of a drill. Prosthesis placement slightly into the vestibule may contribute to the retardation of otosclerotic regrowth.

▶ Mendell Robinson has had much experience in stapedial surgery. This article nicely documents his experience in dealing with regrowth of otosclerosis and will assist surgeons who do stapedectomy but who have less experience. Stapedectomy and the long-term results of stapedectomy will relate to the experience of the surgeon, and this certainly applies in the case of Dr. Robinson and his long-term observations and results.—M.M. Paparella, M.D.

Update of Reparative Granuloma: Survey of the American Otological Society and the American Neurotology Society

Seicshnaydre MA, Sismanis A, Hughes GB (Med College of Virginia, Richmond; Cleveland Clinic Found, Ohio)
Am J Otol 15:155–160, 1994   130-95-4–6

Introduction.—Reparative granuloma (RG), an uncommon complication of stapes surgery, is a formation of granulation tissue involving both the prosthesis and the oval window in a symptomatic patient. Most otologists consider RG to be a cause of sensorineural hearing loss and dizziness. There is no consensus on the appropriate management of RG. The current practice in treating this complication was examined.

Methods.—Members of the American Otological Society and the American Neurotology Society were polled via questionnaire.

Results.—Thirty-eight percent of the 467 questionnaires that were mailed were returned. The average number years of practice was 20, and among the 176 respondents, 277,101 stapedectomies and 42,309 stapedotomies had been performed. The incidence of RG after stapedectomy was .1%, which was significantly greater than the .07% reported with stapedotomy. Seventy-seven surgeons reported having encountered at least 1 RG. Most respondents believed that the cause of RG was foreign body material or infection. Four surgeons doubted the existence of RG. Reparative granuloma appeared most often in stapedectomies using Gelfoam or fat as the grafting material and prostheses made of metal. In the case of stapedotomy, blood clot and Gelfoam were the most common grafting materials and Teflon prostheses most often associated with RG, but the sample size for this group was small. Vertigo was the most frequently reported manifestation of RG. More than half the surgeons who had managed RG reported immediate surgical intervention. Fifty-eight percent favored removal and replacement of the prosthesis and grafting material; 36% removed only the RG. The overall impact on hearing was roughly equal between profound hearing loss, stabilization, and improvement. Improvement was more often associated with immediate surgery and concomitant steroid therapy. Fourteen surgeons reported cases of persistent tinnitus, and 10 reported cases of persistent vertigo.

Discussion.—The nature of this survey required respondents to report from memory and personal impressions, which are inherently biased. A survey requiring retrospective data retrieval probably would have yielded little response. The results indicate that RG can occur with either type of surgery and with any type of prosthesis and grafting material. Other reports have implicated Gelfoam and fat in an increased incidence of RG. At least 1 other study revealed an association between Teflon and RG. Two studies of immediate surgical intervention, each in a small series of patients, reported favorable hearing outcomes, but 1 study of nonsurgical management with steroids, antibiotics, and plasma expanders reported good outcomes as well. Reparative granuloma should be suspected after stapes surgery when vertigo and hearing loss are present and the eardrum appears dull and erythematous. This survey suggests that the best outcomes are achieved with early surgical intervention combined with steroids.

▶ This study is of interest and includes a large population of patients (several hundred thousand) having stapedial cases. The observations largely match my own: it seems I saw RGs several times in former years, but I have not seen one for the past 10, 15, or more years. The complications of stapedectomy include RG. It is also interesting that we do not see as much in the literature regarding perilymphatic fistulas after stapedectomy. Reparative granuloma and perilymphatic fistula after stapedectomy were commonly discussed in the literature and at meetings, and apparently the incidence is reduced, perhaps in relation to improved techniques or the lower incidence of cases treated now compared with decades ago.—M.M. Paparella, M.D.

5 Facial Nerve and Tumors

Glomus Tympanicum in Infancy

Jacobs IN, Potsic WP (Children's Hosp of Philadelphia; Univ of Pennsylvania Medical Ctr, Philadelphia)

Arch Otolaryngol Head Neck Surg 120:203–205, 1994   130-95-5-1

Background.—Glomus tumors, the most common neoplasm of the middle ear, usually occur in middle-aged women. They are very rare in

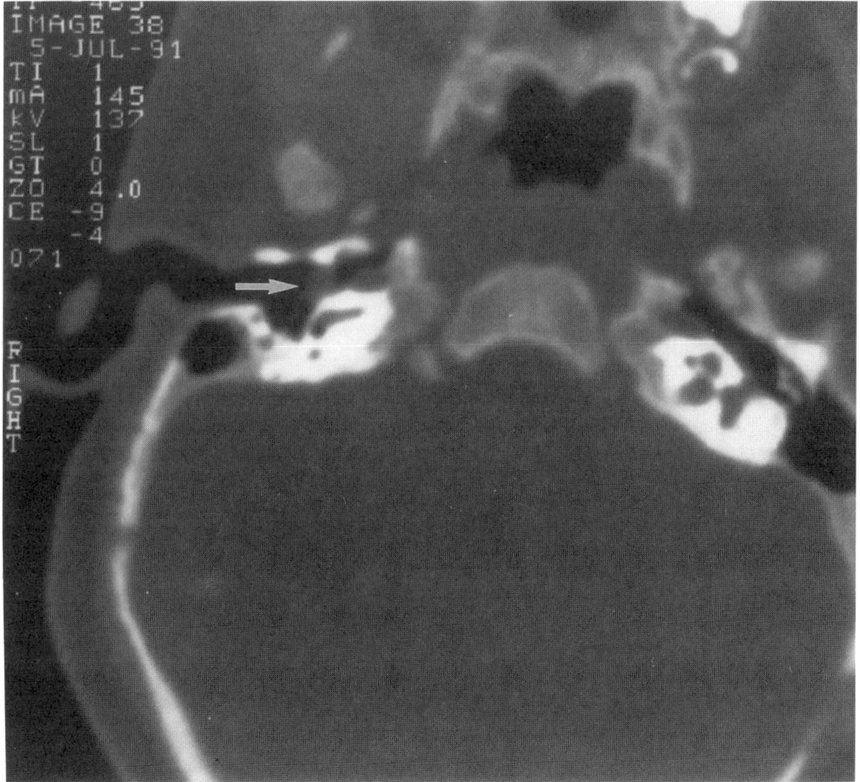

Fig 5–1.—Contrast-enhanced CT scan reveals a small lesion on the cochlear promontory (*arrow*). (Courtesy of Jacobs IN, Potsic WP: *Arch Otolaryngol Head Neck Surg* 120:203–205, 1994.)

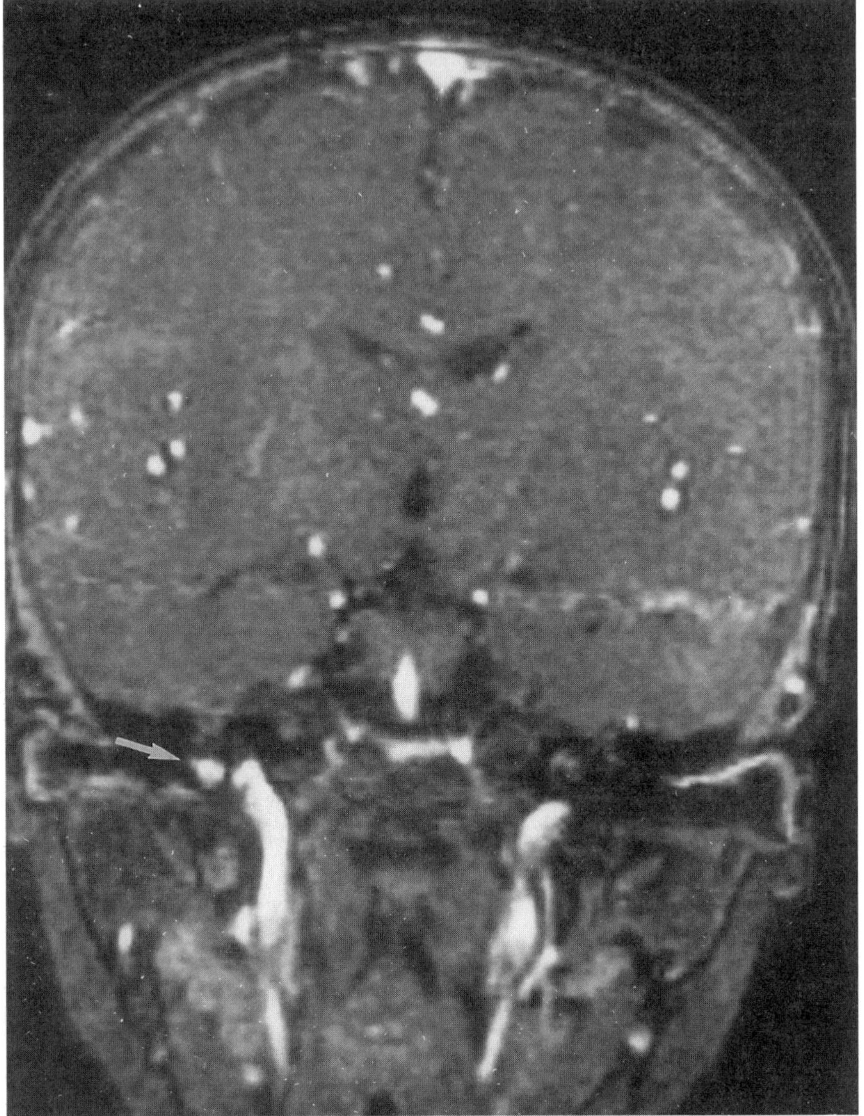

Fig 5–2.—Coronal gadolinium-enhanced MR angiogram reveals a lesion in the mesotympanum (*arrow*). (Courtesy of Jacobs IN, Potsic WP: *Arch Otolaryngol Head Neck Surg* 120:203–205, 1994.)

children. A 6-month-old girl with glomus tympanicum limited to the middle ear was described.

Case Report.—Girl, 6 months, was initially seen with a red mass behind the right anterior tympanic membrane discovered on routine physical examination. She had no history of otologic or neurologic problems, and the results of a

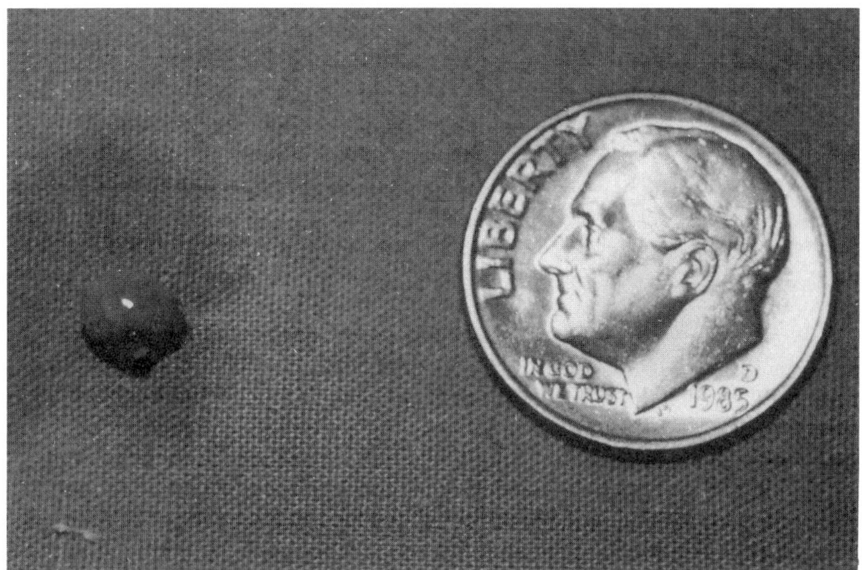

Fig 5–3.—Surgical specimen after excision from the mesotympanum. (Courtesy of Jacobs IN, Potsic WP: *Arch Otolaryngol Head Neck Surg* 120:203–205, 1994.)

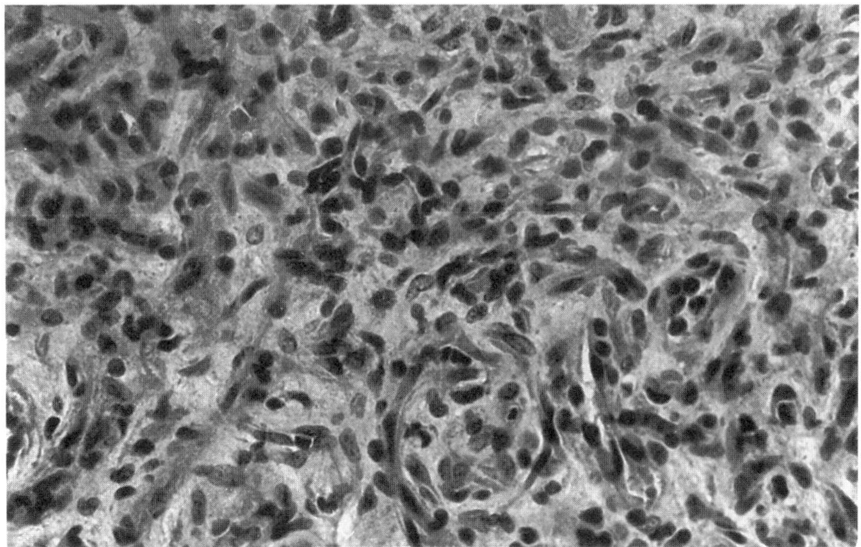

Fig 5–4.—Hematoxylin-eosin stain of glomus tympanicum tumor (original magnification, ×50). (Courtesy of Jacobs IN, Potsic WP: *Arch Otolaryngol Head Neck Surg* 120:203–205, 1994.)

sound-field hearing assessment were normal, except for a flat tympanogram on the right. A vascular lesion on the right cochlear promontory was noted on CT with IV contrast (Fig 5–1). On MR angiography, a lesion in the mesotympanum enhanced greatly after administration of gadolinium (Fig 5–2). A right middle ear exploration through a postauricular approach showed a vascular mass arising from Jacobsen's nerve. This mass extended anteriorly into the area of the eustachian tube and medially to the malleus. The surgeon elevated the tympanic membrane from the malleus and amputated the long process of the malleus to increase surgical exposure. The tensor tympani muscle was then divided to permit complete tumor removal with a surrounding cuff of mucosa (Fig 5–3). Jacobsen's nerve was cut inferiorly and superiorly to the tumor. Hematoxylin-eosin and reticulin staining demonstrated a high degree of cellularity and nests of cuboidal cells surrounded by a connective tissue stroma (Fig 5–4), a histologic appearance consistent with a paraganglioma. The infant's postoperative course was unremarkable. She is being followed up with serial CT scans.

Conclusion.—This patient with glomus tympanicum appears to be the youngest ever reported in the literature. Otolaryngologists must maintain a high index of suspicion in patients with persistent inflammation that fails to respond to standard treatment methods. With a timely diagnosis and improvements in imaging technology, pediatric glomus tumors may be diagnosed at an earlier stage and have a better overall prognosis. Aggressive surgery is needed if the tumor is discovered before significant intracranial or skull base extension occurs. Meticulous postoperative follow-up is important, because the incidence of multicentric tumors is high.

▶ Glomus tympanicum has typically been seen in adults. It is unusual to see it in children, and it is certainly more unusual to find it in an infant. To my knowledge, this is the first such report of this occurrence. Perhaps glomus tympanicum should be looked for more frequently in younger children, and other studies may corroborate a higher incidence in the future.—M.M. Paparella, M.D.

Middle Ear Adenoma and Adenocarcinoma

Amble FR, Harner SG, Weiland LH, McDonald TJ, Facer GW (Mayo Clinic and Found, Rochester, Minn; Mayo Clinic, Scottsdale, Ariz)
Otolaryngol Head Neck Surg 109:871–876, 1993   130-95-5-2

Objective.—Adenomas and adenocarcinomas originating from the middle ear are rare. Eleven previously reported and 5 new cases of middle ear adenoma and adenocarcinomas seen between 1905 and 1992 were described.

Clinical Features.—There were 7 female and 9 male patients, aged 7 to 77 years. The average time from onset of symptoms to diagnosis was 120.8 months (range, 1 to 492 months). The most common symptoms

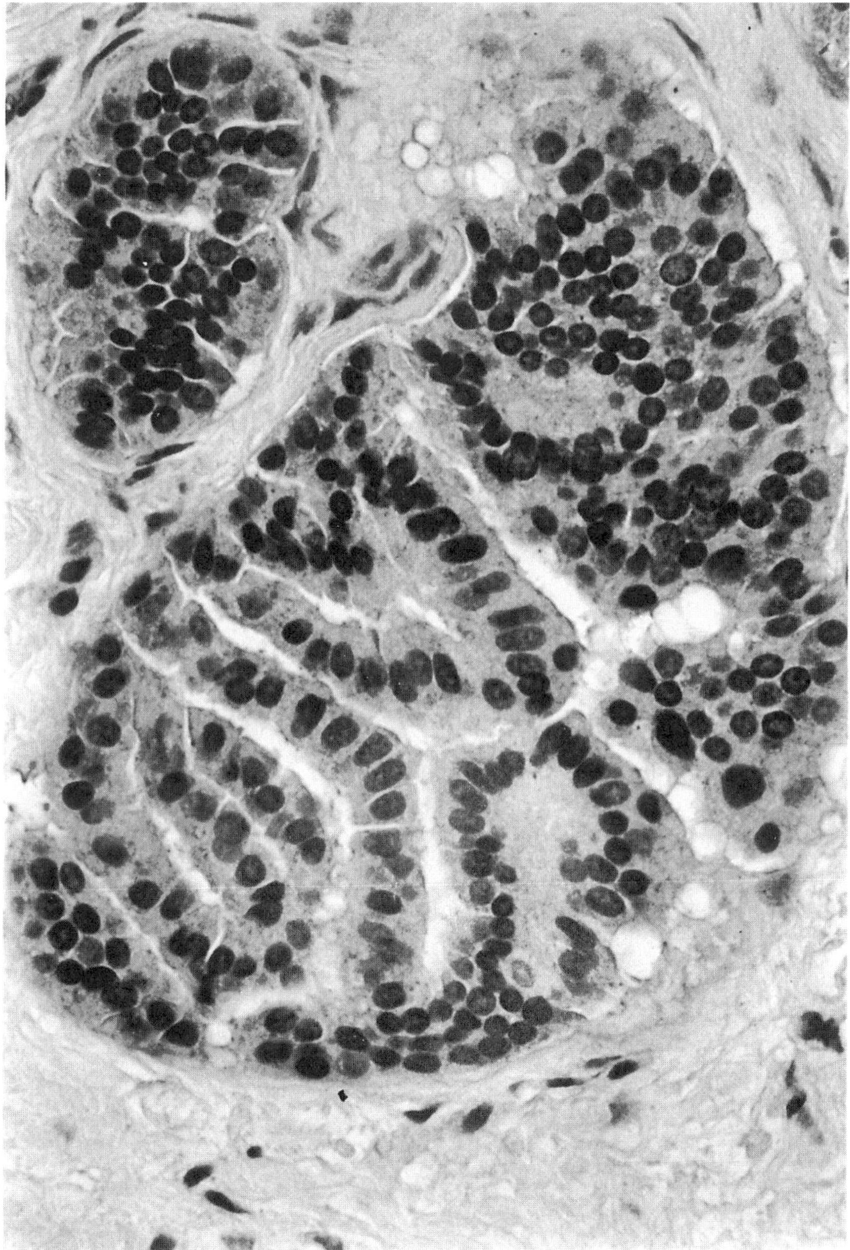

Fig 5–5.—Photomicrograph shows positive staining for keratin. (Immunoperoxidase stain; original magnification, ×400.) (Courtesy of Amble FR, Harner SG, Weiland LH, et al: *Otolaryngol Head Neck Surg* 109:871-876, 1993.)

at presentation were decreased hearing, pain (ear, face, and head), and otorrhea. Five patients had abnormal angiographic findings. Three patients had tumors that extended to the eustachian tube, and 6 had tumors close to the tympanic membrane. None had metastases.

Treatment/Outcome.—Treatment varied greatly. All patients underwent surgery, including biopsy or incomplete removal, or excision, with or without radiation therapy or chemotherapy. Three of 7 patients with facial nerve involvement and 3 of 9 patients who underwent biopsy or incomplete removal of the tumor died. All 7 patients who had tumor excision were alive with no evidence of disease during an average follow-up of 87.4 months after treatment. One patient who underwent radical surgery for an invasive-appearing tumor remained disease-free for 13 years; another patient who received chemotherapy for palliation was alive with disease at 264 months. Overall, 3 patients died of the disease, 1 died of unrelated cause, 5 were alive with disease, and 7 were alive without disease.

Pathology.—The tumors were malignant in 4 patients and benign in 9, with 4 benign tumors showing aggressive features; the other 3 patients had no evaluable slides. All 9 tumors stained histologically were positive for keratin (Fig 5–5), and 6 were positive for chromogranin.

Summary.—Patients with middle ear adenoma and adenocarcinoma frequently present with decreased hearing, otorrhea, and otalgia, but a large percentage have facial nerve involvement by the time of diagnosis; the latter is a poor prognostic factor. It appears that glomus tissue is the most likely origin for these tumors. Because of its relatively slow growth and benign features, surgery and observation similar to that for glomus tumors are warranted.

▶ Adenomas and adenocarcinomas primarily occur in the middle ear cleft. Whenever possible, the treatment is total surgical extirpation. It can be done nicely with an endaural approach and wide removal of the lateral temporal bone and tympanomastoid, if necessary, to extirpate the tumor in toto. Describing their experience with 11 cases, these authors also discuss the pathogenesis of these tumors and the possible origin as occurring in the periganglionic tissue. This site of origin seems plausible and merits considered attention.—M.M. Paparella, M.D.

Congenital Cholesteatoma: Review of Twelve Cases
Huang TS, Lee FP (Chang Gung Med College, Taipei, Taiwan, Republic of China)
Am J Otol 15:276–281, 1994   130-95-5–3

Introduction.—Congenital cholesteatoma was rarely seen in the first half of the century; however, in recent years, more cases have been reported in younger patients. Its pathogenesis is unclear, and its diagnosis is difficult. A review of 12 patients was done to define some previously unrecognized features of the disorder.

Methods.—The records of 12 patients of varying ages with congenital cholesteatoma, chosen as a sample of 1,611 patients with cholesteatoma seen between 1984 and 1992, were reviewed.

Results.—All patients had some type of hearing loss, and 5 had tinnitus. The tympanic membrane was bulging in different quadrants in 8 patients and was normal in 4. Two patients had ear discharge, which came from bony fistulae outside the intact tympanic membrane. Radiologic evidence suggested temporal bone defects in 6 patients and middle ear ossicular defects in 2 patients. Only 4 patients had cystic, contained cholesteatomas; 2 of these patients had multiple cholesteatomas at separate sites in the same temporal bone. The other 8 patients had highly invasive epidermoids. Congenital cholesteatomas were diagnosed in 9 patients, but otosclerosis and the Meniere syndrome were initially diagnosed in 2 and 1 patients, respectively.

Discussion.—Review of 12 patients with congenital cholesteatoma showed several unusual diagnostic features. Patients can have purulent discharge in the external auditory canal with an intact tympanic membrane, which may indicate massive involvement in the mastoid cavity. Symptoms can mimic unilateral otosclerosis, especially among Asians; high-resolution CT should be used to confirm diagnosis. Patients with multicentric involvement in the same temporal bone are more likely than those with single-site involvement to have congenital ossicular abnormalities. Patterns of epidermoid sites in adults and older children often differ from those of very young children, which suggests different modes of pathogenesis.

▶ Congenital cholesteatomas can sometimes be confused with acquired cholesteatomas. This article, which describes 12 cases of cholesteatoma of the middle ear, mastoid, and petrous pyramid in juveniles and adults, helps to identify the difference between the 2 types of tumor. Another point should be mentioned: Cholesteatoma can also be acquired beneath an intact tympanic membrane. We have seen this both in our temporal bone laboratory and in certain patients. Therefore, the continued differential between congenital and acquired cholesteatoma can be difficult.—M.M. Paparella, M.D.

Prevalence of Facial Canal Dehiscence and of Persistent Stapedial Artery in the Human Middle Ear: A Report of 1000 Temporal Bones

Moreano EH, Paparella MM, Zelterman D, Goycoolea MV (State Univ of New York, Stony Brook; Univ of Minnesota, Minneapolis; Minnesota Ear, Head and Neck Clinic, Minneapolis)

Laryngoscope 104:309–320, 1994   130-95-5–4

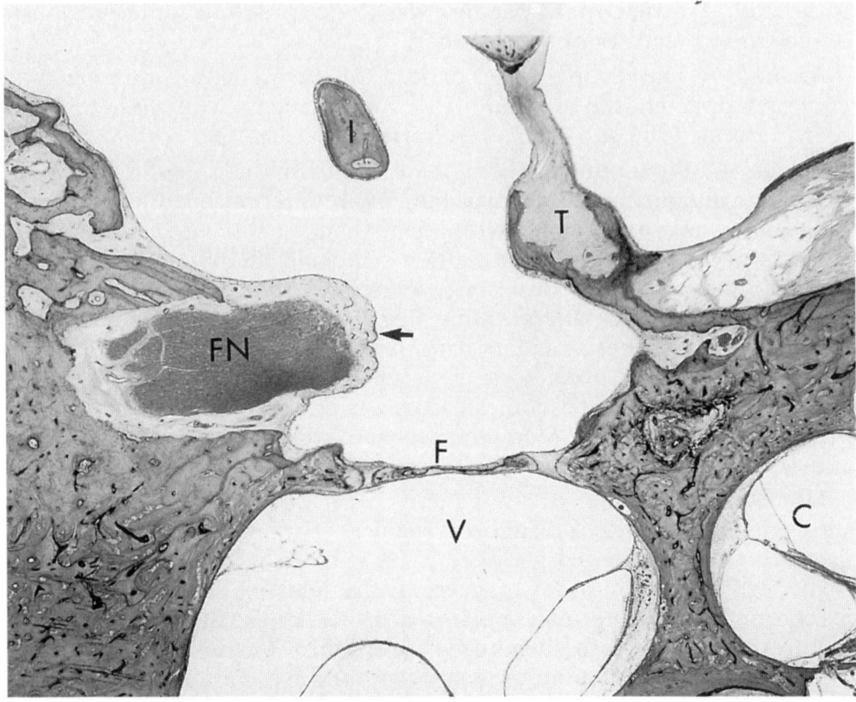

Fig 5–6.—Facial cranial dehiscence (*arrow*) at the oval window in the left ear of a man, 66. *Abbreviations:* FN, facial nerve; *I*, incus; *T*, tensor tympani tendon; *F*, stapes footplate; V, vestibule; C, cochlea. (Hematoxylin-eosin stain; original magnification, ×20.) (Courtesy of Moreano EH, Paparella MM, Zelterman D, et al: *Laryngoscope* 104:309–320, 1994.)

Background.—Although many articles about the anatomical variants in the middle ear cavity have been published, definitive information is limited. A systematic review of 1,000 human temporal bones was done to determine the prevalence of dehiscence of the bony wall of the facial canal and of persistent stapedial artery. These findings were then compared with those reported in the literature.

Methods.—The 1,000 bones had been obtained from 538 individuals. Nine hundred twenty-four were paired, and 76 were unpaired. Age ranges from early childhood to late adulthood were represented.

Findings.—Fifty-six percent of the temporal bones studied contained at least 1 facial canal dehiscence (Fig 5–6). Eighty-one percent of the bones from individuals younger than 2 years of age had a dehiscence compared with 53.7% in bones from persons aged 40 years and older. The prevalence of bilaterality of this canal wall gap was 76.3%. The oval window area was the most common site of dehiscence. A third of the temporal bones had a microdehiscence of the facial canal, found in the oval window area in 74.9% (Fig 5–7). Forty percent of the time, this mi-

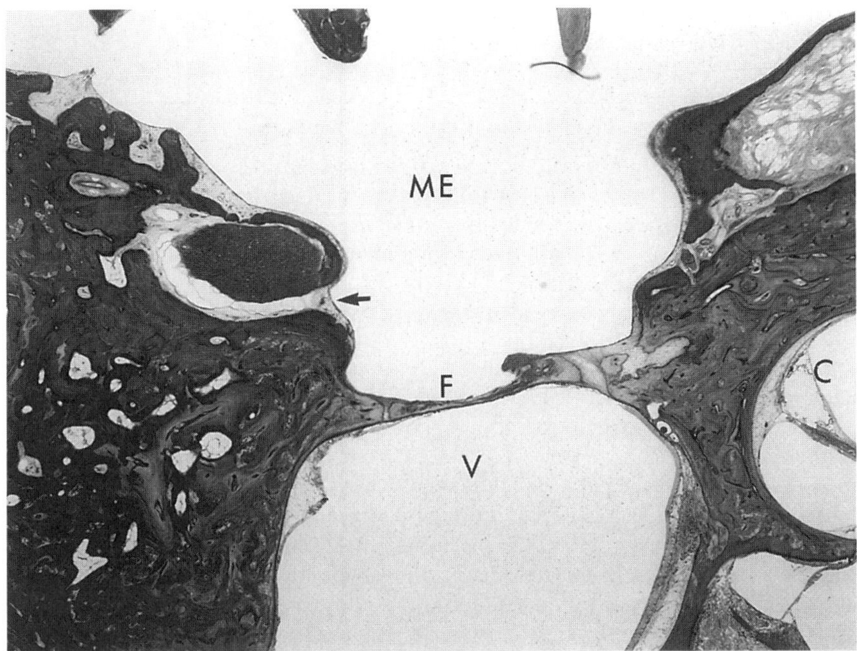

Fig 5–7.—Facial canal microdehiscence (*arrow*) at the oval window in left ear of a woman, 55. *Abbreviations:* ME, middle ear cavity; F, stapes footplate; V, vestibule; C, cochlea. (Hematoxylin-eosin stain; original magnification, ×20.) (Courtesy of Moreano EH, Paparella MM, Zelterman D, et al: *Laryngoscope* 104:309–320, 1994.)

crodehiscence was bilateral. The prevalence of persistent stapedial artery was .48%.

Conclusion.—These findings are consistent with those of the 2 largest temporal bone studies to date, which found a 55% and 57% prevalence of facial canal dehiscence, respectively. The concept of "microdehiscence" was introduced in the current paper. Microdehiscences are too small to be classified as dehiscences but are large enough to result in inflammatory processes that cause compression of the facial nerve, producing facial palsy.

▶ This report of 1,000 temporal bones indicates a percentage of dehiscence of 56%. As we see clinically, the most common site is above the stapes and the area of the oval window. A coincidental finding is that one half of 1% of these patients had a persistent stapedial artery, another structure to consider clinically when treating this area.—M.M. Paparella, M.D.

The Facial Nerve: How to Find It

Pulec JL (Pulec Ear Clinic, Los Angeles)
ENT J 72:677–685, 1993   130-95-5–5

Introduction.—Iatrogenic facial paralysis is one of the most serious complications of temporal bone surgery. The surgeon must recognize the stage in an operation when the facial nerve may be at risk or its orientation may be uncertain. Twelve different surgical techniques for safe exposure and identification of the facial nerve throughout its course through the temporal bone at any stage of an operation were described.

Techniques.—Method 1 is the most common method to identify the facial nerve and involves the direct exposure of the lower half of the mastoid portion. With the low power of the operating microscope, suction irrigation, and a large cutting drill, bone can be removed directly from the lateral part of the mastoid segment inferior to the posterior semicircular canal and superior to the stylomastoid foramen (Fig 5-8). Although more time-consuming, method 2 involves bone removal along the sigmoid sinus inferiorly to the digastric groove and muscle, and then anteriorly until the stylomastoid foramen and facial nerve are exposed. Method 3 is used to accomplish a facial recess approach to the tympanum without disturbing the external auditory canal, ossicular chain, labyrinth, or facial nerve. The facial nerve is identified in the mastoid as in method 1 and is then followed superiorly to the cochleariform process with a small drill and suction irrigation. The area of dissection is rotated as a spiral anteriorly as the dissection progresses in a superior direction to avoid the lateral semicircular canal (Fig 5-9). To identify the tympanic portion of the facial nerve to the geniculate ganglion, the facial nerve is exposed as in method 3, removing bone from the cochleariform process to the geniculate ganglion.

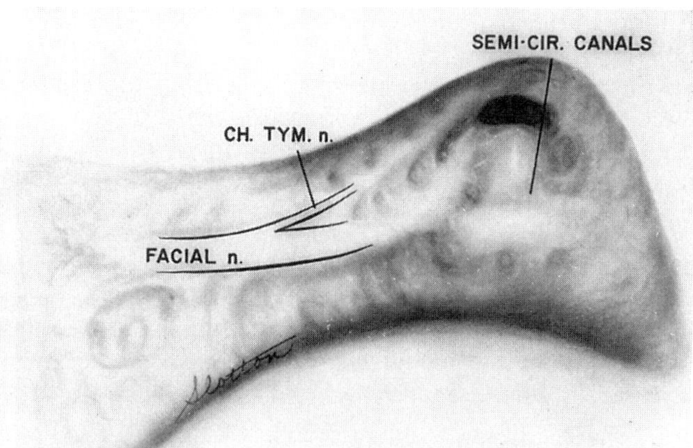

Fig 5–8.—Depiction of the most common method used to find the facial nerve. The lateral part of the inferior half of the mastoid segment is exposed directly with drill. *Abbreviations: CH. TYM. n.,* chorda tympani nerve; *FACIAL n.,* facial nerve; *SEMI-CIR. CANALS,* semicircular canals. (Courtesy of Pulec JL: *ENT J* 72:677–685, 1993.)

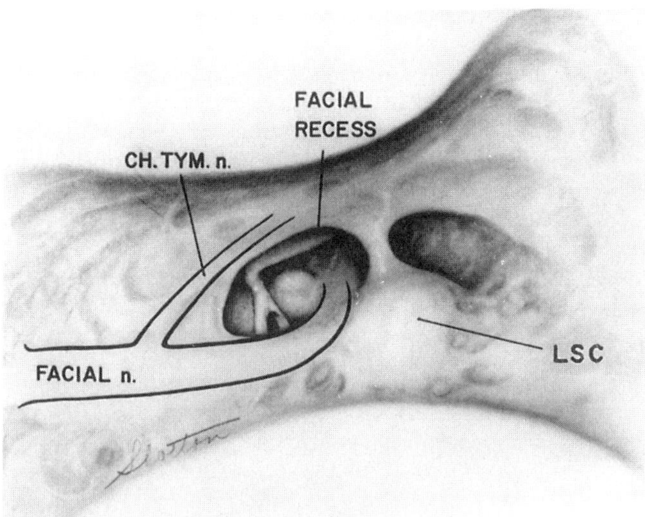

Fig 5–9.—Example of the standard approach through the facial recess for procedures such as facial nerve decompression, intact canal wall tympanoplasty, and glomus tympanicum procedures. *Abbreviations: CH. TYM. n.*, chorda tympani nerve; *FACIAL n.*, facial nerve; *LSC*, lateral semicircular canal. (Courtesy of Pulec JL: *ENT J* 72:677–685, 1993.)

In the presence of a cholesteatoma that extends into the antrum, the facial nerve is identified as in method 1 and exposed superiorly to the cholesteatoma. When surgical dissection begins at the tubotympanum moving posteriorly, the facial nerve can be identified immediately superior to the cochleariform process and posterior superior to the pyramid and stapes. If there is extensive distortion of the anatomy of the tympanum when neither the round nor the oval window are clearly identified, dissection begins at the eustachian tube and posteriorly over the promontory until the tympanic membrane or its groove in the promontory is reached; the nerve or groove is traced superiorly to the cochleariform process. When there is massive destruction of almost all bony landmarks, such as in very extensive cholesteatoma, neglected malignant otitis externa, or radial necrosis of the temporal bone, the anterior external auditory canal or glenoid fossa and condyle is traced medially to the tubotympanum; the tensor tympanic muscle within the semicanal superior to the eustachian tube is traced posteriorly to its tendon and the facial nerve.

In the best method to identify the mastoid and tympanic portions of the facial nerve during a postauricular labyrinthectomy or translabyrinthine approach, the semicircular canals are opened with a cutting drill and bone is removed along with the horizontal semicircular canal in an anterior and inferior direction. To identify the facial nerve with certainty during the translabyrinthine approach to the internal auditory canal, the midportion of the internal auditory canal is exposed by removing bone from posterior to anterior to expose the superior vestibular nerve to its lateral extent; bone is removed over the superior lateral portion of the internal auditory canal at the levels of the medial wall of the vestibule until the fallopian canal is exposed. For total exposure of the labyrinthine portion of the facial nerve, the facial nerve is traced from the stylomastoid foramen to the internal genu, paying careful attention as it makes a very acute angle at the internal genu in its posterior inferior course medially; small diamond drill bits are used to trace the nerve in its labyrinthine portion. For middle cranial fossa approach to the facial nerve, the middle meningeal artery is traced to the foramen spinosum, and the greater petrosal nerve is identified posterior to the foramen as it enters the facial hiatus. Bone is removed from the greater petrosal nerve to the geniculate ganglion and the internal genu, and the facial nerve is exposed to the tympanum and to the internal auditory canal.

▶ Iatrogenic trauma to the facial nerve continues to be one of the most important concerns of the neurotologist. It is helpful to have an experienced neurotologist describe anatomical variations and pathologic conditions found with different surgical techniques to allow the surgeon to safely expose and identify the facial nerve.—M.M. Paparella, M.D.

Idiopathic Facial Nerve Paralysis: A Randomized Double Blind Controlled Study of Placebo Versus Prednisone

Austin JR, Peskind SP, Austin SG, Rice DH (MD Anderson Cancer Ctr, Houston; Univ of Southern California, Los Angeles; Univ of Texas Health Science Ctr, Houston)
Laryngoscope 103:1326–1333, 1993   130-95-5–6

Background.—Idiopathic facial nerve paralysis (IFNP) is a common disease of unknown etiology, although there are many theories. Treatment options are similarly varied. Oral steroids are the most common therapeutic agent for treatment of IFNP, even though there have been

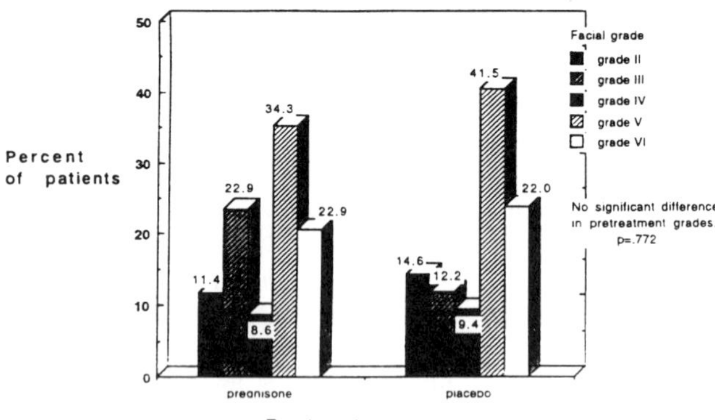

Fig 5–10.—Distribution of facial nerve grade at the time of entry to the study for the 2 treatment groups. (Courtesy of Austin JR, Peskind SP, Austin SG, et al: *Laryngoscope* 103:1326–1333, 1993.)

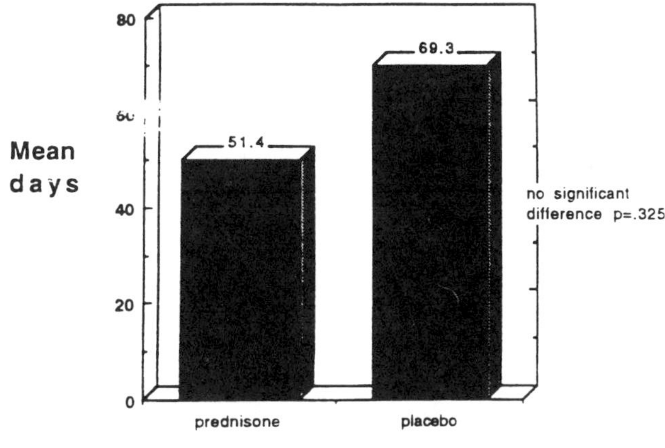

Fig 5–11.—Mean time to resolution of facial nerve paralysis for the 2 treatment groups. (Courtesy of Austin JR, Peskind SP, Austin SG, et al: *Laryngoscope* 103:1326–1333, 1993.)

no randomized controlled studies demonstrating the superiority of steroids over placebo.

Methods.—Over 14 months, 76 patients with IFNP entered the double-blind randomized controlled study and were followed through recovery. Of the 76, 35 received prednisone and 41 received placebo. All patients were evaluated by clinical criteria, laboratory analysis, and neurologic testing. The following measures were used to assess outcome: time to recovery, facial paralysis grade at onset and at recovery, IFNP sequelae, pain, and anxiety level. The facial paralysis was graded by the House and Brackmann scale.

Results.—Initial assessments revealed that the two groups were equivalent in the study's assessment measures. After treatment, there were no differences between the 2 groups in terms of time to recovery, pain relief, anxiety levels, or sequelae, particularly autonomic synkinesis. There was a significant correlation between grade of facial paralysis at onset and time to recovery (Figs 5–10 and 5–11); patients with more severe paralysis had longer recovery times. Prednisone significantly improved the facial grade at recovery, with fewer patients (2 vs. 8) having denervation develop.

Discussion.—Because most of the assessment measures were not changed by prednisone, it is unlikely that patients with mild IFNP disease would significantly benefit from prednisone treatment. However, because prednisone prevents denervation, all patients with more severe paralysis, who are at risk for denervation, should be treated with prednisone.

▶ Although the etiology of facial nerve paralysis is still considered to be idiopathic, there is evidence to suggest that there can be a viral origin with subsequent inflammatory changes. This study indicates, using a double-blind controlled approach, the efficacy of prednisone. Most of us use steroids to treat these patients initially, and this study by Austin and colleagues lends credence to this approach.—M.M. Paparella, M.D.

Facial Nerve Neuromas Presenting as Acoustic Tumors
McMenomey SO, Glasscock ME III, Minor LB, Jackson CG, Strasnick B (Otology Group, Nashville, Tenn; Eastern Virginia Med School, Norfolk, Va)
Am J Otol 15:307–312, 1994   130-95-5–7

Introduction.—Neuromas of the facial nerve are relatively infrequent lesions that most often grow slowly and are benign. A facial neuroma that arises in the cerebellopontine angle (CPA) or internal auditory canal (IAC) may mimic an acoustic neuroma.

Objective.—An experience with 32 facial nerve neuromas diagnosed and treated during 1975 to 1992, 12 of which were considered acoustic neuromas before surgery, was reviewed. The patients were followed for 1 to 18 years.

Findings.—All 12 patients thought to have an acoustic neuroma had sensorineural hearing loss, and half had unilateral tinnitus. None of them had facial nerve weakness, whereas two thirds of patients recognized as having facial neuromas had slowly progressive facial palsy. Three fourths of the patients thought to have acoustic tumors, especially those with larger masses, had abnormal auditory brain-stem responses. The tumors were most often located in the CPA and IAC. Only 4 of the 12 lesions extended as far as the geniculate ganglion.

Management and Outcome.—In 5 patients it was possible to dissect the tumor from the main trunk of the facial nerve, but in 7 cases it was necessary to sacrifice the facial nerve. A hypoglossal-facial nerve anastomosis was performed in 71% of patients. Only 2 patients had primary nerve anastomosis. Patients in whom it was possible to dissect the tumor free had the best functional recovery, but the results were not consistently acceptable. Most of the patients recognized as having facial neuromas were managed by cable grafting the missing nerve segment or anastomosis of the facial to the hypoglossal nerve.

▶ A lesion of the cerebellopontine angle usually suggests the presence of a vestibular schwannoma or an acoustic tumor, but meningiomas and, as this study indicates, facial nerve neuromas can also be present in this region. Until a pathologic diagnosis is established, one cannot be certain of the lesion in this region.—M.M. Paparella, M.D.

Results of Reconstruction of the Facial Nerve

Ferreira MC, Besteiro JM, Tuma P Jr (Univ of Saõ Paulo, Brazil)
Microsurgery 15:5–8, 1994   130-95-5–8

Introduction.—Traumatic injuries to the facial nerve may lead to severe functional and aesthetic deficits when left untreated. There have been few reports of reconstruction of the facial nerve in its extratemporal part, and no convenient method described to assess the results of such reconstruction. A series of 59 patients was reviewed using the authors' own system for evaluating extratemporal facial nerve reconstructions.

Patients and Methods.—All patients had sustained unilateral lacerations to the facial nerve and underwent surgery at periods ranging from 3 weeks to 6 months after trauma. Most had been injured in traffic accidents. Twelve had lesions extending from the trunk up to the main branches of the facial nerve (group 1), 32 had intraparotid lesions with loss of nerve extending from the main branches up to the distal branches (group 2), and 15 had injuries on distal branches only (group 3). In all instances, the sural nerve was used in grafting procedures. The evaluation system compares the normal side with the paralyzed side, assigning scores of 0–2 for each of 6 voluntary contractions, for involuntary mimic actions, and for deformity at rest.

Results.—The grafting procedure resulted in no major complications or worsening of the clinical situation. Patients in group 1 showed an average preoperative score of 10% to 20% of motion on the paralyzed side vs. the normal side. After 1 year, motion had improved to 60% to 70%. Patients in group 2 improved from 30% to 40% preoperatively to 80% to 90% postoperatively. Motion scores in patients with lesions to distal branches (group 3) increased from 70% to 80% before grafting to 85% to 95% postoperatively.

Conclusion.—Previously reported methods for evaluating surgical treatment of facial palsy were designed largely for patients with Bell's palsy. The method described here yields a precise, quantitative estimate of the results of direct nerve reconstruction, cross-face nerve grafting, or several other operations for long-standing facial palsy. Patients who sustained an injury to the facial nerve or its branches and underwent reconstruction with nerve grafting showed significant improvement relative to preoperative motion and lack of symmetry.

▶ This author has a large series of cases: 59 patients who received grafting with a sural nerve. He attempted a quantitative approach to assessment of recovery and found a significant improvement of function in patients with traumatic injuries to the extratemporal facial nerve. Usually, such grafts need to be considered in the temporal bone as well as extratemporally, and one can assume the principles of healing to be similar.—M.M. Paparella, M.D.

Intracanalicular Acoustic Neuroma: Early Surgery for Preservation of Hearing
Haines SJ, Levine SC (Univ of Minnesota, Minneapolis)
J Neurosurg 79:515–520, 1993   130-95-5–9

Purpose.—The availability of gadolinium-enhanced MRI has made it possible to diagnose very small acoustic neuromas of the internal auditory canal. Many of these patients have only minimal unilateral hearing loss, and there is little information on the natural history and prognosis of these lesions. A surgical experience in 14 consecutive patients with intracanalicular acoustic neuroma has been reviewed.

Patients.—Patients with intracanalicular tumors accounted for 12% of the total number of patients who had surgery for acoustic neuroma during a 5-year period. There were 8 women and 6 men, age range 26 to 70 years. Two deaf patients with recurrent tumors were operated on by a translabyrinthine approach. Of the remaining 12, the presenting symptoms included hearing loss, vertigo, or tinnitus; the surgical approach was through the middle fossa in 7 and through the posterior fossa in 5. Eleven patients had functional hearing preoperatively, and 9 retained hearing postoperatively. Postoperative facial nerve function was normal in 12 of 14 patients.

Conclusion.—For patients with intracanalicular acoustic neuroma, current surgical techniques can preserve hearing in about 80% of cases. Pending careful studies of the natural history of untreated neuromas and the recurrence rate of treated tumors, early surgery appears to offer the best chance of hearing preservation.

▶ This article appeared in the *Journal of Neurosurgery,* and these authors appropriately emphasize the importance of early diagnosis and early treatment for small lesions that are intracanalicular. It is encouraging that postoperative serviceable hearing exceeds 80% in this group studied.—M.M. Paparella, M.D.

Technique to Avoid Cerebrospinal Fluid Otorhinorrhea With Translabyrinthine Removal of Acoustic Neuroma
Pulec JL (Pulec Ear Clinic, Los Angeles)
Laryngoscope 104:382–386, 1994   130-95-5–10

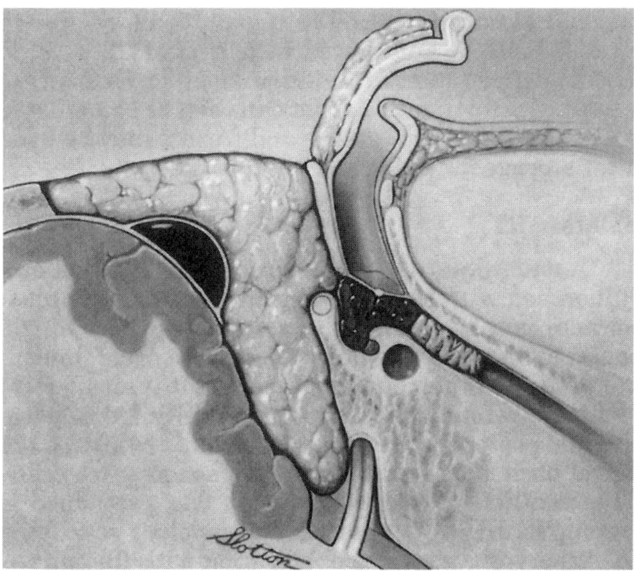

Fig 5–12.—Surgical step 4. A single piece of fat trimmed to a conical shape obliterates the petrous apex and mastoid. (Courtesy of Pulec JL: *Laryngoscope* 104:382–386, 1994.)

Background.—Otorhinorrhea with CSF can accompany the surgical removal of acoustic neuroma. A technique for avoiding CS otorhinorrhea during translabyrinthine removal of acoustic neuromawas described.

Technique.—The technique involves a crescent-shaped incision 2 inches long, placed half an inch behind the postauricular fold. A complete mastoidectomy and labyrinthectomy are performed. After the tumor has been removed completely and the bleeding controlled thoroughly, the facial recess is opened widely between the fibrous annulus of the tympanic membrane and facial nerve. A Yankauer curette is passed through the facial recess, and part of the mucous membrane is removed from the tubotympanum. The mucous membrane is scratched away from half of the circumference of the tubotympanum so that adhesions would be formed to fibrous tissue. A strip of thick, firm, fibrous tissue is excised from the lower edge of the temporalis muscle attachment and packed very firmly into the tubotympanum with significant pressure from a Rosen elevator. A piece of muscle is excised from the temporalis or sternomastoid muscle at the upper or lower edges of the postauricular incision and placed in the middle ear to obliterate the tympanum. An abdominal fat graft is removed and prepared for placement into the mastoid cavity and apex. The surgeon takes care so that the medial extent does not protrude significantly into the posterior fossa (Fig 5–12). A tight closure is obtained (Fig 5–13).

Outcomes.—This technique was used successfully in 100 consecutive patients. There was only 1 case of CSF otorhinorrhea, suggesting that the technique is effective. Morbidity was minimal.

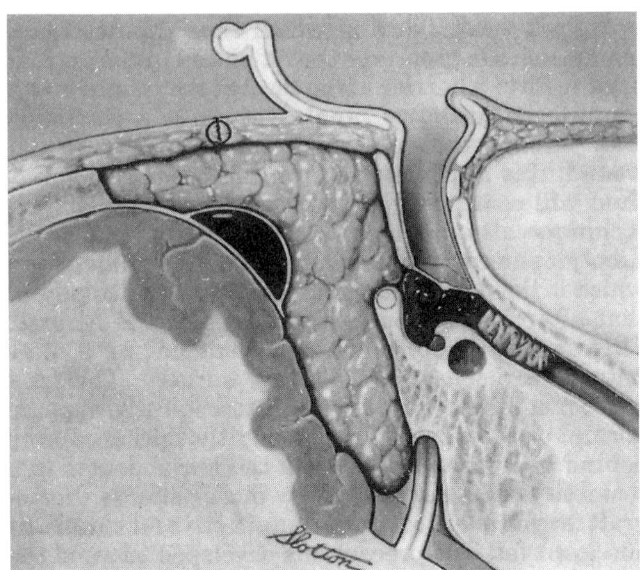

Fig 5–13.—Surgical step 5. Subcutaneous chromic catgut suture closure keeps pressure against the fat plug. (Courtesy of Pulec JL: *Laryngoscope* 104:382–386, 1994.)

Conclusion.—This technique for avoiding CSF otorhinorrhea with translabyrinthine removal of acoustic neuroma involves scarifying the tubotympanum and obliteration with fibrous tissue through the facial recess approach. The procedure can be performed in about 10 minutes. When used with obliteration of the petrous apex and mastoid with fat, this procedure can be used to almost completely eliminate postoperative CSF otorhinorrhea after translabyrinthine acoustic neuroma removal.

▶ This innovative approach—attempting to obstruct the tubotympanum and obliterate the tympanum with fibrous tissue through the facial recess approach—makes sense in terms of helping to control CSF otorhinorrhea. This method acknowledges the importance of the middle ear cleft in its role in this complication of removing an acoustic neuroma.—M.M. Paparella, M.D.

The Effect of Unilateral Chorda Tympani Damage on Taste

Kveton JF, Bartoshuk LM (Yale Univ, New Haven, Conn)
Laryngoscope 104:25–29, 1994   130-95-5–11

Introduction.—Taste sensation is mediated by the interaction of facial, glossopharyngeal, and vagal nerves. Although each nerve contributes separate and limited information, patients with loss of a single nerve within the taste network do not experience a change in overall taste perception. The nerves may have inhibitory effects on each other, and when 1 nerve is lost, another nerve may compensate because it is no longer inhibited.

Methods.—Taste intensities were measured at sites innervated by nerves VII and IX in 8 patients with unilateral nerve VII loss. Solutions representing the 4 taste qualities were touched to either side of the front of the tongue, the foliate papillae, the circumvallate papillae, and the palate. Thermal testing with ice water was done on either side of the tongue.

Results.—Taste response on the side ipsilateral to the nerve VII loss was diminished, particularly at the front of the tongue, but it was not completely absent with any solution at any site. Taste response on the contralateral side was stronger at all sites, particularly at the front of the tongue. There were no significant differences in overall taste sensation from swallow tests.

Discussion.—These findings of asymmetric taste sensation at sites innervated by the nerve IX support the hypothesis that the loss of nerve VII releases inhibition of nerve IX. Unexpectedly, taste function in the palate followed the same pattern, providing evidence that the palate is also innervated by both nerves VII and IX.

▶ The chorda tympani is commonly traumatized during stapedial surgery or other procedures done on the middle ear. These authors studied patients who had acoustic tumors removed and experienced subsequent loss of the ability to taste. The hypothesis that cranial nerve IX is inhibited by cranial nerve VII is of interest. One should not forget that the lingual nerve provides most sensory taste function to the tongue and that when the chorda tympani is disturbed, this is left intact and can compensate over time for the loss of the chorda tympani as well.—M.M. Paparella, M.D.

Indications for Cranial Nerve Monitoring During Otologic and Neurotologic Surgery
Jackler RK, Selesnick SH (Univ of California, San Francisco; The New York Hosp–Cornell Med Ctr, New York)
Am J Otol 15:611–613, 1994   130-95-5-12

Objective.—A panel of experienced otologic surgeons explored the usefulness of contemporary cranial nerve monitoring (CNM) techniques for a variety of otologic and neurotologic procedures. The value of CNM in a given procedure was categorized as proved through outcome analysis, proved through anecdotal experience, promising but as yet unproved, or unhelpful or otherwise not indicated.

Tumors of the Internal Auditory Canal and Cerebellopontine Angle.—It was agreed that facial nerve monitoring (FNM) was of value in removing acoustic neuromas and other tumors involving the internal auditory canal and cerebellopontine angle. Published studies support the value of FNM in these cases. It was also agreed that FNM helps to identify and preserve the facial nerve. Several panelists pointed out that FNM can slow surgery by creating false alarms indicative of FN injury. Panelists agreed that when the FN maintains a low stimulation threshold after tumor removal an excellent functional result is likely, whereas absent electric stimulability is an adverse predictor. Panelists expressed considerably less enthusiasm about the value of auditory nerve monitoring than about FNM.

Tumors of the Cranial Base.—Early experiences have been promising when CNM was used to monitor the lower cranial nerves, in jugular foramen surgery, and the nerves that control extraocular muscle function during surgery of the cavernous sinus and petroclival region. Facial nerve monitoring was useful during rerouting of the facial nerve for enhanced exposure during surgery of the cranial base.

Vestibular Neurectomy and Surgery of Chronic Otitis Media and Cholesteatoma.—The panelists were ambivalent about the value of CNM during vestibular neurectomy and reached no consensus as to its value during chronic ear surgery. Two of 5, however, routinely used FNM during all chronic ear surgeries.

Repair of Congenital Aural Atresia.—Although none of the panelists performed large numbers of reconstructions of atresia, all routinely used FNM during reconstruction of congenital aural atresia.

Conclusion.—The panelists believed that CNM had value in the residency and fellowship training. One expressed the view that FNM reduced the risk of facial nerve injury during surgery proctored by an experienced teacher. Concern was expressed that an inexperienced surgeon could be falsely reassured by the use of FNM. The panelists emphasized that CNM methods cannot substitute for a detailed knowledge of the surgical anatomy of the FN. Each surgeon must make an individual, informed decision as to the selective application of CNM.

Intraoperative Electrophysiological Monitoring of the Facial Nerve: Is It Standard of Practice?

Roland PS, Meyerhoff WL (Univ of Texas Southwestern Medical Ctr, Dallas)
Am J Otolaryngol 15:267–270, 1994   130-95-5–13

Background.—The facial nerve has been monitored electrophysiologically for more than a decade in a number of neurotologic operations, especially those entailing removal of posterior fossa tumors. In addition, some surgeons monitor the nerve during routine otologic operations such as stapedectomy, tympanoplasty, and tympanomastoid surgery.

Objective.—Monitoring practices were surveyed by sending a questionnaire to all 410 members of the American Otological and American Neurotology Societies. Nearly two thirds of the members responded.

Findings.—An overwhelming majority of respondents do not consider intraoperative facial nerve monitoring to be the standard of care. A number of respondents expressed concern over the cost of monitoring. Some noted that use of a monitor is not a substitute for a thorough knowledge of the relevant anatomy, whereas others stated that any surgeon who needed to use a monitor should not perform otologic surgery at all. A few respondents mentioned specifically that they believe monitoring to be necessary, or very useful, during training.

Conclusion.—At present, there are no objective reasons for routinely monitoring the facial nerve during otologic surgery.

▶ These 2 articles (Abstracts 130-95-5–12 and 130-95-5–13) discuss the same subject. With the advent of new technology and relative inexperience on the part of some newly trained neurotologists, there is a greater reliance on intraoperative monitoring to avoid injury to the facial nerve during otologic surgery. Both of these publications indicate that experience and common sense should prevail and that intraoperative monitoring does not constitute a new standard of care; in fact, it can add excessive cost to the hospital bill and, in some instances, may provide too much reliance on technology rather than on anatomical pathologic findings, which remain the keynote in avoiding injury to the facial nerve.

Derlaki, commenting on Abstract 130-95-5–12, stated that "FNM was not needed for experienced surgeons who have performed hundreds or thousands of chronic ear operations with little or no FN morbidity." Certainly, that comment is correct. The study by Roland and Meyerhoff indicates that, of the 410 questionnaires sent to members of the American Otological and Neurotological Society, overwhelmingly the majority of members do not regard intraoperative monitoring of the facial nerve as the standard of care. This does not mean that an individual who finds intraoperative monitoring useful should not use this technique; again, he or she should practice according to his or her experience and what is best for the patient.—M.M. Paparella, M.D.

6 External Ear, Middle Ear, and Mastoid

Otitis Externa: Management of the Recalcitrant Case
Selesnick SH (Cornell Univ Med College—The New York Hosp, New York)
Am J Otol 15:408–412, 1994   130-95-6-1

Introduction.—Trauma is a critical factor disposing to otitis externa. The disorder is characterized by otalgia that may be sharp and may radiate locally. Persistent itching and hearing loss also may develop. Examination shows an erythematous and edematous canal with extreme tenderness within it. The most common pathogen isolated is *Pseudomonas aeruginosa,* which is present in more than 40% of cases.

Management.—Elimination of any predisposing factors, such as a breach in the integrity of the skin, will minimize the risk of optitis externa and enhance the treatment of active infection. It may help to suspend ear drops that might dispose to allergy and to use hypoallergenic cosmetics. Adequate cleaning of the external canal is important and, if necessary, should be done on a daily basis. In recalcitrant cases, cultures are obtained for aerobic and anaerobic bacteria and fungi. Topical antimicrobial therapy will be effective in more than 95% of cases. Multiple antibiotics are routinely administered. Ciprofloxacin is an effective oral agent because it combats *Pseudomonas* species.—Extended treatment may be necessary for treatment-resistant patients. If otitis remains unresponsive, a biopsy is indicated to rule out an occult necrotic tumor.

▶ Recalcitrant or intractable external otitis can be a major clinical challenge and can create great discomfort to the patient on a long-term basis. This article describes aspects of microbiology and immune considerations in patients with diabetes and in others. The advice it provides is certainly useful. There are rare patients who will fail all medical therapy on a long-term basis and will have intractable obstructive pathologic conditions develop. These patients can be treated conservatively and surgically, if all else fails. The procedure is called meatoplasty and canalplasty followed by Thiersch's skin grafting.—M.M. Paparella, M.D.

Effect of Cotton-Tipped Swab Use on Earwax Occlusion

Macknin ML, Talo H, VanderBrug Medendorp S (Cleveland Clinic Found, Ohio)
Clin Pediatr 33:14–18, 1994   130-95-6–2

Background.—Previous studies of the relationship between cotton-tipped swabs (CTS) and cerumen plugs have yielded conflicting findings. Parents' and children's approach to cerumen removal, patients' level of cerumen occlusion, and the relationship between the use of CTS and cerumen occlusions were investigated.

Methods and Findings.—A total of 651 consecutive patients from a general pediatric practice answered a questionnaire with their parents' help. More than half the sample was male. The patient age ranged from 2 weeks to 20 years. Sixty-two percent of the patients said they had used CTS in the preceding 2 months. Clinicians who were unaware of the questionnaire findings reported that 7% of both right and left ear canals were at least 75% occluded by cerumen. This occlusion was associated with use of CTS on the left side but not the right.

Conclusion.—Cleaning the external auditory canal with CTS does not free ear canals of wax. To the contrary, it may be associated with cerumen impaction. In a small percentage of persons, use of CTS may be dangerous.

▶ This study suggests that CTS can be used with accumulation of cerumen, and this is commonly done throughout the world. It is also true, however, that too often cotton-tipped applicators can cause trauma if used inappropriately by the patient. This is a practical, common problem, and this study is of interest to the practitioner in otolaryngology.—M.M. Paparella, M.D.

Long-Term Surgical Results for Congenital Aural Atresia

Shih L, Crabtree JA (Univ of Southern California, Los Angeles)
Laryngoscope 103:1097–1102, 1993   130-95-6–3

Background.—The surgical management of congenital aural atresia remains a major challenge for even the best and most experienced otologic surgeons. Its goals are to achieve functional hearing without a hearing device and to maintain a patent, reconstructed external auditory canal that is free from infection. Lessons learned from examination of long-term results in the postoperative course of patients who underwent this surgery have been outlined.

Method.—In a retrospective review, 39 primary surgical procedures were done in 29 patients with congenital aural atresia. The surgical techniques used differed according to the severity of the condition: mild, moderate, or severe. The results of surgery were reviewed according to functional hearing achieved and the incidence of complications, such as stenosis, infection, lateralized or failed graft, and facial palsy.

Results.—Overall, 64% of the patients achieved serviceable hearing of 40 dB or better. Surgical intervention was seen to be most successful within the mild group, who experienced a hearing gain within 20 dB of the cochlear reserve in the majority of cases. Within the moderate and severe group, the attainment of long-term hearing gain was less successful. Twenty-four percent of these patients failed to gain any significant hearing improvement. Moreover, postoperative complications of stenosis developed more frequently in these groups, particularly with the earlier use of full-thickness skin grafts. Thirty-five percent of moderate cases and 60% of severe cases experienced postoperative stenosis. Poor pneumatization and active bone growth because of the age of the children were major contributing factors in recurrent stenosis. Thirty-one percent of primary cases experienced infection, including problems of trapped squamous epithelium behind stenoses. Epithelitis or the chronic, recurrent weepy cavity and recurrent external otitis were common problems. Of the 12 patients with infections, 3 were in the severe group, 6 were in the moderate group, and 3 were in the mild group. Other complications included lateralized graft in 2 patients, and failed grafts in a further 2. No cases of facial paralysis were reported.

Conclusion.—Surgical correction of mild cases of congenital atresia is generally highly successful. This can be done with a canaloplasty to achieve good hearing results and a low rate of postoperative complications. The results of surgery are more variable in moderate and severe cases, with hearing in the serviceable or near-serviceable levels. Surgical intervention should not necessarily be denied in difficult cases. However, a hearing aid may be necessary to achieve functional hearing. The overall complication rates for all groups for stenosis and infection were 33% and 31%, respectively. Most cases of infection were seen in moderate and severely affected patients. In view of these results, expectations and prognosis for moderate and severe patients must be discussed with patients and family before making the decision to have surgery.

▶ I agree with the suggestions and findings of these authors. Long-term results may differ from short-term results after repair of congenital aural atresia. The middle ear cleft is markedly hypoplastic in congenital atresia compared with a normal mesotympanum, and this small size with a graft applied can encourage osteoneogenesis, fibrosis, and other changes that can create a hearing loss on a long-term basis. The authors' other considerations, such as using split-thickness grafting, are helpful as well.—M.M. Paparella, M.D.

Prevalence of Carotid Canal Dehiscence in the Human Middle Ear: A Report of 1,000 Temporal Bones

Moreano EH, Paparella MM, Zelterman D, Goycoolea MV (State Univ of New York, Stony Brook; Univ of Minnesota, Minn)
Laryngoscope 104:612–618, 1994   130-95-6-4

Background.—Anatomical variations within the middle ear cavity may be involved in the etiology of some forms of ear disease. A bony dehiscence of the internal carotid artery canal may be an important pathogenic anomaly. The prevalence of dehiscence, microdehiscence, and thin bony coverage of the carotid canal wall were examined.

Methods.—One thousand human temporal bones from 538 individuals were paired and subdivided according to age. Dehiscence was defined as the absolute lack of continuity in bone coverage; microdehiscence, as a small gap in the bony coverage; wafer-thin bony coverage, as very thin bony coverage of the carotid canal with no bony gap.

Results.—Overall, 84.9% of bones had an intact carotid canal. A carotid canal dehiscence was found in 7.7% of the bones (Figs 6–1 and 6–2); 15.9% of bones from individuals less than 2 years of age and 6.3% from those 40 or older contained a dehiscence. Carotid canal microde-

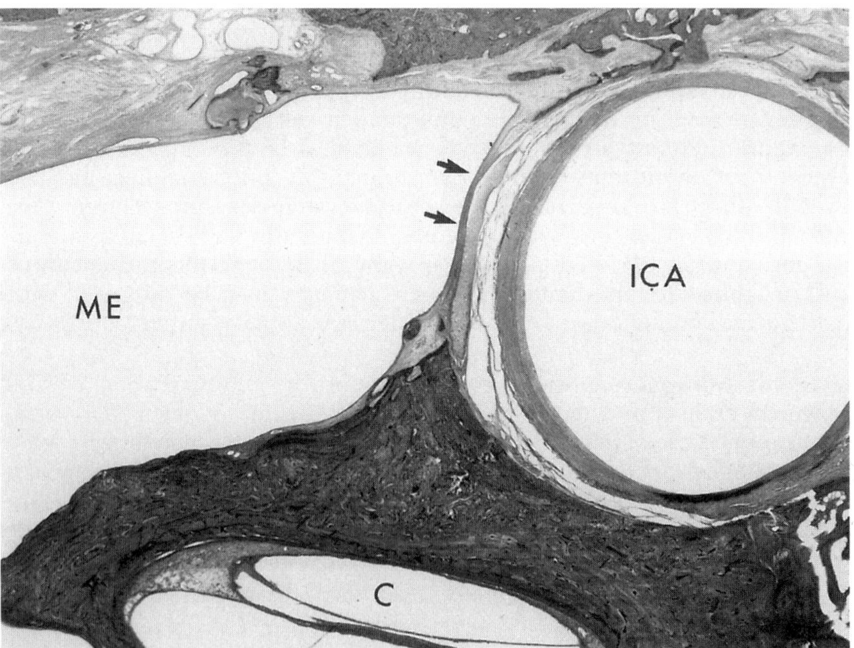

Fig 6–1.—Carotid canal dehiscence (*arrows*). Left ear of a woman, 40. *Abbreviations: ICA,* internal carotid artery; *ME,* middle ear cavity; *C,* cochlea. (Hematoxylin-eosin; original magnification, ×17.) (Courtesy of Moreano EH, Paparella MM, Zelterman D, et al: *Laryngoscope* 104:612–618, 1994.)

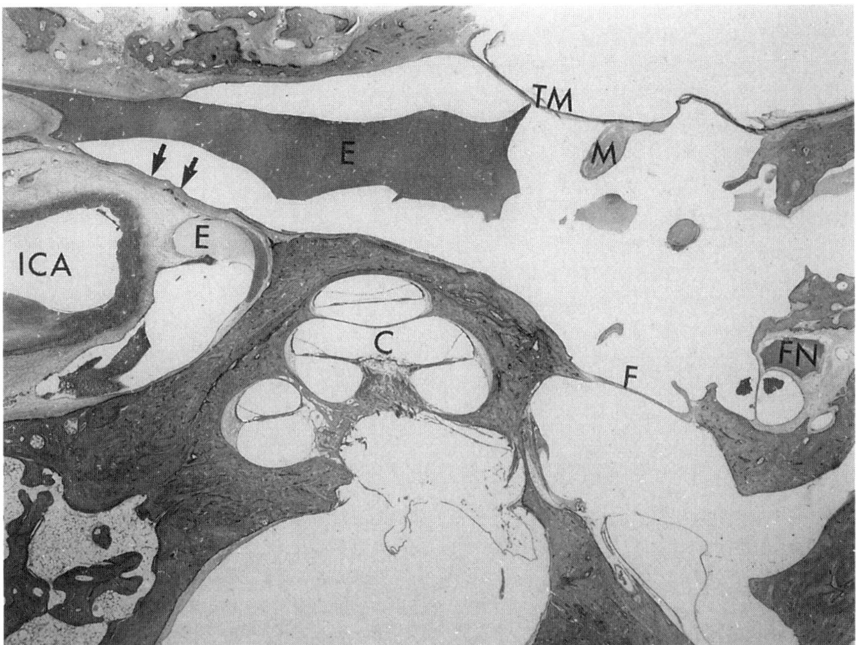

Fig 6–2.—Carotid canal dehiscence (*arrows*). Right ear of a woman, 74. Note that middle ear effusion (*E*) has also accumulated inside the carotid canal adjacent to the wall of the internal carotid artery (*ICA*). *Abbreviations:* *FN*, facial nerve; *TM*, tympanic membrane; *M*, malleus; *F*, stapes footplate; *C*, cochlea. (Hematoxylin and eosin; original magnification, ×9.) (Courtesy of Moreano EH, Paparella MM, Zelterman D, et al: *Laryngoscope* 104:612–618, 1994.)

hiscence was found in 7.4% of all temporal bones, in 11.1% of bones from individuals less than 2 years of age, and in 7.5% of bones from individuals 40 and older. No temporal bone contained both a dehiscence and microdehiscence; 15.1% contained either entity. Bilateral dehiscence was exhibited by 7.5% of temporal bones and bilateral microdehiscence by 12.3%. One hundred thirty-four bones had one gap or the other, and 24 of these were bilateral. Twenty bones had a dehiscence in one ear and a corresponding microdehiscence in the other. Thin bony coverage with neither dehiscence nor microdehiscence was observed in 15.5% of temporal bones. A thin carotid canal was seen in 8.3% of the bones from the younger group and in 17.3% of bones from the older group.

Conclusion.—As temporal bone age increases, the prevalence of carotid canal dehiscence and microdehiscence decreases, and the prevalence of thin coverage increases.

▶ This study indicates a 7.7% incidence of dehiscence of the carotid canal, which is surprisingly high. This is a large series that is being evaluated, and the study findings will be helpful to the surgeon working on the middle ear to avoid trauma to the carotid artery. Apparently, this is the first such study of the histologic sections of a large number of temporal bones to look at these findings. I recall a few patients who had chronic otitis media and aneurysms or bulging of the carotid artery in the protympanum, which led to obstruction of the eustachian tube. Therefore, this is an important consideration for the neurotologic surgeon to keep in mind.—M.M. Paparella, M.D.

Congenital Cholesteatoma
Friedberg J (Univ of Toronto)
Laryngoscope 104:S1–S24, 1994   130-95-6-5

Introduction.—Forty patients with congenital cholesteatoma have been followed prospectively since the late 1970s. All of them have had surgical and pathologic confirmation of the diagnosis. Thirty-eight other cases have been encountered at the same otolaryngology department. These patients had a mean age of $4^1/_2$ years, and the degree of involvement was directly related to age. Most often cholesteatoma was limited to part of the mesotympanum, usually the anterosuperior portion, but one fourth of the patients were seen with extensive mesotympanic disease, and a comparable number had extension beyond the mesotympanum.

Pathogenesis.—Bony erosion seems to develop when osteolytic enzymes are released by inflammatory cells and granulation tissue. Bone destruction is a relative late feature of the disease. It is believed that cholesteatoma is more aggressive in children. Squamous metaplasia secondary to chronic otitis media has not been convincingly related to cholesteatoma. Ingrowth of ectoderm from the external into the middle canal has been proposed as a pathogenetic factor, as has the presence of embryonic-cell rests.

Diagnosis.—The history usually is not very contributory. Extension is most likely to develop inferiorly and posteriorly before the epitympanum and attic become involved. Extension into the posterior mesotympanum often is associated with erosion of the ossicles and hearing loss. The diagnosis of congenital cholesteatoma is primarily clinical. A biopsy is indicated only if the nature of a lesion is seriously in doubt.

Management.—Prompt surgical removal of cholesteatoma from the middle ear is especially important for young patients. Suggested procedures range from simple myringotomy, sleeve autografting, and tympanotomy to radical mastoidectomy. There probably is little indication for a classic radical mastoidectomy in children with congenital cholesteatoma. Patients should be followed for at least 2 years even when initial disease is confined to the middle ear. Those who require some form of mastoidectomy should be followed indefinitely.

▶ This comprehensive study of congenital cholesteatoma is of interest. The author has seen a large series and has done a careful review of the literature regarding this pathologic entity. As mentioned earlier, the difficulty lies in differentiating congenital cholesteatoma from acquired cholesteatoma, because even an acquired cholesteatoma can, in certain instances, occur beneath an intact tympanic membrane as an example of so-called silent chronic otitis media. We have evidence to that effect from temporal bones.—M.M. Paparella, M.D.

Localization of Function in the Eustachian Tube: A Hypothesis
Sando I, Takahashi H, Matsune S, Aoki H (Univ of Pittsburgh, Pa)
Ann Otol Rhinol Laryngol 103:311–314, 1994   130-95-6–6

Background.—The eustachian tube has 3 major functions: ventilation, clearance, and protection of the middle ear. Recent morphometric studies were used to discuss a hypothesis for localization of these functions in different portions of the eustachian tube.

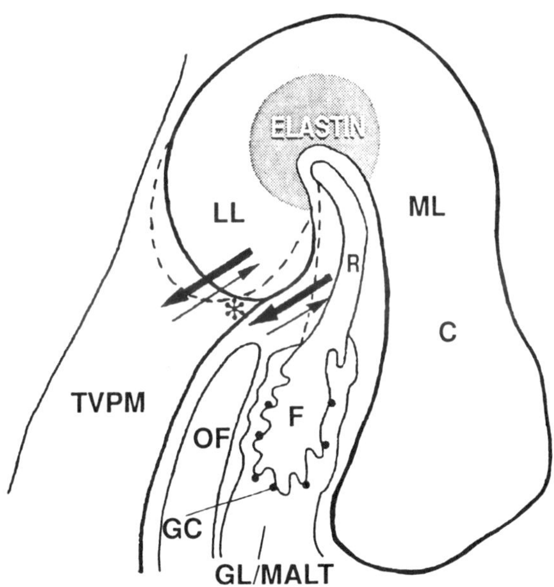

Fig 6–3.—Drawing of a cross section through the midcartilaginous portion of the eustachian tube and the hypothesized actions involved in tube function. The thick arrows indicate the direction of movement of the lateral lamina (*LL*) and lateral epithelial lining of the tube move away from medial lamina (*ML*) of the eustachian tube cartilage and medial epithelial lining of tube, respectively, when the tensor veli palatini muscle (*TVPM*) contracts. *Dashed lines* indicate the resultant position of LL and the lateral epithelial wall of the roof (*R*) portion of the eustachian tube. *Thin arrows* indicate passive movement of previously mentioned structures, mediated by action of the elastin in the hinge portion of the cartilage, to their resting positions when contraction of TVPM ends. *Asterisk,* the tendon of the TVPM inserts into the perichondrium at the tip of LL of eustachian tube cartilage (*C*) at a right angle. Also, goblet cells (*GC*), tubal glands (*GL*), mucosa-associated lymphoid tissue (*MALT*), and Ostmann's fatty tissue (*OF*) are mainly located close to the floor (*F*) portion of the eustachian tube. (Courtesy of Sando I, Takahashi H, Matsune S, et al: *Ann Otol Rhinol Laryngol* 103:311–314, 1994.)

Ventilation Function.—Ventilation of the middle ear is known to take place through active opening of the eustachian tube, mediated largely by contraction of the tensor veli palatini muscle (TVPM). In normal anatomy, the contraction of this muscle moves the lateral lamina of the eustachian tube inferolaterally away from the medial lamina, offering an efficient mechanism for active opening of the eustachian tube. The C-shaped or concave shape of the roof of the eustachian tube lumen allows for considerable expansion laterally with inferolateral movement of the lateral lamina consequent to contraction of the TVPM, thus bringing smooth active opening of the eustachian tube. However, the floor portion of the eustachian tube may be resistant to opening because it is surrounded by glandular and fatty tissue. This points to the possibility that active opening of the eustachian tube for ventilation of the middle ear is principally the result of inferolateral movement of the lateral lamina and the lateral epithelial lining of the roof portion of the eustachian tube (Fig 6–3).

Clearance Function.—Mucociliary action in the eustachian tube is largely responsible for clearance of the middle ear. Ciliated cells appear to be more abundant in the lower portion of the eustachian tube than in the roof. The fact that there is a greater distribution of both goblet cells and eustachian glands on the floor than the roof, as well as more mucosal folding, indicates that more active clearing occurs on the floor. Active mucociliary flow is a functional advantage to eustachian tube clearance, and the mucosal folding provides an increased surface area of tubal mucosa and protects its surface from airflow, thus aiding the smooth transport of secretion from the middle ear to the nasopharynx.

Protective Function.—A thick, meshlike distribution of elastin is present on the luminal side of the intermediate portion of the tubal cartilage between the medial lamina and the lateral lamina, serving to protect the roof portion of the eustachian tube. Further mechanical protection is provided by Ostmann's fatty tissue, which is thought to prevent the floor portion of the eustachian tube from opening by exerting static pressure on the lumen. Numerous mucosal folds in the floor once again help close the eustachian tube and thus protect the middle ear from secretions ascending from the nasopharynx. Mucosa-associated lymphoid tissue, which consists mainly of lymphocytes grouped around a germinal center, is also thought to have a protective function. Furthermore, mucus secreted by the glands and goblet cells of the floor of the eustachian tube is rich in immunoglobulin and anti-infectious enzymes.

Conclusion.—It is likely that anatomically localized changes in eustachian tube morphology can selectively affect ventilation, clearance, and protection of the middle ear of patients with otitis media. This hypothesis provides a testable framework for correlating physiologic and morphological studies of eustachian tube function, and for correlating pathophysiologic and histopathologic studies of eustachian tube dysfunction associated with otologic diseases such as otitis media.

▶ These authors create an interesting hypothesis: The roof of the eustachian tube is involved mainly with ventilation, and the floor is mainly involved with clearance. From the point of view of gravity, this would make physiologic and phylogenetic sense. I think this hypothesis has merit, and the authors certainly provide support with some scientific data.—M.M. Paparella, M.D.

Middle Ear Symptoms While Flying: Ways to Prevent a Severe Outcome
Brown TP (Whiting Field Naval Air Station, Pensacola, Fla)
Postgrad Med 96:135–137, 141–142, 1994   130-95-6–7

Introduction.—Pressurized cabins in airplanes prevent most serious forms of pressure-related changes during flying; however, some passengers occasionally experience severe middle ear blocks. The causes of barotrauma, its prevention, and treatment were reviewed by a physician who has treated military pilots.

Effects of Barometric Changes.—The eustachian tube equalizes the pressure of the middle ear with that of the surrounding environment. Airplane ascent does not usually cause a problem, but equalization difficulties are not uncommon during descent. Passengers experience discomfort at a pressure differential of 60 mm Hg. At about 90 mm Hg, the eustachian tube becomes locked; pressure differentials of 100 mm Hg and above rupture the tympanic membrane and may cause vomiting, hearing loss, dizziness, and vertigo.

Prevention of Ear Block.—Flying should be avoided when symptoms of upper respiratory tract infection are present. Middle ear pressure can be equalized by yawning, swallowing, or chewing, especially during ascent. If these attempts fail, the Valsalva maneuver is an option. The maneuver consists of taking a small breath, pinching off the nose, and attempting to force air through the pinched-off nostrils. When repeated during descent and as soon as fullness is noted in the ears, passengers should be able to stay ahead of the pressure differential. Other options include nasal spray decongestants inhaled 1 hour before takeoff and 30 minutes before descent, oral decongestants started 1 to 2 days before the flight, and antihistamines for passengers with allergies. Infants and toddlers can be given liquids during ascent and descent. Decongestants and the bulb syringe are also useful in children.

Treatment.—Severe or persistent ear block may require use of the Politzer bag or a myringotomy. The Politzer bag is similar to a nasal bulb syringe used in pediatric patients. With 1 naris occluded, the flange of the bag is placed in the other naris and the patient rapidly repeats aloud the letter *k* while compressing the hand-held bulb. A few minutes with this method clears 50% of ear blocks. If other methods fail, myringotomy should produce dramatic relief.

Conclusion.—The most important preventive measure for middle ear block is to avoid flying during an upper respiratory tract infection. Pressure can be relieved by yawning, chewing, or swallowing; other options are antihistamines, decongestants, and the Valsalva maneuver. Persistent or severe cases may require the Politzer bag or a myringotomy.

▶ Because flying has become commonplace for all our patients, symptoms in the middle ear while flying are a bigger problem than they used to be. Patients who have ear disease with a variety of pathologic correlates are especially affected by flying. Middle ear diseases of various pathologic types are particularly affected by flying. The other question is: When can patients fly, subsequent to otologic surgery? The ideas presented by Dr. Brown are helpful, and I believe they are used by most of us in advising our patients to prevent barotrauma, especially during descent.—M.M. Paparella, M.D.

Adenotonsillectomy in the Treatment of Secretory Otitis Media
Austin DF (Idaho Falls, Idaho)
ENT J 73:367–369, 373–374, 1994   130-95-6–8

Introduction.—On the basis of the belief that secretory otitis media in children is a manifestation of recurrent or chronic catarrhal disease of the upper respiratory tract whose epicenter usually lies in the nasopharynx, a physician's treatment for patients with persistent effusion has been tonsillectomy and adenoidectomy (TA) or adenoidectomy rather than insertion of ventilating tubes into the middle ear. Eighty-three patients who were followed for at least 1 year were reviewed.

Methods.—In the early years of the experience, both ears were cleared of effusion when a ventilation tube was inserted in only a single ear. Intubation of the middle ear was then abandoned, and TA was performed instead for catarrhal otitis media. In a preliminary study of 31 patients, the operated and unoperated ears showed no significant differences. Twenty-nine of the patients benefited by at least short-term unilateral improvement of hearing. Children with persistent effusion despite adequate treatment are advised to have TA without intubation.

Results.—A comparison of hearing test results of the 83 patients who had TA alone and the 31 patients who had TA with unilateral tube insertion yielded only 1 significant difference: those treated with TA alone had a better hearing result. Only 8 of the 83 patients had recurrent episodes after TA and 2 required 1 tube insertion each.

Conclusion.—Children with chronic catarrhal disease or with chronic tonsillitis and adenoiditis should be evaluated thoroughly for environmental, immunologic, infectious, and nutritional factors. Medical treatment, nutritional supplements, and improvement of nasal hygiene may resolve the catarrhal process in many cases. Far too many ears undergo intubation, a procedure that may be unnecessary and may lead to complications.

▶ Austin has experience dealing with these problems and provides practical know-how in managing patients who have otitis media with effusion and who have adenotonsillitis. We would all agree that if patients have symptoms of tonsillitis and adenoiditis or adenoid hypertrophy, treatment certainly benefits recovery or resolution of otitis media with effusion. In my opinion, the importance of this study is that it emphasizes that to practice good otology one has to be mindful of what traditionally has been known as the ear, nose, and throat. One can add that patients who have septal obstruction or sinusitis will have inflammatory disease of the middle ear (this is true in children as well as in adults), and so it is important to pay attention to the nose, sinuses, and throat and, as this case indicates, to the adenoids and tonsils as well, when dealing with patients who have otologic and related diseases.—M.M. Paparella, M.D.

The Medical Appropriateness of Tympanostomy Tubes Proposed for Children Younger Than 16 Years in the United States
Kleinman LC, Kosecoff J, Dubois RW, Brook RH (Harvard Med School, Boston; RAND Health Science Program, Santa Monica, Calif; Univ of California, Los Angeles)
JAMA 271:1250–1255, 1994   130-95-6–9

Background.—Two thirds of American children are given a diagnosis of otitis media by the age of 2 years. When episodes of acute otitis media or persistent middle ear effusion recur, physicians often consider placing tympanostomy tubes in the ear. In 1988, about 670,000 operations to insert tympanostomy tubes were performed in the United States. Data concerning the efficacy of the operation are contradictory, and reports of complications are frequent. The appropriateness of the clinical reasons given for inserting tympanostomy tubes was analyzed.

Methods.—Nurse reviewers conducted telephone interviews with staff members who had patients' charts at hand. An interactive computer program based on a smart-logic branching algorithm developed by a national utilization review firm guided the interviews. If the reasons given for recommending the operation were found inappropriate, a physician reviewer discussed the patient's data with the otolaryngologist.

The records were reviewed of 6,611 children (age, 22 days to 15.9 years) from 49 states and Washington, D.C., who were recommended for tympanostomy tubes from January 1990 to July 31, 1991. Appropriateness criteria were developed by a panel of 5 pediatricians and 4 otolaryngolgists using the RAND/UCLA 2-round modified Delphi method.

Results.—Of 6,429 children proposed to undergo operation because they had recurrent otitis media or persistent otitis media with effusion

(97% of the 6,611), 2,627 (41%) were found to have had appropriate indications for tympanostomy tube placement, 2,078 (32%) had equivocal indications, and 1,724 (27%) had inappropriate indications. All of the appropriate indications were found in children with documented effusions lasting more than 90 days.

These authors believe that approximately one-quarter of all tympanostomy tube operations proposed for children in the United States should not have been performed and that an additional one third of the proposed operations were of questionable value.

Conclusion.—Physicians are urged to defer operations for children with uncomplicated cases of recurrent acute otitis media or otitis media with effusion for at least 90 days or until effusion continues through a course of antibiotic therapy or children with recurrent episodes have an episode while receiving antibiotics. Parents of children with equivocal indications should be informed of the equivalent risks and potential benefits of a tympanostomy tube operation.

▶ As managed medical care grows disproportionate to societal need and as the fallacious concept of "the gatekeeper" and "outcome studies" become central tenets in the future of managed care, studies such as this, which affect society deleteriously and create harm that will take years to correct, will continue. This study has been criticized by many of our leading colleagues and by editors of our journals. In sum, this is a flawed study containing bias and conflict of interest. It certainly discredits tympanostomy tubes, without displaying any understanding or accountability for the pathologic conditions, the pathogenesis, or the experience that has been well established in literally thousands of patients during the past few decades.

This study had remarkable coverage in the lay media and created such harm that the best we can do is try to get back to basics in terms of what is best clinically and to stress the pathogenesis and the pathologic findings in these conditions. For example, I have approximately 600 human temporal bones in my laboratory, all of which have varying forms of otitis media, and if one looks at otitis media with effusion for any period, one quickly sees that it is not innocuous fluid, such as water sitting in a glass, but, rather, can be considered a mild poison that causes damage over time. In 12 temporal bones from infants who died of *Hemophilus influenzae* meningitis, in 1 infant, 6 months old, who had some granulation tissue as well as mucopurulent fluid, one could see that the incus was literally destroyed in that short a period. It is hoped that, in the future, we will be able to get back to basics and help our patients, and that such studies as this one will not be undertaken. However, in this new day of cost-control and managed care, that is probably hoping for too much.—M.M. Paparella, M.D.

The Effect of Water Exposure After Tympanostomy Tube Insertion
Parker GS, Tami TA, Maddox MR, Wilson JF (Eastern Virginia Med School,

Norfolk; Univ of Cincinnati, Ohio; Naval Hosp, Newport, RI; et al)
Am J Otolaryngol 15:193–196, 1994   130-95-6–10

Background.—Authorities disagree about the role of unprotected water exposure in the development of otorrhea in patients with tympanostomy tubes. Although most otolaryngologists advise patients to avoid swimming or to restrict exposure of the ears to water while swimming, evidence suggests that such practices may not affect the infection rate.

Methods and Findings.—Two hundred twelve consecutive patients who were undergoing the placement of tympanostomy tubes were randomly assigned to swimming and nonswimming groups. No ear plugs, canal occlusion, or antibiotic drugs were used in either group. One hundred seven patients were followed for 1 year. The incidence of otorrhea and the number of episodes of otorrhea did not differ significantly between groups.

Conclusion.—Swimming apparently is not contraindicated in patients with tympanostomy tubes. Precautions to avoid water exposure do not reduce the incidence of otorrhea.

▶ My experience in patients has been similar to these authors' experience. In many patients who have typanostomy tubes, swimming can be encouraged; however, common sense advice, such as keeping the head above water or not too much water, is helpful. This study is practical and useful to the otolaryngologist who is commonly faced with questions of this type.—M.M. Paparella, M.D.

Swimming and Grommets: A Prospective Survey
Gilbert JG (Timaru Hosp, New Zealand)
N Z Med J 107:244–245, 1994   130-95-6–11

Introduction.—Recent studies have challenged the long-held belief that patients with grommets are at increased risk of having infections if they swim or swim without ear protection. Nevertheless, many otolaryngologists still advise their patients not to swim, or to wear ear plugs while swimming. The incidence of otorrhea or otalgia in patients with grommets in situ who were allowed to swim was determined.

Methods.—During a 4-month period, 19 children with bilateral patent grommets were allowed to swim with 1 ear protected with cotton wool and petroleum jelly covered by a bathing cap, which was pulled up to expose the other ear. Parents recorded every instance of swimming with the head immersed, as well as every episode of pain or otorrhea. The patency of the grommets was confirmed every 6 weeks.

Results.—The children swam with the head immersed a total of 551 times. Each child swam between 3 and 101 times, with an average of 29 times. Most (16) of the children had Shepard grommets; the other 3 had

T-tubes. One of the children with T tubes had bilateral otorrhea 1 day after swimming, which was diagnosed as acute otitis media. Ear pain was present in 3 other instances, with no evidence of infection; 2 occurred in protected ears and 1 in an unprotected ear.

Discussion.—During the summer months, children with grommets in situ have a very low incidence of otorrhea and they can safely swim without ear protection. However, they should be advised that it is preferable not to dive or to swim more than 3 feet under the water. These findings may not be applicable during the winter months, when there might be a higher incidence of otorrhea, or with Polynesians, who have different middle ear and eustachian tube anatomy and physiology.

▶ This study, like that outlined in Abstract 130-95-6–10, also indicates a low incidence of otorrhea or infection in children who swim with ventilation tubes in place. As both of these studies indicate, however, this does not mean that swimming or exposure to water cannot cause difficulty but, rather, that it can be safe with the proper consideration.—M.M. Paparella, M.D.

Adult-Onset Otitis Media With Effusion

Finkelstein Y, Ophir D, Talmi YP, Shabtai A, Strauss M, Zohar Y (Tel Aviv Univ, Israel)
Arch Otolaryngol Head Neck Surg 120:517–527, 1994   130-95-6–12

Background.—Otitis media with effusion (OME) is believed to be rare in adults, typically occurring secondary to neoplastic diseases of the nasopharynx or other head and neck tumors. However, OME has been the presenting symptom in 23% of adults with chronic sinusitis, suggesting a higher prevalence. The prevalence and etiology of adult-onset OME were investigated.

Methods.—One hundred sixty-seven patients who were given a diagnosis of OME underwent intranasal and nasopharyngeal endoscopy. Computed tomography of the skull base, neck, and paranasal sinuses was performed in 65 patients.

Results.—Paranasal sinus disease caused OME in 110 patients; smoking-induced nasopharyngeal lymphoid hyperplasia and adenoidal hypertrophy, in 15; head and neck tumors, in 8; and undetermined factors, in 3. Wegener's granulomatosis was diagnosed in 1 patient with a 2-year history of polyarthritis who had purulent intermittent bloody rhinorrhea, headache, left ear fullness, and hearing loss of 3 weeks' duration. Physical examination revealed granulation tissue on the nasal septum and medial conchae, purulent discharge, and green crusts. Nasendoscopy showed granulations on an eroded left torus tubarius (Fig 6–4) and on the hyperemic nasopharyngeal mucosa. Yellow sticky fluid was aspirated during myringotomy. Computed tomography revealed adenoidal hypertrophy, irregular tori tubarii, and sinuses filled with soft tissue.

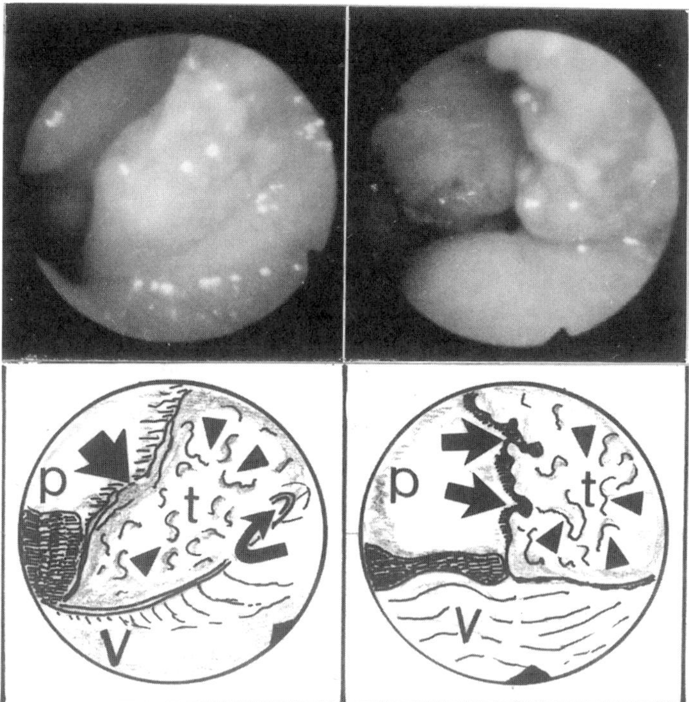

Fig 6–4.—Endoscopic view of the left eustachian tube orifice in a patient with Wegener's granulomatosis. **Left,** contralateral view. **Right,** ipsilateral view. *Arrows* indicate erosions; *arrowheads,* granulations; and *curved arrow,* edematous tubal orifice. *Abbreviations: p,* posterior pharyngeal wall; *t,* torus tubarius; V, velum. (Courtesy of Finkelstein Y, Ophir D, Talmi YP, et al: *Arch Otolaryngol Head Neck Surg* 120:517–527, 1994.)

Symptoms resolved with aggressive steroidal and cytotoxic treatment, but persistent middle ear effusion prompted insertion of a ventilation tube. After 1 year, the patient had contralateral OME develop. Nasendoscopic examination revealed a purulent discharge from the ipsilateral infundibulum. The OME resolved after antibiotic treatment.

Conclusion.—Adult-onset OME is relatively common. Although it is most often caused by sinusitis, there is a high correlation between nasopharyngeal abnormalities and middle ear disease. Therefore, diagnosis and treatment of adult-onset OME requires thorough endoscopic examination of the intranasal and nasopharyngeal structures and CT examination to rule out neoplastic disease.

▶ Otitis media with effusion can occur in adults as well as in children. This paper describes the careful diagnostic approach to this problem. This study indicates that attention should be paid not only to the nasopharynx and to function or dysfunction of the eustachian tube but, also, to the nose and sinuses, which are adjacent to the eustachian tube and can either complicate or help cause OME. Although it is rare, the clinician should always consider the possibility of nasopharyngeal carcinoma or other tumors as possible etiologic agents as well.—M.M. Paparella, M.D.

Cytokeratin Patterns of Normal Middle Ear Epithelia in Humans, Cats, and Chinchillas
Sano S-I, Schachern PA, Haruna S-I, Paparella MM (Jikei Kai Med College, Tokyo; Univ of Minnesota, Minneapolis)
Ann Otol Rhinol Laryngol 103:227–234, 1994   130-95-6–13

Introduction.—Virtually all epithelia contain the intermediate-size filaments called cytokeratins. Approximately 19 human cytokeratin polypeptides have been recognized, and their antibodies have been used in tissue recognition studies and to diagnose tumors.

Objective.—Cytokeratin patterns were examined in epithelia from the tympanic orifice, tympanic cavity, and mastoid cavity of humans, cats, and chinchillas. The results were compared with those obtained in tracheal epithelium and the epidermis of the external auditory canal. The cytokeratins were examined by use of indirect immunofluorescence technique with the avidin/biotin-peroxidase-complex method.

Findings.—Epithelia from all sites in the middle ear stained for some type of cytokeratin. Broad-spectrum anticytokeratin antibodies stained epithelium of the middle ear cleft, tracheal epithelium, and the external canal epidermis in all 3 species. Studies with specific antibodies demonstrated species differences in staining patterns in the middle ear and tracheal epithelia. The same staining pattern usually was observed in epithelia of the middle ear and trachea. No monospecific cytokeratin antibody reacted with the epidermis of the external ear canal.

Conclusion.—A knowledge of cytokeratin patterns in middle ear epithelia should prove helpful in assessing the hyperplastic and metaplastic changes of otitis media, but caution is required when making comparisons between species.

▶ Otitis media is characterized by many hyperplastic and metaplastic changes in the mucoperiosteum. Patterns of cytokeratin in epithelium of the middle ear can be helpful in understanding these pathologic changes that can happen rather rapidly in the middle ear cleft of patients. Interestingly, for comparative purposes, this study included humans and cats as well as chinchillas. Further such studies are warranted to help us gain a better understanding of the pathogenesis of otitis media, especially how otitis media with effusion (mucoid otitis media) can and does become chronic otitis media and chronic mastoiditis characterized by intractably pathologic tissue, either granulation tissue, cholesterol granuloma, and/or cholesteatoma.—M.M. Paparella, M.D.

Lymphocyte Migration to the Middle Ear Mucosa

Kato H, Watanabe N, Bundo J, Mogi G (Oita Med Univ, Japan)
Ann Otol Rhinol Laryngol 103:118–124, 1994   130-95-6–14

Background.—After enhancement of the mucosal immunity, antigen-specific immunoglobulin (Ig) A–forming cells appear in the inflamed mucosa of the middle ear cavity and eustachian tube. To clarify the mechanism of selective migration and localization of antigen-specific IgA-forming cells in the middle ear mucosa, the antigenic effects and influences of T cells from various lymphoid tissues on lymphocyte migration into the middle ear mucosa were studied using a reconstitution technique of lymphocytes in radiated chimera recipients of guinea pigs.

Methods.—Antigen-specific lymphocytes of IgA and IgG classes were induced in guinea pigs according to a previously described immunization strategy. From those animals, lymphocytes of Peyer's patches and spleen were labeled with chromium 51 and transferred to radiated chimera recipients. The right tympanic cavity was inoculated with dinitrophenylated ovalbumin as antigenic stimulation; the left ear, acting as control, received an injection of hydroxypropyl cellulose solution. To induce nonantigenic inflammation to the mucosa, another group of animals received intratympanic inoculation with live bacteria of *Streptococcus pneumoniae* biotype 3.

Results.—The mean levels of radioactivity in the middle ears with antigenic and nonantigenic stimulation were significantly higher than those of the control ears. Radioactivity levels of the middle ears were not influ-

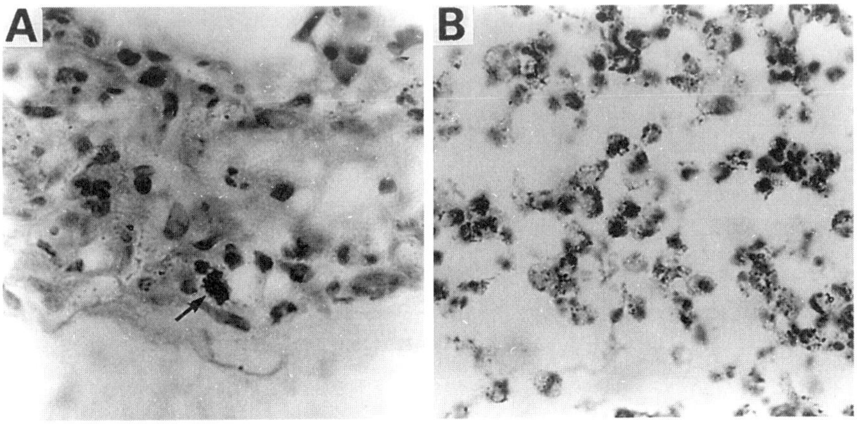

Fig 6–5.—Autoradiographs. **A,** middle ear mucosa. Some lymphocytes labeled with tritium-labeled thymidine (*arrow*) from Peyer's patches of animals with mucosal immunization are found scattered in inflamed mucosa. **B,** middle ear effusion. Many labeled cells of Peyer's patches from animals with mucosal immunization are observed in effusion of recipients with nonantigenic stimulation on middle ear mucosa. (Courtesy of Kato H, Watanabe N, Bundo J, et al: *Ann Otol Rhinol Laryngol* 103:118–124, 1994.)

enced by the origin and subsets of transferred cells nor by antigenic stimuli to the mucosa. Many labeled cells were observed in the middle ear effusions, whereas few were scattered in the inflamed mucosa (Fig 6–5).

Summary.—In the early stage of inflammation of the middle ear mucosa, circulating lymphocytes, including antigen-specific T and B cells, may be recruited from the blood circulations to the inflamed middle ear mucosa by nonspecific inflammatory processes that may mask antigen-specific factors in lymphocyte migration.

▶ Lymphocytes, including antigen-specific T and B cells, can be recruited from circulating blood to the inflamed mucosa of the middle ear. This finding and studies of this type, which should be continued, provide insight into the role of immunology in the pathogenesis of otitis media.—M.M. Paparella, M.D.

Micropathologic Changes of Pars Tensa in Children With Otitis Media With Effusion

Sano S, Kamide Y, Schachern PA, Paparella MM (Univ of Minnesota, Minneapolis; Minnesota Ear, Head, and Neck Clinic, Minneapolis; Jikeikai Med College, Tokyo)
Arch Otolaryngol Head Neck Surg 120:815–819, 1994   130-95-6–15

Background.—Past studies have reported a relationship between otitis media with effusion (OME) in children and chronic otitis media in adults. However, relatively little is known about the histopathologic changes in the tympanic membrane in OME. Such changes in the pars tensa resulting from the chronic inflammatory processes of OME were investigated, and the potential consequences of the degeneration of the lamina propria of the pars tensa were discussed.

Method.—Thirty children between 4 and 10 years of age who did not show improvement after 3 months of conservative therapy for OME were given general anesthesia for insertion of ventilation tubes. Sixty 1 × 2-mm biopsy specimens were removed from the intermediate zone of the anteroinferior quadrant of the tympanic membrane. Sixteen complete samples were available for histologic analysis. Control specimens were obtained from the temporal bone of 4 subjects at autopsy: twins at 33 weeks after conception, a 3-month old infant, and a 30-year-old adult.

Results.—The most notable histopathologic finding in the patients with OME was an increase in the thickness of the pars tensa as a result of edema and fibrosis. An increase in the thickness of the subepidermal layer was also found, but to a lesser degree. Rich vascularization was seen in both the submucosal and the subepidermal layers. Inflammatory cells were more localized in the submucosal layer than in the subepidermal layer. Overall slight edema was seen in the fibrous layer, which resulted in some cases in wave-like distortions of the fibers, and created ultrastructural spaces between the fibrous bundles in the outer radial layer, and between typical collagen fibrils in the inner circular layer. Few inflammatory cells were found in the fibrous layer, and new vascularization was poor in this area. In some cases the fibrous layer in the tympanic membrane was absent and replaced by connective tissue in which edema, irregular collagen fibrils, fibrinoid degeneration, elastic bundles, and fibroblasts were seen. The tympanic membranes of the OME group were significantly thicker than those of the control group. The lamina propria of the tympanic membrane was thicker in the OME group than in controls. However, when the thickness of the epidermal, subepidermal, fibrous, submucosal, and mucosal layers was compared, only the thickness of the submucosal layer showed a substantial difference to the control group. Thus, the thickness of the tympanic membrane in OME was found to depend on the thickness of the submucosal layer, which was increased as a result of edema and fibrosis.

Conclusion.—The tissue response of the tympanic membrane in otitis media with effusion is edema and subsequent fibrosis of the submucosal layer. Edema in the fibrous layer leads to spaces between the fiber bundles and the degeneration of the fibrous framework. Repeated inflammation brings more serious degeneration, such as the growth of nonelastic fibrous tissue and scar tissue, resulting in lost elasticity of the membrane. Although the incidence of OME decreases after the age of 12 years, the pathologic changes that have already occurred in the tympanic membrane during childhood can render it more vulnerable to perforation or other sequelae, such as retraction pockets or cholesteatoma in later life.

▶ The tympanic membrane, especially its subepithelial portion, which is contiguous with the mucoperiosteum of the middle ear, certainly plays a role in otitis media. In fact, the tympanic membrane, through otoscopy or pneumatic otoscopy and microscopy, allows us a portal or window to assess the pathologic changes of otitis media; therefore, it is relevant to look at light microscopic and electron microscopic studies of the tympanic membrane in patients who have these diseases, as done in this study.—M.M. Paparella, M.D.

Tympanic Membrane Perforation in Survivors of a SCUD Missile Explosion
Patow CA, Bartels J, Dodd KT (85th Evacuation Hosp and 207th Evacuation Hosp of the US Army, Dhahran, Kingdom of Saudi Arabia; Walter Reed Army Inst of Research, Washington, DC)
Otolaryngol Head Neck Surg 110:211–221, 1994   130-95-6–16

Background.—On February 25, 1990, in Dhahran, Kingdom of Saudi Arabia, a single Iraqi SCUD missile exploded inside a warehouse constructed of steel girder frame and light aluminum siding. The building housed military personnel of the United States during Operation Desert Storm. A systematic survey of individuals who were near the impact site at the time of the blast was conducted to assess the blast injury to the ear. Tympanic membrane (TM) perforation was used as the clinical marker for aural blast injury.

Findings.—One hundred seventy-two service members were near the impact site at the time of the blast. Of these, 34 had unilateral TM perforations and 28 had bilateral TM perforations. Of the 86 patients who sustained sufficient injury to be hospitalized, 59 of 84 patients examined (70%) had TM perforations. Of the 90 TM perforations, 39% were estimated to be 25% or less of total TM surface area, 36% were 26% to 50% of TM surface area, 16% were 51% to 75% of TM surface area, and 10% were greater than 75% of TM surface area. The majority of TM perforations (84%) were curvilinear central perforations, and 13% were radial and triangular in shape. Relative protection from TM perforation was afforded by being distant from the blast, being in open doorways, or wearing headphones. Service members within 50 feet of the blast had a 75% incidence of TM perforation; bilateral TM perforations occurred most frequently among those within 30 ft of the explosion. Based on a grading system developed by Griffin, one third of TMs estimated to be within 10 feet of the blast had perforations of 50% or more of the TM surface area, and only 11% of TMs had no visible damage. Likewise, for bilateral TM perforation, the greatest damage occurred at 10 feet or less, and the greatest incidence of damage occurred between 10 and 30 feet from the blast. Symptoms consisted mainly of changes in hearing and mild tinnitus.

Discussion.—The ear is particularly vulnerable to damage from blast overpressure because it intensifies the force of the blast wave and contains one of the most delicate tissues of the human body, the TM. Among the survivors of a SCUD missile explosion, those who were closest to the blast had the most severe TM injury, including the highest proportion of bilateral TM perforation. In addition to the distance from the blast, the extent of injury varied based on the position of the individual, the presence of energy absorbent materials, and the complex pattern of blast wave pressure in the building. Historical nuclear blast data were used to estimate the SCUD blast waveform based on the measurement of the SCUD impact crater. A mathematical model based on the estimated waveform characteristics was constructed to estimate the pressure load on the TM of the individuals. When validated against the actual field data of the proximity and incidence of TM perforations, the calculated blast overpressure of the SCUD missile blast and the actual pattern of TM perforations were compatible. This model can be used as a tool for future reserach in the prevention and therapy of blast injury to the ear.

▶ Of 172 individuals, 34 had perforation of the tympanic membrane develop as a result of the explosion of a SCUD missile. Injuries of this type during wartime are not considered by the average otolaryngologist in daily practice. Nevertheless, such problems do occur, and they do provide information that will allow us to assess a variety of injuries that do occur in our patients and in our practices.—M.M. Paparella, M.D.

Repair of Chronic Tympanic Membrane Perforations Using Epidermal Growth Factor: Progress Toward Clinical Application

Lee AJ, Jackler RK, Kato BM, Scott NM (Univ of California, San Francisco)
Am J Otol 15:10–18, 1994   130-95-6–17

Background.—Preliminary studies of the use of epidermal growth factor (EGF) in healing of chronic tympanic membrane (TM) perforations in the chinchilla show promising results. The original protocol requires rimming of the perforation's epithelial edge, placement of a paper patch over the perforation to act as a scaffold, placement of a Gelfoam pledget in the middle ear canal to act as reservoir for the drug, and administration of EGF solution (1 mg of EGF per mL of phosphate-buffered saline (PBS). This method allowed 81% healing of EGF-treated TM perforations compared with healing in only 25% of the controls. A simplified protocol was devised in an attempt to develop a simple outpatient method of healing chronic TM perforations.

Method.—The chinchilla model of chronic TM perforations was used. Without disrupting the perforation's edge or using a paper patch, a large Gelfoam pledget was placed over the chronic perforation in contact with the residual TM (Fig 6–6). Then, 50 µL of .5-mg EGF/mL PBS was applied to the Gelfoam pledget. In control ears, 50 µL of PBS was applied

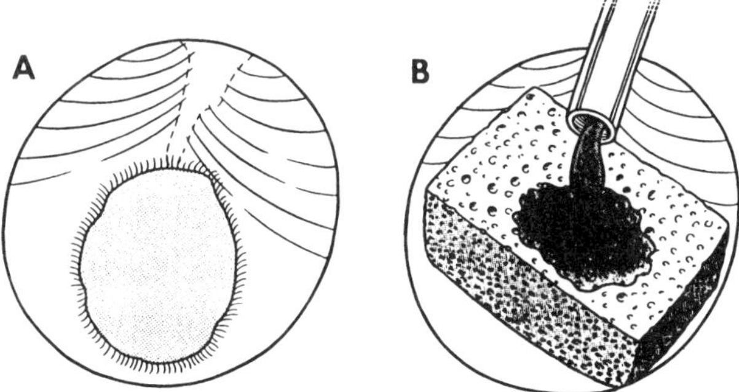

Fig 6–6.—Schematic view of experimental tympanic membrane (TM) methodology. **A,** stable, subtotal, noninfected TM perforation with mature epithelial margin. **B,** large Gelfoam pledget is placed over the TM perforation in contact with residual TM and the medial ear canal, and epidermal growth factor is applied to Gelfoam via a micropipette. (Courtesy of Lee AJ, Jackler RK, Kato BM, et al: *Am J Otol* 15:10–18, 1994.)

to the Gelfoam pledget. Treatment was administered every other day for 3 doses.

Outcome.—In the modified protocol, 80% of EGF-treated ears achieved complete closure of TM perforations, compared with only 20% of control ears. These results were similar to those achieved with the original method. At 4 to 9 months after treatment, EGF-healed TMs gradually achieved an overall thickness and relative proportionality of the 3-component layers similar to those of normal TMs. The squamous and mucosal layer appeared essentially normal, whereas the middle fibrous layer became more densely fibrous. In the three control TMs that healed spontaneously, the regenerated membranes had less than half the thickness of normal TMs. In the dose ranging studies, EGF at 50% and 25% lower concentrations than the original protocol were equally effective in inducing chronic TM perforations to heal. In an ototoxic screening study, surface preparations of the entire organ of Corti and cross-sections of the basal turn of the organ of Corti revealed no significant cochleotoxicity after topical application of EGF to the middle ear (total dose, 75 µg).

Conclusion.—Neither the excision of the perforation's epithelial margin nor placement of a structural scaffold is essential for EGF efficacy for the repair of chronic TM perforations. Because the biological action of EGF requires continuous contact with the target tissue for at least 5 hours, Gelfoam or some other spongelike substance is probably necessary for EGF efficacy. The quality of the healed EGF-treated TM is histologically similar to that of normal TMs. There are no significant ototoxic effects of EGF when used as prescribed in the treatment protocol. Clinical trials of EGF in the management of chronic TM perforations are being initiated.

▶ This interesting and careful study in an animal model indicates that EGF may be promising in the management of chronic perforations of the tympanic membrane. Studies of this type will better allow us to assess this possibility in clinical application in the future.—M.M. Paparella, M.D.

Type 1 Tympanoplasty in Children
Kessler A, Potsic WP, Marsh RR (Children's Hosp, Philadelphia; Univ of Pennsylvania, Philadelphia)
Arch Otolaryngol Head Neck Surg 120:487–490, 1994   130-95-6–18

Background.—The use and timing of tympanoplasty in young children continues to be controversial. Some recommend that the procedure be performed as soon as middle ear status has stabilized, whereas others, who are fearful of the likelihood of recurrent middle ear disease and eustachian tube dysfunction in younger children, prefer to delay it until a certain age. The factors affecting the surgical success rate and reperforation rate in type 1 tympanoplasty were investigated.

Method.—Between 1985 and 1989, 183 children underwent type 1 tympanoplasty in either one or both ears, amounting to a total of 209 operations. Most patients were 6 to 12 years old at the time of surgery, but 37 operations were done on patients younger than 6 years. The children were followed up for a minimum of 6 months and a mean of 25.5 months. Surgical success was defined as an intact graft at least 6 months after surgery. Long-term success included patients with an intact eardrum at the end of follow-up. Cases were defined as failures if perforation recurred within 6 months of surgery or if perforations occurred after 6 months when the eardrum was known not to be intact at 6 months.

Results.—Of the 209 operations performed, 16 failures were encountered, 12 of which happened in the first 3 months after surgery. Later reperforations occurred in 11 other patients. The overall short-term success rate was 92% with 87% of ears remaining free of reperforation to the end of follow-up. Age appeared to have no apparent relation to short-term surgical success. Neither was the condition of the contralateral ear an indicator of outcome. No significant differences for surgical success were found for the size of the perforation or for the quadrants involved. Grafts tended to fail more frequently in patients with marginal perforations that in those with central perforations.

Conclusion.—These results indicate that even in young patients, type 1 tympanoplasty can have a high success rate. Factors such as age, size of quadrants of the perforation, and status of the contralateral ear were not found to have statistical significance in predicting short-term surgical success. Even for factors associated with reduced success rates—marginal perforation, age younger than 6 years, or contralateral otitis—a 75% or greater success rate was seen. Therefore, age is not of itself a contraindication to tympanoplasty.

▶ Many might disagree with the conclusion of this study, i.e., that tympanoplasty can be considered at any age, even in very young children. As always, I think the indication of surgery will depend on the clinical pathologic findings plus the experience of the otolaryngologist in dealing with this problem. One also wants to assess the nature of the perforation of the tympanic membrane, e.g., whether it is marginal and whether it has a chance of leading to more serious pathologic conditions of chronic otitis media.—M.M. Paparella, M.D.

Xenograft Versus Autograft in Tympanoplasty

Callanan VP, Curran AJ, Gormley PK (Univ College Hosp, Galway, Republic of Ireland)
J Laryngol Otol 107:892–894, 1993   130-95-6–19

Introduction.—In the early years of tympanoplasty, skin grafts were used. However, these grafts sometimes perforated or developed cholesteatoma. More recently, other autografts, in which vein, temporalis fascia, or tragal perichondrium are used, have been more successful. Xenografts, including porcine dermis (Zenoderm), have also been used in tympanoplasty, but their efficacy has not been established. In retrospective study, the results of tympanoplasty using either Zenoderm or temporalis fascia autograft were compared.

Methods.—Fifty-three tympanoplasty operations were done by the same surgeon over 3-years. Temporalis fascia autografts were used in 43 procedures, and Zenoderm was used in 10. The success rate and other patient characteristics in the 2 groups were compared.

Results.—The success rate for tympanoplasty with temporalis fascia autograft was 95%; with Zenoderm xenograft, the success rate was 40%. The patients with failed xenografts were regrafted with temporalis fascia autografts; all of these procedures were successful. There were no significant differences in patient age, type of tympanoplasty, tympanic membrane perforation, or the condition of the contralateral ear. Bone conduction was not changed by surgery in either group. However, air conduction was significantly improved in the patients receiving autografts and was unchanged in the patients receiving xenografts.

Discussion.—The success rates for tympanoplasty significantly differed, with patients receiving Zenoderm xenografts experiencing poor results. The differences could not be explained by any patient characteristics. It was therefore concluded that Zenoderm should not be used for tympanoplasty.

▶ A xenograft is tissue transplanted between members of different species. This author found that an autograft (i.e., a graft, such as temporalis fascia, removed from the patient) is far more successful than tissue removed from another animal species. The rate of success using xenografts was very low, and the author appropriately suggests that this is not a suitable grafting material for tympanoplasty. At the same time, an appropriate xenograft may be developed in the future; if so, this would enhance our ability to do tympanoplasty. Moreover, it would be nice if a collagen graft that could be taken off the shelf could be developed particularly for cases that have acute perforations and do not require comprehensive tympanoplasty.—M.M. Paparella, M.D.

Management of Chronic Suppurative Otitis Media: Superiority of Therapy Effective Against Anaerobic Bacteria
Brook I (Georgetown Univ, Washington, DC)
Pediatr Infect Dis J 13:188–193, 1994   130-95-6–20

Objective.—Many previous studies on the bacterial etiology of chronic suppurative otitis media (CSOM) do not establish the role of anaerobic bacteria in the infection. The aerobic and anaerobic microbiology and management of CSOM were determined retrospectively in 69 children.

Methods.—Exudates were collected through direct middle ear aspirations through the perforation in the tympanic membrane, and inoculated into aerobic and anaerobic media.

Bacteriology.—A total of 103 anaerobic and 85 aerobic isolates were recovered. Anaerobic bacteria alone were isolated from 16% of isolates; aerobic bacteria only in 30%; and mixed aerobic and anaerobic flora, in 54%. Therefore, anaerobes were isolated from 70% and aerobes from 84% of the patients. The most common bacteria isolated were anaerobic gram-positive cocci, *Prevotella* sp, *Bacteroides* sp, *Staphylococcus aureus*, *Pseudomonas aeruginosa*, *Klebsiella pneumoniae*, and *Fusobacterium* sp. More than half (58%) of the patients harbored β-lactamase-producing bacteria, including 15 anaerobes and 30 aerobes.

Clinical Outcome.—Patients treated with clindamycin responded most rapidly (mean, 8.3 days), compared with those treated with ampicillin (12.0 days), erythromycin (16.5 days), and cefaclor (14.6 days). Furthermore, resolution of the infection was achieved in 80% of patients treated with clindamycin, compared to 50% of those treated with ampicillin, 46% with erythromycin, and 33% with cefaclor. Of the 31 patients who failed to respond to therapy, 26 harbored organisms resistant to the antimicrobials given, including 21 anaerobic and 15 aerobic organisms.

Conclusion.—These findings illustrate the importance of resistant aerobic and anaerobic organisms in the polymicrobial etiology of CSOM and the superiority of antimicrobial therapy that provide adequate coverage against anaerobic bacteria. Further studies are needed to investigate and conclusively establish the optimum therapeutic approach of CSOM.

▶ In treating children and adults who have suppurative otitis media, whether acute or chronic, it is important to consider the role of aerobic as well as anaerobic organisms. This study considers their relative roles and makes suggestions concerning methods of management.—M.M. Paparella, M.D.

Long-Term Results of Mastoid Cavities Grafted With Cultured Epithelium Prepared From Autologus Epidermal Cells to Prevent Chronic Otorrhea

Premachandra DJ, Woodward B, Milton CM, Sergeant RJ, Fabre JW (Kent and Sussex Hosp, Tunbridge Wells, Kent, England; Queen Victoria Hosp, East Grinstead, Sussex, England)

Laryngoscope 103:1121–1125, 1993   130-95-6–21

Introduction.—One third of patients who undergo mastoidectomy experience recurrent discharge from a mastoid cavity, and no satisfactory treatment has been found for chronic otorrhea and infection. Most of the methods used to arrest otorrhea involve major surgery. A simple procedure that was developed to solve the problem of postoperative otorrhea was evaluated in 26 patients who were followed for 10 to 18 months.

Patients and Methods.—The patients all had uncontrollable otorrhea resulting from failure of epithelialization of the mastoid cavity. Their mastoid cavities had failed to heal despite regular outpatient care and meticulous use of topical antibiotic treatment. Average age of the patients was 42 years; duration of otorrhea ranged from 2 to 32 years. The treatment uses autologous cultured keratinocyte layers grafted onto the unepithelialized open mastoid cavities. Local anesthesia is used for the skin biopsy, but the outpatient procedure is otherwise completed without anesthesia. The treatment protocol requires 4 visits over several weeks.

Results.—Seventeen of 28 grafted mastoid cavities had no discharge after the protocol was completed. Clinical examination showed complete epithelialization with no evidence of granulation tissue. Seven mastoid cavities were initially improved but had areas that failed to epithelialize, and discharge continued during respiratory infections. In the 3 patients in whom there was no improvement, the procedures were considered to have failed.

Conclusion.—Otorrhea has a disabling effect on patients, many of whom require cotton wool plugs during the day and special pillowcases at nighttime. Epithelialization of the mastoid cavity was achieved in most of these cases by application of cultured keratinocyte layers to the cavity. In 17 of the 28 cavities treated, the ears were completely dry during up to 18 months of follow-up. The technique is not applicable when discharge is the result of a high facial ridge or a small meatal opening.

▶ In this study, the use of cultured epithelium prepared from autologous epidermal cells is of interest. In similar situations, I would have used Thiersch's grafting—perhaps with equal success. Of course, Thiersch's grafting represents autologous tissue taken from the patient being treated. Nevertheless, this study is of interest, and if it can be confirmed by others, it may become a clinically useful tool.—M.M. Paparella, M.D.

Tympanomastoidectomy for Chronic Suppurative Otitis Media of Irradiated Ears of Nasopharyngeal Carcinoma Patients
Yuen PW, Wei WI (Univ of Hong Kong)
J Otolaryngol 23:302–304, 1994   130-95-6–22

Background.—Radiotherapy, the primary treatment for nasopharyngeal carcinoma (NPC), commonly causes otologic complications. Chronic suppurative otitis media (CSOM) develops in approximately 25% of patients who experience complications after radiotherapy. Despite long periods of active conservative treatment, most of these patients will continue to have chronic otorrhea. Therefore, surgical intervention has been adopted for patients who do not respond to conservative management. The results of tympanoplasty, with or without mastoidectomy, were reported for 16 patients.

Methods.—The patients had all received radiation (60 to 66 cGy) for NPC and were free of recurrent malignancy at the time of operation. The median age of the group was 55 years, and the median time between radiotherapy and operation was 4 years. All had tubotympanic disease with central perforation. Myringoplasty was performed using the temporalis fascia underlay technique. Ossiculoplasty was not attempted in any patient. The median duration of follow-up was 18 months.

Results.—Twelve of the 16 patients required cortical mastoidectomy in addition to myringoplasty to clear up the inflammatory mastoid air cells. The tympanic membrane was intact at the latest follow-up in 11 patients (69%). Those with successful myringoplasty had no secretory otitis media, indicating a functioning eustachian tube. Eight of the 11 had no more otorrhea after the operation, whereas 3 had persistent otorrhea because of exposed residual osteoradionecrotic bone in the external ear canal. The remaining 5 patients had reperforation of the eardrum and persistent otorrhea.

Conclusion.—Tympanomastoidectomy is recommended for patients with NPC and active CSOM who fail to respond to conservative treatment. Despite adverse factors in this series of patients, 50% had no more otorrhea after operation. Osteoradionecrosis is usually localized to the external ear, and temporal bone resection is not required. Repeated operation may be needed in some cases, however, when the extent of osteoradionecrosis is not evident at the initial operation.

▶ We have had an experience similar to that described by these authors: When the temporal bone is irradiated, osteoradionecrosis can result. This can occur if the temporal bone is intact or, in some instances, if the patient has already received a tympanomastoidectomy. These patients require particularly meticulous long-term care and should be followed at least twice a year, if not more frequently, to prevent topical irritation or inflammations from becoming more penetrative.—M.M. Paparella, M.D.

Prevention of Recurrence of Cholesteatoma in Intact Canal Wall Tympanoplasty

Yanagihara N, Gyo K, Sasaki Y, Hinohira Y (Ehime Univ, Japan)
Am J Otol 14:590–594, 1993   130-95-6–23

Background.—Since 1965, an intact canal wall tympanoplasty (ICWT) has been used for the treatment of cholesteatoma, but the incidence of recurrence was high (41%). A planned staged ICWT and reestablishment of the aeration of the tympanic cavity are required to eradicate possible causes of recurrence, cholesteatoma residue, and retraction pocket.

Techinque.—In the first-stage operation, the facial recessus, tympanic sinus, and anterior attic are opened wide to ensure total removal of the cholesteatoma and to facilitate communication between the eustachian tube and tympanomastoid cavity (Fig 6–7). A .5-mm Silastic sheet is placed in the tympanic cavity supported by a silicon rubber drain tube. The eardrum is reconstructed with a piece of fascia temporalis using the conventional underlaying technique. To close the large bony defect at the tympanic scute, a piece of artificial dura is attached to the bone of the external auditory canal using fibrin glue. The second-stage operation is performed between 9 and 12 months later. The Silastic sheet and residual cholesteatoma are removed, and 1 of 3 operations is performed according to the grade of aeration and healing of the mucosal disease (Fig 6–8). With type S1, only ossiculoplasty is indicated in a well-aerated middle ear lined by well-healed mucosa and without defective tympanic scute. With type S2, scutumplasty and ossiculopasty are indicated for the ear with a defective tympanic scute but with a well-aerated middle ear cavity. Type S3 operation includes mastoid obliteration with porous hydroxyapatite grains, scutumplasty, and ossiculoplasty for either the ear with a retraction pocket or a defective tympanic scute and poorly aerated middle ear cavity.

Outcome.—Between 1979 and 1991, 95 adults and 39 children without previous surgery underwent the planned stage ICWT. During an average follow-up of 37 months (1 to 11 years), cholesteatoma recurred in 2.2% and all occurred in children (7.6%). In 1 child, the ICWT was repeated without further recurrence. Therefore, overall, the external ear canal was preserved in 132 of 134 (99%) patients. Deep retraction pockets developed in 15% of adults and 23% of children. The incidence of deep retraction pocket was lowest in adults with type S1 operation and highest in children with type S3 operation, but, regardless of the type of

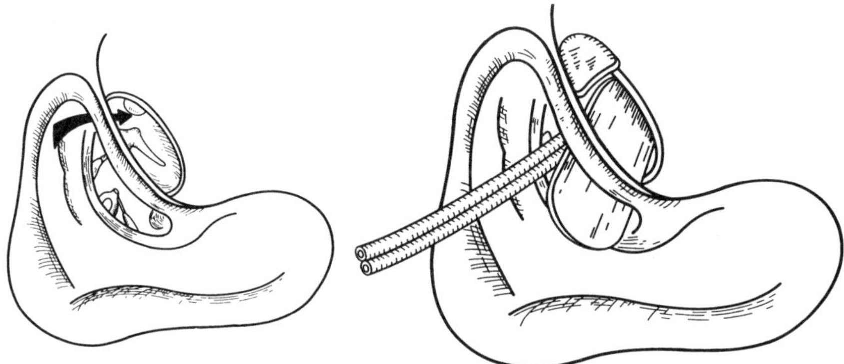

Fig 6–7.—Planned staged intact canal wall tympanoplasty. **Left,** the facial recessus, tympanic sinus, and anterior attic are opened wide (*arrow*) to ensure total safe removal of cholesteatoma and to facilitate communication between the eustachian tube and the tympanomastoid cavity. **Right,** a Silastic sheet (*shaded area*) is placed in the tympanic cavity and supported by a silicon rubber tube. (Courtesy of Yanagihara N, Gyo K, Sasaki Y, et al: *Am J Otol* 14:590–594, 1993.)

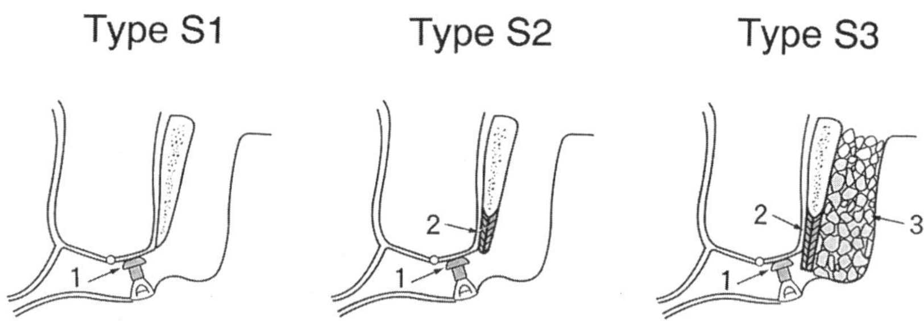

Fig 6–8.—Three types of operations performed in the second stage of planned staged tympanoplasty. *Abbreviations:* S1, only ossiculoplasty; S2, scutumplasty and ossiculoplasty; and S3, mastoid obliteration, scutumplasty, and ossiculoplasty. (Courtesy of Yanagihara N, Gyo K, Sasaki Y, et al: *Am J Otol* 14:590–594, 1993.)

operation at the second stage, the incidence of deep retraction pocket was always higher in children.

Conclusion.—The goal of surgical treatment of cholesteatoma can be achieved by combining ICWT with new surgical techniques. The ICWT allows preservation of the important structures and function of the ear without recurrence of cholesteatoma, as long as aeration of the middle ear is secured. Hence, a functional eustachian tube is a prerequisite of the successful ICWT. However, because of the high incidence of deep retraction pocket, further surgical improvement is needed to maintain aeration of the tympanic cavity.

▶ Recurrent cholesteatoma after intact canal wall tympanomastoidectomy is an all-too-common problem. These authors describe their technique and experience in trying to avoid this complication. Their ideas are helpful and of interest. At the same time, if there is any question of residual disease, one should not hestitate to consider open cavity tympanomastoidectomy with circumferential saucerization; lowering or reduction of the mastoid cavity by removal of mastoid cortical bone; and careful grafting, which may be essential to avoiding recurrent disease.—M.M. Paparella, M.D.

Total and Partial Ossicular Replacement Prostheses in Children
Kessler A, Potsic WP, Marsh RR (Children's Hosp, Philadelphia; Univ of Pennsylvania, Philadelphia)
Otolaryngol Head Neck Surg 110:302–303, 1994   130-95-6–24

Background.—Ossicular reconstruction in children carries some risk of failure resulting in recurrent middle ear disease. Nevertheless, the procedure presents an opportunity to restore binaural hearing during school years, when hearing is critical. A series of 45 ossicular reconstructions with total and partial ossicular replacement prostheses (TORPs and PORPs) in children was described.

Methods.—Forty-five children (mean age, 9.8 years) underwent ossicular reconstruction with TORPs or PORPs. Cartilage was placed between the tympanic membrane and prosthesis head. Ossicular reconstruction was delayed and replaced with another procedure in cases of cholesteatoma. Children were followed for a mean of 2.7 years after surgery.

Results.—None of the grafts placed in conjunction with tympanoplasty failed. Three PORPs and 3 TORPs extruded or became dislodged, producing a surgical success rate of 87%. A mean 2.1 years lapsed between surgery and detection of failure. The average age of patients at prosthetic failure was not significantly different from the average age of patients with successful prosthetic placement. Most patients achieved satisfactory hearing results. Among the 39 surgical successes, 29 had air-bone gaps of 30 dB or less; 21 had air-bone gaps of 20 dB or less. Speech reception thresholds were at least 30 dB in 74% of cases in which this measure was available, and 20 dB or better in 22.

Conclusion.—The value of early reconstruction was supported. When performed as soon as middle ear status is stable, early reconstruction gives children binaural hearing during the school years when it is critical to academic success.

▶ The authors report a good result using TORPs and PORPs in children. The age of the child and the nature of the disease will dictate whether the result will be good. For example, if the child has chronic otitis media and chronic mastoiditis, the TORP or PORP becomes a minor consideration; more important is control of the pathologic condition and the disease itself. On the other hand, if a somewhat older child, e.g., a 12- or 14-year-old, has an injury to the ear and loss of the incus, a TORP or PORP will work very well. Therefore, the first priority is proper diagnosis of the disease and concentration on control of the pathologic condition.—M.M. Paparella, M.D.

Experiences With the New Audiant XA-II Implant and the Behind-the-Ear (BTE) Device
Tange RA, Zuidema T, Berg RVD, Dreschler WA (Academical Med Centre, Amsterdam)
ORL J Otorhinolaryngol Relat Spec 56:78–82, 1994   130-95-6–25

Background.—Some patients with large conductive hearing loss who cannot tolerate conventional air conduction or bone conduction hearing aids may benefit from an implantable bone conductor device. Bone-anchored systems consist of an implantable titanium skull screw and an external sound processor unit. Problems with earlier systems were addressed with the modified Audiant screw-type XA-II implant, a newly developed behind-the-ear (BTE) processor, and a new transducer coil with variable magnetic strength. Ten patients were selected for an evaluation of this sytem.

Methods.—Strict inclusion criteria were the following: conductive hearing loss of at least 40 dB, bone conduction PTA not worse than 25 dB HL, air conduction speech discrimination scores of 80% or better, air conduction PTA worse than 40 dB HL, and air conduction speech reception thresholds worse than 40 dB HL. In addition, patients had failed to benefit from conventional air conduction hearing aids, had permanent and inoperative otorrhea or atresia, could not use ear plugs, and showed good motivation. Patients received implants while under general anesthesia. A final choice of processor was made during an adjustment period of 4 to 12 weeks. Audiometric tests used were standard audiometry, functional gain measurements, and speech audiometry using monosyllabic words.

Results.—Patients ranged in age from 29 to 72 years. All had ear disease of long duration. The XA-II implant was successfully fixed in the temporal bone in all cases, and patients started to use the hearing aid 8 weeks after implantation. The skin healed well with no reactions. Seven patients continue to use the Audiant bone conductor, but 3 found it to be less powerful than their previous hearing aid. The Audiant system was judged comfortable by all patients and was effective in compensating the air-bone gap almost completely at the higher frequencies. Speech intelligibility was improved both in quiet and in background noise.

Conclusion.—The 3 patients who failed to benefit from the system were borderline cases with regard to the selection criteria. The maximum output of the system appears to limit its usefulness in perceptive losses beyond 20 dB (PTA), not the 25 dB suggested by the manufacturer. However, with proper patient selection, the Audiant XA-II implant and the BTE device offer clear sound, good wearing comfort, and a simple apparatus.

Clinical Results of Percutaneous Implants in the Temporal Bone
Mylanus EAM, Cremers CWRJ, Snik AFM, van den Berge NW (Univ Hosp Nijmegen, The Netherlands; Diaconessenhuis, Eindhoven, The Netherlands)
Arch Otolaryngol Head Neck Surg 120:81–85, 1994   130-95-6–26

Introduction.—When the aural canal blockage required by an air-conduction hearing aid is not tolerated, a bone-conduction hearing aid can be used. A new bone-conduction hearing aid, involving a percutaneous implant anchored to the mastoid process, was recently made available. The implantation depth and stability and skin reactions were studied in patients treated with this new system.

Methods.—The bone-anchored hearing aid (BAHA) was implanted in 68 ears in 65 patients, including 8 adolescents, who had either chronic otitis media, chronic otitis externa, or an inoperable congenital anomaly. The percutaneous titanium implant placement and transpositioning of autologous skin was performed in 2 stages separated by 4 months. The depth of the implantation drilling was recorded. After an additional month, the BAHA was attached. The patients were evaluated every 3 to 4 months for 8 to 45 months.

Results.—Implantation depth was 4 mm in 5 of the 8 adolescents and 46 of the 60 adults. In 2 adolescents and 10 adults, the implantation depth was 3 mm, because the temporal bone was thin. The fixtures were securely retained in the skull in 66 of 68 cases. Only 9 of the patients experienced skin reactions that threatened the retention or the percutaneous abutment; all were adequately resolved with local cleaning, local or systemic antibiotic therapy, and excision of granulation tissue. Skin reactions occurred at any time during the 2 years after implantation. Unfavorable skin conditions at the abutment site, including thick or diseased skin, were associated with increased occurrence of skin reactions. Two additional patients lost the abutments and were successfully reimplanted.

Discussion.—The fixtures were successfully anchored in 97% of the procedures and caused no serious skin reactions in 86%. There was a low risk of percutaneous complications. Unfavorable skin conditions at the abutment site should be prevented or promptly treated.

▶ The first of these 2 articles (Abstracts 130-95-6–25 and 130-95-6–26) describes the use of the BTE processor as a new complement to the Audiant device. Such studies will be of interest to see whether this gains general clinical acceptability. The second article discusses percutaneous implants in which the bone-anchored hearing aid is coupled to a percutaneous titanium implant placed in the mastoid process in 2 surgical stages. The device would appear to be efficacious, and again the question is whether this will gain clinical acceptability with the American public in particular, from both a cosmetic point of view and an auditory function view.—M.M. Paparella, M.D.

HEAD AND NECK SURGERY

G. RICHARD HOLT, M.D., F.A.C.S.

Introduction

We must continue to be vigilant in our use of universal precautions against the transmission of hepatitis and AIDS viruses in our practices. As we see in this section, reliance on the integrity of single-gloving during a surgical procedure is to be questioned. Double-gloving may be more protective, but it is also more costly.

Advances continue to be made in respiratory airway surgery, both in biomaterials available for implantation and in techniques. Open laryngeal framework surgery and open laryngeal procedures for tumor excision continue to be espoused. New research into the use of vascularized pedicle flaps for tracheal reconstruction seems promising. More home-monitoring for obstructive sleep apnea is recommended, with a reduction in equipment costs and overhead.

Burnout among head and neck surgeons may be related more to the frustrations of insurance bureaucracy than to long hours and survival disappointments. Quality-of-life issues are studied as a means of focusing the attention of health care professionals on this issue and of developing a team approach to support.

Pediatric *Haemophilus influenzae* infections may be reduced in frequency and severity through the use of vaccinations, and these need to be considered for more widespread use. Tuberculous cervical adenitis may be on the upswing, particularly along the border and in large cities where children are exposed to pulmonary tuberculosis. We must maintain a high index of suspicion for these diseases. Other environmental health issues are also reviewed.

I believe you will learn a great deal from these 134 articles, as I surely did, and if you know the authors, be sure to congratulate them on their work.

G. Richard Holt, M.D., F.A.C.S.

7 Advances in Head and Neck Surgery Research

Distraction Osteogenesis in the Irradiated Canine Mandible
Gantous A,Phillips JH, Catton P, Holmberg D (Hosp for Sick Children, Toronto; Toronto Bayview Regional Cancer Centre; Ontario Veterinary College, Toronto)
Plast Reconstr Surg 93:164–168, 1994   130-95-7–1

Background.—There has been some success but significant morbidity with the use of reconstruction plates and free vascularized flaps to reconstruct mandibular defects after ablative head and neck surgery and radiotherapy. Distraction osteogenesis has successfully been used to reconstruct long bones, but it has not been used in patients with head and neck cancer because its efficacy in irradiated bone is not known. This technique was tested in the reconstruction of canine mandibular defects after irradiation.

Methods.—Five dogs with 1 toothless hemimandible underwent a course of irradiation that would be appropriate in the treatment of a human with oral carcinoma. After 6 months, 20 mm of bone was removed, a reconstruction plate was applied to stabilize the mandible, and the transport disk and lengthening apparatus were applied to the defect proximally. Distraction of the transport disk began after 10 days and continued for 30 days. The lengtheners were removed after another 30 days. The mandibles were removed and evaluated after 4 to 5 weeks. The dogs were assessed with weekly radiography.

Results.—There was complete bone regeneration in 4 of the 5 dogs. Although the new bone could be palpated at 4 weeks, it could not be visualized radiologically until 7 weeks. Histologic evaluation confirmed that the defects were replaced with new bone.

Discussion.—Irradiation did not prevent osteogenesis. Further studies are necessary to replicate these results. However, these results indicate that the distraction osteogenesis technique can be used to reconstruct defects after radiation therapy for cancer treatment and, in some cases, could replace free tissue transfers and their attendant morbidity as the treatment of choice.

▶ I think this is exciting information. We do not yet know how much deformation/reformation of the facial skeleton can be done with distraction osteogenesis. It would be interesting to see whether the rate of closure could be accelerated in irradiated bones while administering concomitant hyperbaric oxygen.—G.R. Holt, M.D., F.A.C.S.

Comparison of CT Imaging Artifacts From Craniomaxillofacial Internal Fixation Devices

Fiala TGS, Novelline RA, Yaremchuk MJ (Massachusetts Gen Hosp, Boston)
Plast Reconstr Surg 92:1227–1232, 1993　　　　　　　　　130-95-7-2

Background.—Imaging after craniomaxillofacial surgery may be needed to assess the status of hard and soft tissues. However, artifacts from implanted metallic devices can reduce the quality of the image, adversely affecting screening after surgery. The artifacts resulting from craniomaxillofacial internal fixation devices in CT images were examined.

Methods.—The plate and screw systems studied were mandibular reconstruction and miniplate systems of titanium, Vitallium, and stainless steel; microplate systems of titanium and Vitallium; and 28-gauge stainless steel wire. These devices were placed on a nylon grid and submerged in water, and CT images were acquired with both bone and soft tissue window settings.

Findings.—The severity of the "starburst" artifact was associated with the physical size of the fixation hardware and its composition. Titanium hardware produced the least amount of artifact. Except for interfragmentary wiring, Vitallium and stainless steel fixation devices resulted in significantly more artifact.

Conclusions.—When postoperative imaging is important in patients undergoing craniomaxillofacial surgery, clinicians should use the least amount of implant material necessary to achieve stable fixation. Clinicians should also consider the proximity of implant material to the region of interest. Compared with Vitallium and stainless steel implants, titanium implants create less artifact.

▶ Any metal that can be magnetized (steel, iron, including bullets, can be a problem for MRI. On the other hand, nonmagnetizing metals, such as titanium, have great biomechanical and biocompatible properties, yet they produce little artifact on MRI and CT.—G.R. Holt, M.D., F.A.C.S.

Vascularized Bone Flaps in Oromandibular Reconstruction

Moscoso JF, Keller J, Genden E, Weinberg H, Biller HF, Buchbinder D, Urken ML (Mount Sinai Med Ctr, New York)
Arch Otolaryngol Head Neck Surg 120:36–43, 1994　　　　　　130-95-7-3

Background.—Oral cavity reconstruction has greatly benefited from the successful transfer of vascularized bone and sensate soft tissue as microvascular free flaps. Donor sites were identified from which vascularized bone could be harvested to accept osseointegrated implants of the minimum dimensions needed to ensure long-term implant stability.

Methods.—The most commonly used donor sites for vascularized bone in oromandibular reconstruction were studied in 28 cadavers. The ipsilateral fibula, iliac crest, radius, and lateral border of the scapula were harvested and sectioned at multiple predetermined sites. For each section, implantability was determined based on measurements of height, width, and cross-sectional area using computer planimetry.

Findings.—The most consistently implantable donor site was the iliac crest, with 83% of the sections satisfying the criteria for implantability. The corresponding percentages for the scapula, fibula, and radius were 78%, 67%, and 21%. At each donor site except the scapula, consistent regional differences in implantability were noted.

Conclusions.—These findings objectively confirm the clinical impression that the iliac crest is the most uniformly implantable source of vascularized bone for mandibular reconstruction. Unexpectedly, the lateral scapular border was the statistical equivalent of the iliac crest for overall implantability. The radius was the least reliable donor site, especially in female cadavers.

▶ If possible, a vascularized mandibular graft is the preferred choice for reconstruction and subsequent osseointegrated implantation. However, as we have found, the implants do quite well in free cancellous grafts after bone reformation has occurred.—G.R. Holt, M.D., F.A.C.S.

Unilateral Palatal Adhesion for Paralysis After High Vagal Injury

Netterville JL, Vrabec JT (Vanderbilt Univ Med Ctr, Nashville, Tenn)
Arch Otolaryngol Head Neck Surg 120:218–221, 1994   130-95-7-4

Introduction.—Tumor involvement of the vagus nerve at the level of the jugular foramen causes significant morbidity after skull-base surgery. Vocal cord medialization has significantly improved the resulting dysphagia and dysphonia, but most procedures addressing hypernasality and nasal reflux caused by velopharyngeal incompetence have been inadequate. A new, relatively easy, 1-stage procedure to improve the symptoms of velopharyngeal incompetence secondary to vagal sacrifice was described.

Technique.—The first incision is a full-thickness incision of the palate following the palatal crease and curving slightly inferolaterally (Fig 7–1). A second incision is made in the posterior wall of the nasopharynx, directly beneath the first incision. The nasopharyngeal incision is undermined at the level of the prevertebral fascia (Fig 7–2). The posterior palate is approximated to the nasopharyngeal

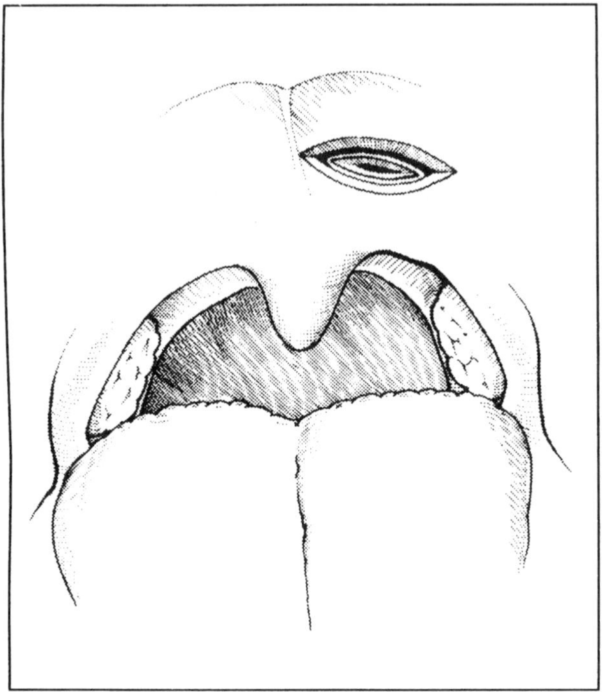

Fig 7–1.—Full-thickness palatal incision, parallel to palatal crease. (Courtesy of Netterville JL, Vrabec JT: *Arch Otolaryngol Head Neck Surg* 120:218-221, 1994.)

wall, making sure to include the palatal muscle and full-thickness posterior pharyngeal wall to achieve effective approximation. Finally, the anterior palatal mucosa is reapproximated, taking care to avoid complete closure of the ipsilateral nasopharynx. A small opening (3 mm) is preserved to prevent stasis of secretions above the adhesion (Fig 7-3). Figure 7-4 provides a schematic of the palatal adhesion.

Outcome.—Eight patients underwent palatal adhesion. All 8 patients noted correction of their hypernasality, with improvement in speech intelligibility. All 6 patients with nasal reflux improved. None of the patients reported symptoms of obstructive sleep apnea, and none experienced hyponasality or otitis media.

Conclusion.—Vagal injury at or above the level of the jugular foramen yields paralysis of the palate and pharyngeal constrictors, resulting in atonia of the lateral wall on the affected side. The procedure described herein addresses this specific deficit, allowing for satisfactory improvement of hypernasality and nasal reflux. The optimal time for performing this procedure is yet to be defined, but 3 months of observation after vagus nerve sacrifice are recommended to allow the patient an opportunity to compensate for the deficit.

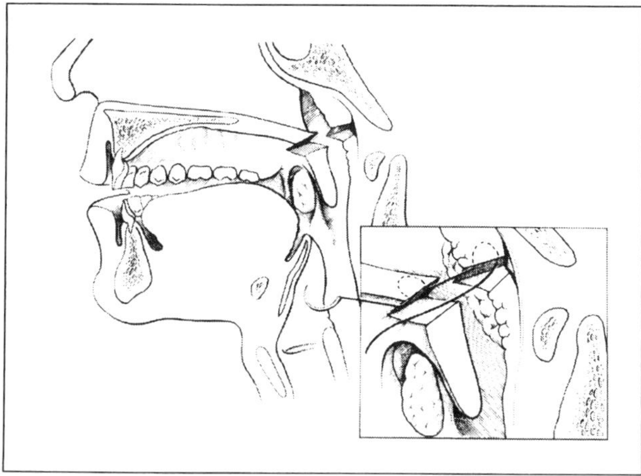

Fig 7–2.—Pharyngeal muscle is undermined at the level of the prevertebral fascia. **Inset,** mattress suture closure. (Courtesy of Netterville JL, Vrabec JT: *Arch Otolaryngol Head Neck Surg* 120:218-221, 1994.)

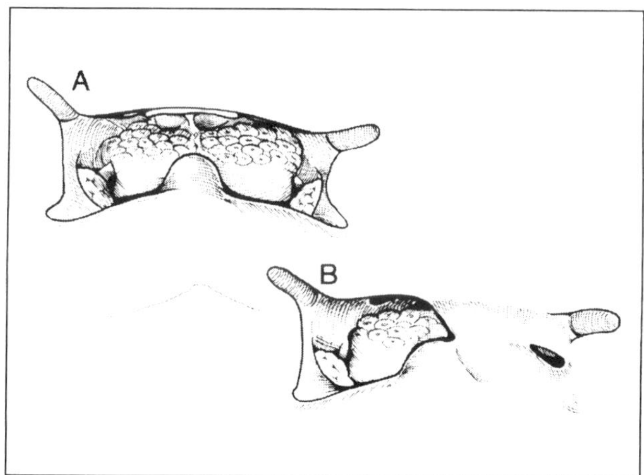

Fig 7–3.—Diagram of the normal nasopharynx (**A**) in comparison with the adhesion (**B**). (Courtesy of Netterville JL, Vrabec JT: *Arch Otolaryngol Head Neck Surg* 120:218-221, 1994.)

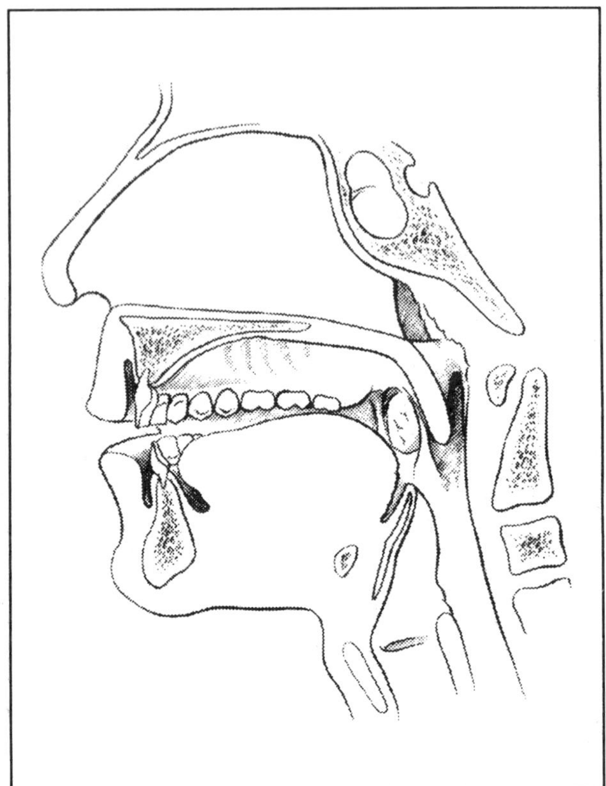

Fig 7–4.—Schematic of palatal adhesion in the sagittal plane. (Courtesy of Netterville JL, Vrabec JT: *Arch Otolaryngol Head Neck Surg* 120:218-221, 1994.)

▶ This is a very nifty innovation by excellent clinicians. The technique would seem to be less morbid than a pharyngeal flap, and it would be technically easier to perform.—G.R. Holt, M.D., F.A.C.S.

Natural Ostiotomy vs. Inferior Antrostomy in the Management of Sinusitis: An Animal Model
Benninger MS, Kaczor J, Stone C (Henry Ford Hosp, Detroit)
Otolaryngol Head Neck Surg 109:1034–1042, 1993   130-95-7–5

Background.—There have been few controlled comparisons of inferior vs. middle meatal antrostomies in the management of chronic maxillary sinusitis. The effect on maxillary sinus mucosa after obstruction of the natural ostia and subsequent inferior antrostomy vs. reopening the natural ostia was studied in a rabbit model.

Methods and Findings.—Sinusitis was induced in 15 rabbits by surgically occluding the natural maxillary sinus ostia. In a subsequent operation, the sinuses were entered, and the natural ostia were reopened on 1 side in each animal. An inferior antrostomy was performed on the opposite sinus. When the sinuses were assessed 8 weeks later, there were no differences in antrostomy patency rates. Gross evidence of acute and chronic inflammation was also comparable. Light and electron microscopic findings between sinuses with natural osteotomy and those with lower antrostomy did not differ between sinuses.

Conclusions.—After the natural ostia of the maxillary sinus in rabbits were occluded, there were no significant differences in gross, light microscopic, or electron microscopic results between inferior antrostomy and natural ostiotomy. The inferior antrostomy group had slightly greater patency rates. Natural osteotomy and inferior antrostomy are both generally effective in treating sinusitis in rabbits.

▶ If our patients were rabbits, this study would support the naysayers of endoscopic sinus surgery meatoplasty. However, it is difficult to extrapolate some of the data to humans, particularly in the face of complicating human disorders such as vasomotor rhinitis, smoking, allergic rhinitis, environmental pollution, and so forth. Nevertheless, this observation does not detract from the importance of this report.—G.R. Holt, M.D., F.A.C.S.

Correlations Between Flow Resistance and Geometry in a Model of the Human Nose
Schreck S, Sullivan KJ, Ho CM, Chang HK (Univ of Southern California, Los Angeles)
J Appl Physiol 75:1767–1775, 1993   130-95-7–6

Background.—Although several models have been developed to express the relationship between flow rate and resistance, there have been none in which resistance is expressed in terms of flow rate and nasal geometry. The relationship between nasal geometry and flow were investigated, and the important geometric features that determine the flow field and nasal resistance were identified.

Methods.—A 3:1 scale model based on MR images of a healthy man was used. Pressure measures, flow visualization, and hot-wire anemometry studies were done at flow rates corresponding to in vivo flows from .05 to 1.5 L/sec. The effect of nasal congestion and the collapse of the external nares were assessed using modeling clay to simulate local constrictions in the cross-section.

Findings.—A dimensionless analysis of pressure losses in 3 sections of the airway showed the influence of various anatomical dimensions on nasal resistance. The exterior nose region acted as a contraction-expansion nozzle in which the pressure losses were a function of the smallest cross-section area. Losses in the interior nose looked like those associated with channel flow. The nasopharynx was modeled as a sharp bend in a circular duct, and good correspondence was noted between the predicted and actual pressure losses under conditions simulating local obstructions and congestion.

Conclusions.—The complex geometry of the nasal passages can be reduced to the simpler geometries of similar flow resistance. The model provided a useful tool for predicting flow resistance based on flow rate and the geometry of the nose. The effects of differences in nose geometry among individuals were predicted using similarity laws. The effects of congestion and swelling of the mucosa on the pressure drop across the nasal passages were also predicted. These predictions correlated well with findings in studies of humans.

▶ It would be dynamite if the authors could get respiratory mucosa to grow in this model! As it is, it looks very good for basic research studies. This one provides a nice start.—G.R. Holt, M.D., F.A.C.S.

Elevated IGF-II and TGF-β Concentrations in Human Calvarial Bone: Potential Mechanism for Increased Graft Survival and Resistance to Osteoporosis
Finkelman RD, Eason AL, Rakijian DR, Tutundzhyan Y, Hardesty RA (Loma Linda Univ, Calif; Jerry L. Pettis Mem Veterans Hosp, Loma Linda, Calif)
Plast Reconstr Surg 93:732–738, 1994   130-95-7–7

Background.—The survival of calvarial bone grafts as donor tissue may be greater than that of bone from other sites. Calvarial bone is also resistant to osteoporosis. Calvarial bone may be enriched in 1 or more of the growth factors that regulates bone repair.

Methods and Findings.—Bone samples were obtained from 10 men, 64 years of age and older, at autopsy. Three skeletal sites—the calvaria, iliac crest, and vertebral body—were sampled. Bone was cleaned, extracted by demineralization, and assayed for the growth factors insulin-like growth factor I (IGF-I), insulin-like growth factor II (IGF-II), and transforming growth factor β (TGF-β). Concentrations of the latter 2 substances were significantly greater in the calvaria than in the iliac crest or vertebral body. Calvarial bone also had more IGF-I, but not significantly so.

Conclusions.—Calvarial bone from men contains significantly greater levels of IGF-II and TGF-β than does bone from the iliac crest or vertebral body. Because growth factors in bone are thought to play an important part in mediating bone repair and stimulating compensatory bone formation after resorption, increased levels of growth factor in calvarial bone suggest a heightened capacity for repair in this tissue.

▶ Although still elusive, the role that growth factors play in bone resorption and formation coupling must be important. We need to continue to address growth factors in basic biocompatibility and biosurvival studies.—G.R. Holt, M.D., F.A.C.S.

The Role of Pressure on Regulation of Craniofacial Bone Growth

Buchman SR, Bartlett SP, Wornom IL III, Whitaker LA (Univ of Pennsylvania, Philadelphia)
J Craniofac Surg 5:2–10, 1994   130-95-7–8

Introduction.—Knowledge of the regulatory factors involved in craniofacial development might allow growth to be used as an adjunct to reconstructive surgery in the attempt to restore facial form. An experimental model was designed to determine whether the graded application of pressure could achieve alteration and reshaping of the facial skeleton.

Methods.—Eighteen mixed-gender 8-week-old kittens were randomly assigned to 3 surgical groups. All were anesthetized and underwent surgical evisceration of an orbit. In group 1 (control), no further manipulation of the orbit was performed. Kittens in group 2 underwent placement of a 2-mL Silastic implant in the evacuated orbit. The implant approximated the orbital volume of an 8-week-old kitten. Kittens in group 3 received a specially designed orbital tissue expander. Groups 1 and 2 had no subsequent treatments. In the animals in group 3, the port was tunneled through the soft tissues above the zygomatic arch and positioned in a subcutaneous pocket on the cranium. During a 16-week period, these animals underwent a graded orbital expansion designed to reproduce normal growth patterns. On the first and third postoperative weeks, 1 mL of normal saline was injected into the expander via the port. An additional .5 mL was added on the fifth week and every 2 weeks thereafter. All animals were sacrificed at 24 weeks, when full craniofacial maturity was reached.

Results.—In response to evisceration, orbital length decreased by 13.7% in group 1. The use of an implant significantly reduced the change in size to 6.8%, whereas use of an expander brought the orbital length to within 2.2% of the contralateral nonoperated side. Orbital width differed even more notably between groups. In comparison with the nonoperated side, group 3 showed a slight increase (.4%) in the size of the affected orbit. Groups 1 and 2, however, showed significant reductions in size (23.4% and 9%, respectively). Orbital depth decreased by 8.7% in the control group, 6.1% in the implant group, and only 1.9% in the expander group. Use of an expander significantly improved the zygomatic midfacial deformity resulting from orbital evisceration, and it restored normal anatomical features and symmetry. Expanded bone also exhibited all the microscopic determinants appropriate to normal growing and developing bone.

Conclusion.—Orbital evisceration caused severe asymmetry and constriction in the orbital and midfacial region of the growing kitten. The graded application of pressure appeared to exert a trophic influence, helping to normalize craniofacial bone growth in these animals.

▶ This paper really appealed to me because of its application of the principles of tissue expansion to bone remodeling. Can something similar be accomplished after facial growth has ceased? This could be very interesting.—G.R. Holt, M.D., F.A.C.S.

An Animal Model for Subperiosteal Tissue Expansion

Tominaga K, Matsuo T, Kuga Y, Mizuno A (Nagasaki Univ, Japan)
J Oral Maxillofac Surg 51:1244–1249, 1993   130-95-7–9

Objective.—Tissue expansion, a procedure that has developed fairly recently, has been used in the breast and other areas of the body for reconstruction purposes. However, there have been few studies of the clinical aspects of subperiosteal tissue expansion. Subcutaneous tissue expansion in the dog model was examined.

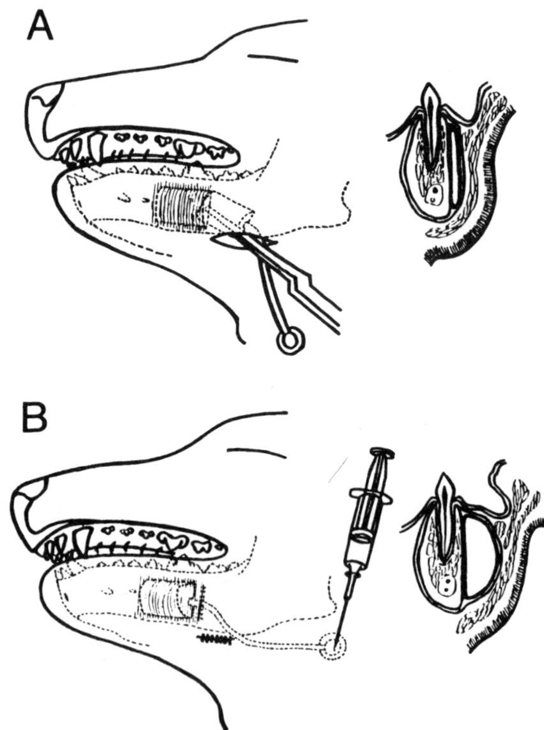

Fig 7–5.—Schematic representation of subperiosteal tissue expansion model. **A,** insertion of the expander. **B,** inflation of the expander. (Courtesy of Tominaga K, Matsuo T, Kuga Y, et al: *J Oral Maxillofac Surg* 51:1244–1249, 1993.)

Methods.—Two hemicylindrical tissue expanders of each size, 4, 7, or 10 mL in volume, were implanted in pockets along the mandibles of twenty-one 15-kg mongrel dogs, aged 2 years (Fig 7–5). After 1 week, in experiment 1, inflation with 1 mL of saline every 4 days was begun through injection domes placed in the anterior neck. In experiment 2, two dogs received 4 injections of 1 mL of saline every 4 days; 2 dogs received 2-mL injections on day 1 and day 13; and 2 dogs received four 1-mL injections every other day. In experiment 3, 16-mL expanders were implanted under the skin at the midline of the breast and inflated with 4 mL of saline every 4 days, 4 times. The animals were observed for as long as 1 month. Optimum expander size, optimum inflation regimen, and histologic changes were determined.

Results.—The 10-mL expander became exposed shortly after full inflation. Three weeks after full inflation in experiment 1, medium expanders caused severe thinning of the alveolar mucosa. No problems were seen with the smallest expanders during the observation period. In experiment 2, there was little resistance to inflation in group 1. The expander was surrounded by fibrous connective tissue. In group 2, exposure occurred with 2 implants, and alveolar mucosal ulcerations were observed with 2 implants. In group 3, 1 implant had ulceration and 1 had severe thinning. In experiment 3, all implants were surrounded by fibrous connective tissue and coarse collagen fibers. After 1 month, bone resorption underneath the implants was observed.

Conclusion.—Subperiosteal tissue expansion leads to more rapid capsule formation than does subcutaneous expansions and has fewer side effects. More studies will be done in this model to determine whether stretched periosteal tissue has osteogenetic potential.

▶ If viable expanded and pedicled periosteum could be used to cover a mandibular graft, perhaps bone healing and remodeling would be facilitated by its apparent osseoinductive properties.—G.R. Holt, M.D., F.A.C.S.

Tracheal Reconstruction Using an Epithelial Equivalent
Duff BE, Wenig BL, Applebaum EL, Yeates DB, Wenig BM, Holinger LD (The Univ of Illinois, Chicago; The Armed Forces Inst of Pathology, Washington, DC; Childrens Mem Hosp Med Ctr, Chicago)
Laryngoscope 104:409–414, 1994   130-95-7–10

Background.—The management of tracheal stenosis resulting from such causes as trauma, inflammation, and tumors remains a challenge. Effective methods to prevent and reconstruct areas of injury have been elusive. The use of a vascularized epithelial equivalent to inhibit wound contraction and tracheal stenosis was investigated.

Methods.—Using dogs, an animal model was developed. A total of 8 dogs were studied: 4 controls and 4 experimental. Abdominal skin punch biopsy specimens were taken from the animals and cultured to form a contracted fibroblast-collagen lattice. An opening was then made in the anterior tracheal wall of each animal. In the control animals, healing occurred by secondary intention, whereas in the experimental group, the autologous fibroblast lattices were placed on the injury at the time of surgery. Three weeks after the surgery, mucosal flow velocity was determined by tracking the movement of a radioactive tracer instilled into the distal trachea. The animals were then sacrificed for examination.

Findings.—Mucosal flow rates in the experimental group showed uniform tracheal transport rates. Two of the 4 controls could not be evaluated because severe stenosis prevented catheter insertion. In the remaining 2 controls, mucosal flow velocity was slower than in the experimental animals. During gross and microscopic examination, all controls showed severe ($\geq$ 95%) stenosis. The experimental group showed very mild ($\leq$ 20%) stenosis. Histologic examination showed marked formation of granulation tissue nearly obliterating the lumen in the control group. The experimental group showed granulation tissue of varying thickness underlying focal areas of epithelial regeneration, and the lumen was patent.

Conclusions.—Near-normal mucosal flow rates were seen after the use of vascularized, precontracted autologous epithelial equivalent for reconstruction of soft tissue stenosis in animals. Further research is needed on the applicability of the technique in humans and at other soft tissue stenoses.

▶ I like the possibility of using the patient's own tissue for reconstruction. Would it be possible to bond (with fibronectin?) cultured mucosal cells with the fibroblast-collagen network to provide an even better stratum for healing?—G.R. Holt, M.D., F.A.C.S.

The Intrinsic Response of the Cricoid Cartilage to Vertical Division

Senders CW, Tinling SP (Univ of California, Davis)
Int J Pediatr Otorhinolaryngol 28:33–39, 1993   130-95-7–11

Background.—Children with acquired or congenital subglottic stenosis may be treated with anterior vertical division of the cricoid cartilage, which enlarges the subglottic lumen. The intrinsic response of cricoid cartilage to anterior vertical division was studied using whole organ in vitro cultures of juvenile gerbil cricoid cartilages.

Methods.—Thirty-four male, 35-day-old gerbils were randomly assigned to 1 of 3 groups—histologic control, experimental control, and experimental. The larynx and the 5 to 6 inferior tracheal rings were harvested from each gerbil after euthanasia. The tissues from the histologic control group were fixed in Karnovsky's solution, whereas tissues from the experimental control and experimental animal groups were placed into sterile dishes and photographed with a referenced ruler. Cricoid tissues from the experimental animals then had anterior vertical division of the cricoid cartilage and were again photographed with a referenced ruler. After the specimens had been cultured in test tubes with 10 mL of culture medium for 70 hours (SD, 2 hours), they were rinsed in Karnovsky's solution for approximately 5 seconds, rephotographed with a referenced ruler, and permanently fixed in Karnovsky's solution. Morphogenic area and distance were measured with a digitalizing tablet and a computer program. Evidence of the viability of cells was evaluated histologically.

Results.—Immediately after the cricoid cartilage was divided, the mean separation was .39 ± .19 micrometers, whereas after the 72-hour culture, this separation significantly increased to a mean of 1.76 ± .81 micrometers. Immediately after division, the mean subglottic lumen area increased by 68%; after 72 hours of culture, it increased by 363%. In the group that did not have vertical division, the mean subglottic area did not significantly change after culture, whereas in the group that received treatment, significant main effects were shown.

Conclusions.—Cricoid cartilage of gerbils separates after vertical division, independent of external factors. The tendency to separate appears to be intrinsic to the cartilage and not to the viability of individual cells. The in vitro increase of 363% after 72 hours is markedly greater than that seen in other in vivo animal models, suggesting that the overall effect of extrinsic factors is to limit the degree of enlargement in the subglottic area after cricoid division.

▶ Nonarticular cartilage has some magical and mysterious biomechanical properties that we still do not fully understand. Why else do we continue to see septal cartilage redeviate after a septoplasty and costal cartilage curl up when it is released from the rib cage? This interesting study may lead to a better understanding of the unique properties of cartilage.—G.R. Holt, M.D., F.A.C.S.

Phrenic Nerve Reinnervation of the Cat's Larynx: A New Technique With Proven Success

Doyle PJ, Westerberg BD, Chepeha DB, Schwarz DWF (St Paul's Hosp, Vancouver, Canada; Univ of British Columbia, Vancouver, Canada)
Ann Otol Rhinol Laryngol 102:837–842, 1993   130-95-7–12

Background.—Reinnervation of the posterior cricoarytenoid (PCA) muscle should lead to vocal cord abduction on inspiration as well as passive adduction to promote phonation. Although previous studies have demonstrated that reinnervation is possible, clinical results have not been promising. It is not yet clear whether successful reinnervation occurs as a result of the transplanted nerve or by an ingrowth of adjacent nerves. To identify the source of reinnervation, the phrenic nerve was

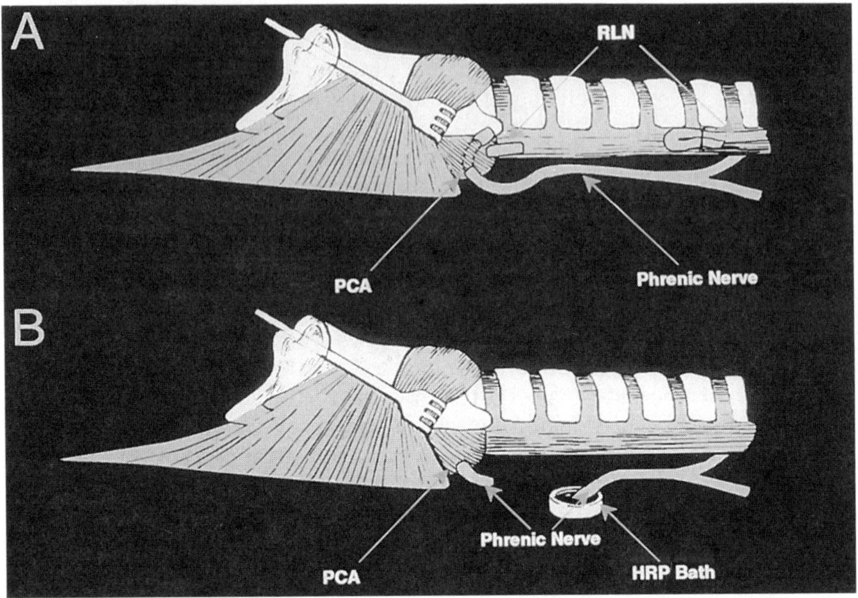

Fig 7–6.—Diagrammatic representation of the laryngeal reinnervation procedure. **A,** sectioned recurrent laryngeal nerve (*RLN*) and phrenic nerve implanted in the posterior cricoarytenoid muscle (*PCA*) **(B).** The cut end of the phrenic nerve exposed to a horseradish peroxidase (*HRP*) bath. (Courtesy of Doyle PJ, Westerberg BD, Chepeha DB, et al: *Ann Otol Rhinol Laryngol* 102:837–842, 1993.)

transplanted directly into the PCA muscle in 12 cats. Fibrin glue was used to prevent nerve trauma and retraction of the nerve from the PCA muscle.

Methods.—Twelve healthy cats weighing between 2 and 3.5 kg were used. The experiment was conducted in 5 stages. These included transection of the left recurrent laryngeal nerve and implantation of the left phrenic nerve in the PCA muscle, followed by direct laryngoscopy to verify vocal cord paralysis. At 4 to 8 months, direct laryngoscopy was repeated to evaluate reinnervation. Reexploration, electromyography (EMG) of the PCA muscle, and retrograde labeling of the phrenic motoneurons using horseradish peroxidase were performed at 6 to 8.5 months after attempted reinnervation. Finally, histologic verification of reinnervation by phrenic motoneurons was conducted (Fig 7–6).

Results.—Successful reinnervation was defined as normal vocal cord abduction on inspiration, reinnervation of the PCA muscle, and demonstration of horseradish peroxidase labeling of the phrenic nerve nucleus. Functional reinnervation was noted in 9 of the 12 cats. In the remaining 3 animals, partial or complete failure was caused by retraction of the nerve from the muscle.

Conclusions.—The phrenic nerve can be used to reestablish coordinated vocal cord abduction. Implanting the nerve directly into the PCA muscle helps prevent synkinesis and poor functional reinnervation. Trials of this procedure are warranted in humans.

▶ Abductor paralysis of the larynx remains a difficult problem. Because the phrenic nerve "fires" during inspiration, it is logical to also attempt to reinnervate the PCA muscle, which is the main inspiratory muscle of the larynx. We will await further studies.—G.R. Holt, M.D., F.A.C.S.

Secretion of a Fibronectin-Like Substance From Head and Neck Carcinomas

Sakumoto M, Tsukuda M, Mochimatsu I, Yago T, Kokatsu T (Yokohama City Univ, Kanagawa, Japan)
ORL J Otorhinolaryngol Relat Spec 56:213–216, 1994   130-95-7–13

Background.—Since fibronectin was discovered more than 20 years ago, many researchers have studied the cell attachment factors of tumor and normal cells. The secretion of cell attachment factors from cultured cell lines of head and neck carcinomas was reported.

Methods and Findings.—Fourteen cell lines of head and neck squamous cell carcinomas were studied. These carcinomas were located on the tongue in 5 cases; the oropharynx in 3; the maxillary sinus in 2; and 1 each in the oral floor, nasopharynx, hypopharynx, and larynx. Positive cell attachment activity occurred in the supernatant of 8 of the cell lines. Supernatant cell attachment activity did not vary among primary tumor cell sites. Laminin was not found in the supernatants, but fibronectin was observed in all 14 tumor cell cultures. The fibronectin concentration in the supernatant was positively correlated with cell attachment activity. The addition of antifibronectin monoclonal antibody, but not antivitronectin monoclonal antibody, inhibited cell attachment activity.

Conclusions.—The fibronectin produced by cancer cells is most likely 1 of the potent mediators of cell attachment. Assay with an antifibronectin antibody showed that the supernatant with cell attachment activity contained fibronectin, and cell attachment activity was clearly inhibited by the addition of a monoclonal antibody to fibronectin.

▶ Would it be possible to culture a patient's tumor cell line, isolate its fibronectin, and produce a monoclonal antibody to it? If tumor cell adhesion were diminished, would it be less likely to invade or metastasize?—G.R. Holt, M.D., F.A.C.S.

Coordination of Oral Cavity and Laryngeal Movements During Swallowing

Gay T, Rendell JK, Spiro J, Mosier K, Lurie AG (Univ of Connecticut, Farmington)
J Appl Physiol 77:357–365, 1994   130-95-7-14

Introduction.—There have been relatively few studies of the mechanism of swallowing, a biological function that involves the actions of the oral, pharyngeal, esophageal, and laryngeal systems. An imaging and analysis technique was developed to quantitatively track the movements of the various structures of the oral cavity and the larynx during swallowing.

Methods.—The subjects were 10 normal adults, 5 men and 5 women, with a mean age of 27.4 years. Tiny lead pellet markers were attached with gel, adhesive, or sutures to the upper and lower lips, tongue, mandible, soft palate, hyoid, and larynx; and their movements were tracked in relation to a similar reference pellet affixed to the upper central incisors. The movements of the oral cavity and laryngeal structures during swallowing of 12 mL of tap water were imaged using standard videofluoroscopic techniques. Each subject produced 10 swallows of tap water followed by 5 swallows with a bite block placed between the molars. The data were input to a computer for the measurement process.

Results.—The upper and lower lips moved synchronously to close off and seal the oral cavity anteriorly after liquid intake. There was considerable variability in lip onset and mandible onset times. With one excep-

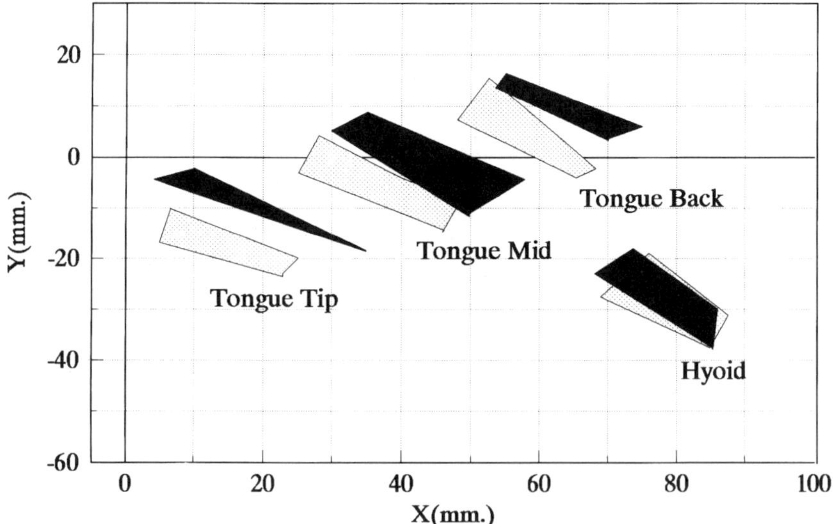

Fig 7–7.—The *x*- and *y*-coordinate movement zones for normal (*solid*) and bite block (*stippled*) swallows for 1 subject. (Courtesy of Gay T, Rendell JK, Spiro J, et al: *J Appl Physiol* 77:357–365, 1994.)

tion, all tongue pellets (tip, mid-tongue, and back) began moving before hyoid elevation. In 6 subjects, the body of the tongue moved as a unit rather than segmentally toward the hard palate. Considerable variability was observed in the interval between attainment of tongue/hard palate closure and peak hyoid elevation. The onset times for palatal elevation varied widely both within and among subjects, thereby suggesting that control of palatal movement is not tightly linked to the movements of other oral cavity and laryngeal structures. The bite block did not affect lip movements but, rather, reduced lip onset time relative to hyoid onset time. The bite block also caused a different pattern of tongue body/hard palate contact in men: the tongue contact zones for the bite block swallows were displaced anteriorly to those of normal swallows, a pattern illustrated in 1 subject (Fig 7–7).

Conclusion.—Movements of the structures of the oral cavity and larynx showed considerable temporal overlap in timing, widespread individual variability in coordination patterns and movement trajectories, and selective effects of the bite block. These findings support the existence of individual adaptive strategies in swallowing movements rather than sequential or immutable patterns.

▶ It is easy either to take for granted the complex, coordinated efforts related to swallowing or to view them as being much too complicated to understand. These researchers have helped us by providing a visual demonstration of the position of the tongue during the swallowing process.—G.R. Holt, M.D., F.A.C.S.

Hyperbaric Oxygen Improves Wound Healing in Normal and Ischemic Skin Tissue

Uhl E, Sirsjö A, Haapaniemi T, Nilsson G, Nylander G (Ludwig-Maximilians Univ, Munich; Univ Hosp, Linköping, Sweden)
Plast Reconstr Surg 93:835–841, 1994   130-95-7–15

Background.—Impaired wound healing often is secondary to inadequate blood supply, which leads to inadequate oxygenation. Therefore, hyperbaric oxygen (HBO) has been used to treat problem wounds. Using a standardized experimental wound healing model in mice, the influence of HBO on wound healing was evaluated in normal and ischemic tissue. The wound surface area and microvascular blood flow, measured using a laser Doppler perfusion imager (LDI), were assessed.

Methods.—The ears of hairless mice were wounded with or without prior induction of ischemia. Animals were treated within 2 hours of wounding and then twice daily with HBO.

Results.—In normal wounds, as compared with controls, HBO significantly accelerated healing. In ischemic tissue, HBO was an even more significant factor in the speed of wound healing. There was no difference in the tissue blood flow between treated and untreated animals.

Conclusion.—Therapy with HBO improves wound healing in both normal and ischemic tissue. This effect is not associated with changes in microvascular perfusion, as measured by LDI. Therefore, the benefit is a result of increased arteriolar oxygen and local diffusion.

▶ It may be a common misconception that HBO is not helpful in healing so-called "normal" wounds. This study, as well as anecdotal clinical experience, provides a different viewpoint. Hyperbaric oxygen can also be of benefit for the slow-healing wound in otherwise normal tissue.—G.R. Holt, M.D., F.A.C.S.

CT-Guided Stereolithography As a New Tool in Craniofacial Surgery
Anderl H, Zur Nedden D, Mühlbauer W, Twerdy K, Zanon E, Wicke K, Knapp R (Univ Hosp, Innsbruck, Austria; Klinikum Bogenhausen, Munich)
Br J Plast Surg 47:60–64, 1994   130-95-7–16

Introduction.—The recent introduction of CT-guided stereolithography makes it possible to produce an exact and comprehensive acrylic model that replicates the original structure. This method was developed during research on the 5,300-year-old "Ice Man" discovered at the Tyrolean-Italian border in 1991 (Figs 7–8 and 7–9) and was applied during surgical correction of craniofacial malformations.

Method.—A Siemens Somatom plus CT-scanner turns around the head to be modeled, producing multiple 2-mm-thick axial slices of the skull. Data are processed in an image-analyzing system to provide the slices of 1 mm thickness that are required to construct a special three-dimensional image of the skull. The stereolithographic apparatus guides a laser beam over the surface of an ultraviolet light–sensitive liquid photopolymer, generating a point-by-point polymerization from the surface to the bottom in .25-mm-thick layers. This procedure results in a model that exactly replicates the original bony subject.

Clinical Application.—An 8-month-old infant with facial bipartition had a model of her skull produced before surgical correction was undertaken. By using the model, surgeons were able to determine the osteotomy lines and measure how much movement of both halves of the face would be required to build up a normal midface. With direction from the stereolithographically produced model, potential damage to the optic nerve was avoided. The infant had a very good functional and esthetic result and showed normal development at 6-month follow-up.

Conclusion.—These results show that CT-guided stereolithography can be used to reduce surgical risk in patients with certain craniofacial malformations. The model is valuable for planning the reconstructive procedure, completing the surgery, and documenting healing and

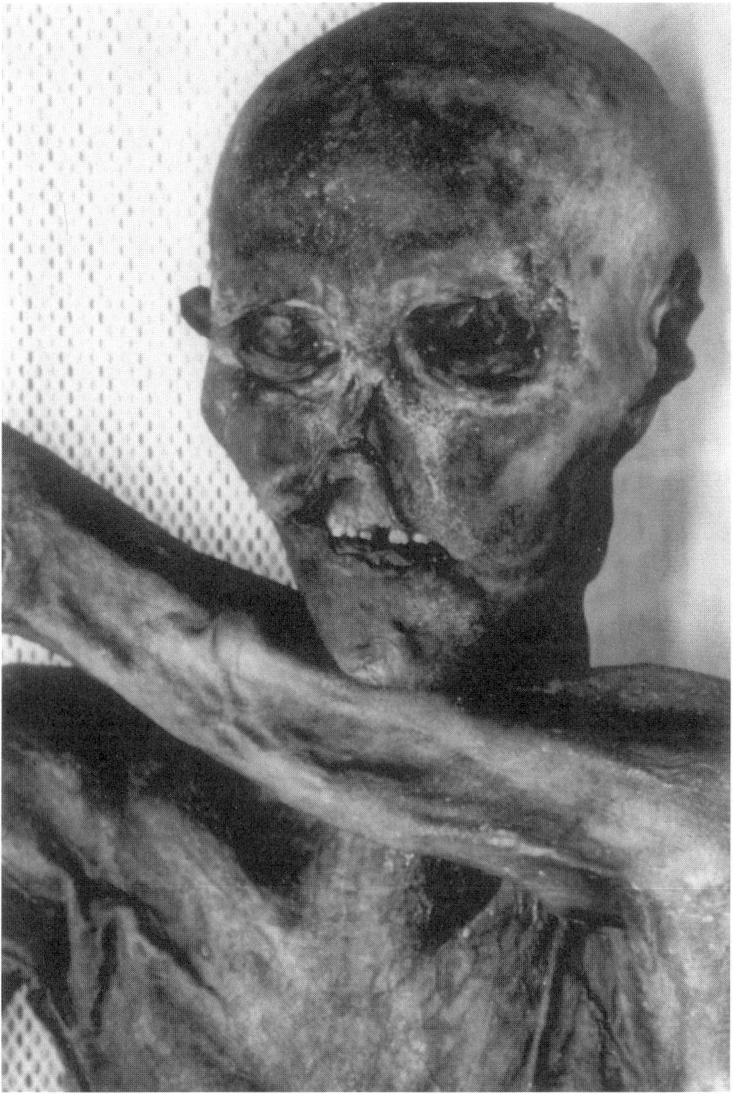

Fig 7–8.—The 5,300-year-old "Ice Man". (Courtesy of Anderl H, Zur Nedden D, Mühlbauer W, et al: *Br J Plast Surg* 47:60–64, 1994.)

growth in follow-up studies. At the present time, however, costs of CT-guided stereolithography are quite high when an entire structure is replicated.

▶ Although it currently is very expensive, this technique can be an extremely valuable resource for difficult reconstruction cases. Because most head and

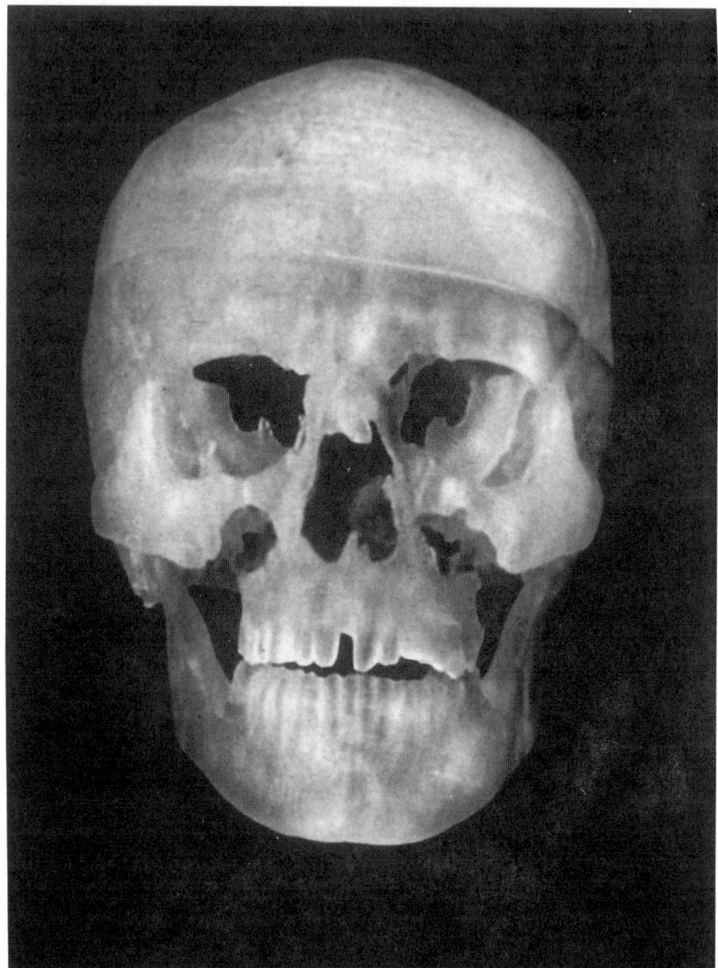

Fig 7–9.—The stereolithographic-produced acrylic skull of the "Ice Man." (Courtesy of Anderl H, Zur Nedden D, Mühlbauer W, et al: *Br J Plast Surg* 47:60–64, 1994)

neck surgeons are visually oriented (left-handers are exceptionally good here!), such scans are nearly as helpful as seeing the deformity in real time.—G.R. Holt, M.D., F.A.C.S.

Evidence for Capsule Gene Sequences Among Pharyngeal Isolates of Nontypeable *Haemophilus influenzae*

St Geme JW III, Takala A, Esko E, Falkow S (Washington Univ, St Louis, Mo;

Natl Public Health Inst, Helsinki; Stanford Univ, Calif)
J Infect Dis 169:337–342, 1994   130-95-7–17

Introduction.—*Haemophilus influenzae*, a common commensal organism of the respiratory tract, is an important cause of localized and systemic disease. Most isolates from the respiratory tract are nonencapsulated and serologically nontypeable, whereas those from systemic sites usually have a polysaccharide capsule. It seems likely that these 2 types of strains share a common heritage. Genetic analyses were performed to determine whether nontypeable strains of *H. influenzae* evolved from encapsulated organisms.

Methods.—The investigators obtained 123 pharyngeal isolates of serologically nontypeable *H. influenzae* from healthy 3-year-old Finnish children during a 4-year period. These strains were examined for capsule gene sequences by using Southern hybridization with pU038, a plasmid that contains 1 complete set of *cap* genes from a type b strain of *H. influenzae*.

Results.—Homology with capsule-specific sequences was demonstrated in 20% of the isolates studied. Eighteen of these 24 isolates, as well as 14 of the rest, showed evidence of the insertion element IS *1016*, which is associated with encapsulation. The 38 isolates hybridizing with pU038 appeared to segregate into at least 35 separate clones, which is consistent with the reported diversity among epidemiologically unrelated isolates of nontypeable *H. influenzae*.

Conclusion.—The presence of capsule gene sequences among nontypeable strains of *H. influenzae* suggests that these strains arose from an encapsulated ancestor. The evolutionary loss of encapsulation may be related to the disadvantages associated with encapsulation during colonization of the respiratory tract. It is possible but uncertain that encapsulation conferred a selective survival advantage for primitive *H. influenzae*.

▶ Although *H. influenzae* vaccines are helping to control epidemics, more research into the adaptation and genetic sequencing of significant bacteria must be undertaken to avoid being caught without treatment for evolving antibiotic-resistant strains.—G.R. Holt, M.D., F.A.C.S.

Tongue Reinnervation by Hypoglossal-Lingual Nerve Transfer
Weinberger JM, Houlden D, Mackinnon SE, Evans PJ (Queensway Gen Hosp, Etobicoke, Ont, Canada; Sunnybrook Health Science Ctr, Toronto; Washington Univ, St Louis, Mo; et al)
Laryngoscope 104:215–221, 1994   130-95-7–18

Objective.—An attempt was made in monkeys to learn whether a proximal hypoglossal-distal lingual transfer is able to functionally reinnervate the uninvolved anterior tongue after glossectomy for carcinoma of the tongue base.

Methods.—The anatomy of the hypoglossal and lingual nerves was studied in dissections of 3 monkey cadavers. Four monkeys then underwent a proximal hypoglossal-to-distal lingual nerve transfer. The submandibular gland was removed, and the right hypoglossal nerve was transected just proximal to its point of arborization in the base of the tongue. The lingual nerve was mobilized as far proximally as possible before being transected. The microsurgical nerve repair used 10–0 nylon sutures. Three animals received an ipsilateral tongue "fillet" 7 months after the nerve transfer. The anterior two thirds of the tongue were divided transversely to the midline, and the flap was resutured in its original site.

Results.—Normal potentials were recorded in the tongue base 7 months after the transfer. There were complex reinnervation motor unit potentials in the mid-tongue and denervation potentials in the tongue tip. Motor potentials were present in all areas of the side of the tongue a year after transfer. The tip exhibited a minor degree of atrophy and exhibited lower-amplitude motor responses. Motor responses to hypoglossal nerve stimulation remained below normal in the tongue base and mid-tongue at 18 months, but they were of normal amplitude in the tongue tip. No denervation potentials were recorded at this time. Reinnervation via the nerve transfer was confirmed by blocking the normal hypoglossal nerve.

Conclusion.—The hypoglossal-lingual nerve transfer appears to be an effective way of functionally reinnervating the anterior part of the tongue in patients who require removal of the tongue base.

▶ This technique offers a hope of success, but it must be confirmed with further laboratory studies. Unfortunately, it was not clear whether the implanted hemitongue had increased clinical physiologic function compared with the controls. This will need to be determined before human studies are conducted.—G.R. Holt, M.D., F.A.C.S.

A New Skin Equivalent: Keratinocytes Proliferated and Differentiated on Collagen Sponge Containing Fibroblasts
Maruguchi T, Maruguchi Y, Suzuki S, Matsuda K, Toda K-I, Isshiki N (Kobe City Gen Hosp, Japan; Kyoto Univ, Japan)
Plast Reconstr Surg 93:537–544, 1994   130-95-7–19

Introduction.—Most skin equivalents developed for coverage of skin defects produced by burns or trauma have served as temporary substitutes. Three types of artificial skin containing keratinocytic components were produced and tested for comparison in an experimental study.

Procedure for Preparation of Artificial Skin Dermis

1. Homogenize 0.3% atelocollagen in a hydrochloric acid solution of pH 3.0 for 60 minutes at 1800 to 2000 rev/min with refrigerated homogenizer.
2. Pour bubbled solution into mold, and freeze rapidly at $-40°C$.
3. Freeze dry for 48 hours.
4. Dry at 105°C for 24 hours under vacuum.
5. Cross-link the collagen sponge in 0.2% glutaraldehyde–0.05 M acetic acid for 24 hours at 4°C.
6. Rinse with phosphate-buffered saline.
7. Soak in 15% ethanol.
8. Freeze rapidly at $-135°C$.
9. Freeze dry for 48 hours.
10. Sterilize with ethylene oxide gas.

(Courtesy of Maruguchi T, Maruguchi Y, Suzuki S, et al: *Plast Reconstr Surg* 93:537–544, 1994.)

Methods.—Normal adult volunteers provided skin samples for primary culture of keratinocytes and fibroblasts. Keratinocytes were cultured on the artificial skin dermis (collagen sponge), using the air-liquid interface culture method (table). To create continuous keratinocyte layers on the artificial skin dermis, pores of its uppermost layer were filled with type I collagen gel, Matrigel, or fibroblasts.

Results.—After incubation for 3 days on collagen gel-coated artificial skin dermis, a band of keratinocytes consisting of 2–6 cell layers was formed. Keratinocytes were cuboidal in shape on the lowest layer and became rather flattened in the upper layers. When cells were cultured for over 5 days, the collagen gel layer started to dissolve and some keratinocytes dropped into the lower artificial skin dermis layer. After incubation for 3 days, keratinocytes cultured on Matrigel-coated artificial skin dermis were piled up into about 20 cell layers. Neither the addition of 10% fetal calf serum nor incubation for an additional 3 days had any remarkable effect on the histologic appearance of the cells. Fibroblasts cultured on artificial skin dermis proliferated slowly, although the cell density increased remarkably after incubation for 4 weeks. Keratinocytes cultured on artificial skin dermis containing fibroblasts exhibited differentiation similar to that of epidermis in vivo. The cells enucleated into cornified materials in the uppermost layer. Cell number decreased after incubation for 2 weeks, and the proportion of cornified materials increased.

Conclusion.—Keratinocytes cultured on the artificial skin dermis containing fibroblasts offered the best skin equivalent. After incubation for 7 days, the thickness of the keratinocytic band became almost equal to that of normal epidermis. Unlike other skin equivalents, keratinocytes and fibroblasts are in direct contact in this method, and direct contact is essential to promote growth of keratinocytes and production of cytokine.

▶ This study nicely demonstrates the important inductive/symbiotic relationship between keratinocytes and their colleagues, the fibroblasts. As in healing of a wound, the fibroblast stratum must be present before adequate epithelialization can occur.—G.R. Holt, M.D., F.A.C.S.

Motion Observed Across Maxillary Continuity Defects Stabilized With Plates and Screws

Funk GF, Stanley RB Jr, McKellop HA (Univ of Southern California, Los Angeles)

Arch Otolaryngol Head Neck Surg 120:187–194, 1994   130-95-7–20

Objective.—The use of plates and screws to stabilize maxillary fractures or elective osteotomies of the maxilla is intended to eliminate the need for 4 to 6 weeks of jaw immobilization. Fresh cadaver skulls were used to estimate the degree of fixation achieved with these devices under conditions of functional loading.

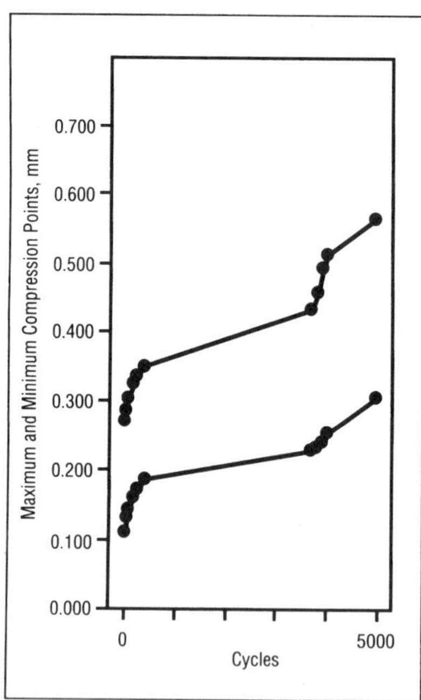

Fig 7–10.—Graphic representation of motion recorded at the anterior transducer adjacent to the failed zygomaticomaxillary buttress plate in skull 2. A sudden increase in both maximum compression and pistoning amplitude can be seen at approximately 4,000 cycles. (Courtesy of Funk GF, Stanley RB Jr, McKellop HA: *Arch Otolaryngol Head Neck Surg* 120:187–194, 1994.)

Methods.—The skulls were embedded in bone cement in a computer-controlled servohydraulic steel test frame allowing both static and sinusoidal loads to be applied. Micromotion transducers were placed in notches cut into the maxilla near the zygomatic buttresses on either side and into the pterygoid plate posteriorly. Bilateral osteotomies were made through the anterior and lateral antral walls and the pterygoid plates and fixed with 5-hole, 2-mm steel miniplates that were attached at near-right angles to the line of the osteotomy.

Observations.—Micromotion was recorded across the level of LeFort I osteotomies even when fixation appeared to be grossly stable (Fig 7–10). In general, the motion recorded at transducer sites took the form of compression of the osteotomy gap. The deformation was chiefly elastic in nature, and its extent appeared to be predictable from the average stability of the screws used in each plate. Most or all of the screws in a 2-plate system were of supertorque quality. Only when 2- and 4-plate systems predicted to be less stable were compared was there greater motion for the 2-plate system.

Implications.—Fixation of maxillary continuity defects with plates and screws is not truly "rigid." If the overall stability of fixation is tenuous, the motion that occurs could lead to resorption and remodeling of bone about the screws and consequent permanent deformation.

▶ Even though the authors express their concerns about micromotion leading to screw loosening and permanent deformation, there also is the possibility that micromotion may be salutory, leading to biological remodeling and response of the bone to physiologic pressures at the fracture site.—G.R. Holt, M.D., F.A.C.S.

Oral and Laryngeal Muscle Coordination During Swallowing
Gay T, Rendell JK, Spiro J (Univ of Connecticut, Farmington)
Laryngoscope 104:341–349, 1994   130-95-7–21

Objective.—In an electromyographic study, the relative contributions and activity patterns of the muscles during the oral phase of swallowing, one of the most important of all human biological functions, were defined.

Methods.—Studies were performed in 6 young adults (mean age, 26 years) of each gender. All had normal oral structures and a complete dentition. Hooked-wire or stick-on surface electrodes were used to study the orbicularis oris inferior, masseter, palatal elevator, genioglossus, mylohyoid, anterior digastric, and vocalis muscles. The study subjects swallowed 15 mL of water with the head placed against a head rest. Studies were repeated with a 12-mm bite block in place between the molar teeth.

Findings.—All the muscles studied were actively involved in the process of swallowing, but analysis of integrated electromyographic signals revealed that swallowing varied among individuals with respect to the particular muscles utilized and how their activities were coordinated. Genioglossus activity, for instance, exhibited a wide range of onset times and durations. The rage of onset times was most narrow for the suprahyoid muscles. Introduction of the bite block altered the pattern of muscle coordination in half the subjects. In some cases, overall muscle activity increased as temporal stability was maintained. In others, temporal relationships were reorganized, with or without changes in muscle activity.

Implications.—Normal individuals exhibit highly variable patterns of swallowing function. Different individuals use differing motor strategies to compensate for a mechanical obstruction to swallowing. It may be that swallowing is more dependent on higher-level brain functions than was formerly thought, rather than being strictly a rigid, lower-level reflex activity.

▶ To substantiate this study, just go to your favorite cafeteria and observe people chewing and swallowing. What a variety of facial, mouth, and throat motions!—G.R. Holt, M.D., F.A.C.S.

Repeated Use of the Same Myocutaneous Flap in Difficult Second Operations of the Head and Neck

Havlik R, Ariyan S (Yale-New Haven Hosp, Conn)
Plast Reconstr Surg 93:481–488, 1994   130-95-7–22

Background.—Repeat surgery for tumor occurrence, a formidable task, is often complicated in the head and neck by previous regional lymphadenectomy and/or postoperative radiotherapy to the surgical field. The treatment of 7 patients with particularly difficult secondary head and neck reconstructive problems was discussed.

Patients.—The patients were 4 men and 3 women, aged 55 to 70 years. Tumor sites included the floor of the mouth, piriform sinus, lower lip, tongue and hypopharynx, arytenoepiglottic carotid exposure, and preauricular skin. Recurrence sites were the infratemporal fossa, tonsillar fossa and lateral pharynx, reconstructed esophagus, orocutaneous fistula, buccal area, and floor of the mouth and tongue. In all cases, the surgeon completely re-elevated the pectoralis major flap on its thoracoacromial vascular pedicle and repositioned it in an alternate site. In 5 cases, the pectoralis major flaps had been irradiated after the initial surgery. Even these flaps were reused successfully.

Conclusions.—The pectoralis major myocutaneous flap is so reliable that, in these selected cases, it was completely re-elevated, isolated, and transposed to a new reconstructive site in the head and neck. This flap "recycling" can be done safely, even after the flap has had a full course of external-beam radiation therapy.

▶ I have used a musculocutaneous flap for "second duty" in some patients, and have benefited from its flexibility and robust quality. Enough time must be allowed for the primary flap to obtain blood supply from its new bed before disturbing it further.—G.R. Holt, M.D., F.A.C.S.

The Roles of Revascularization and Resorption on Endurance of Craniofacial Onlay Bone Grafts in the Rabbit
Chen NT, Glowacki J, Bucky LP, Hong H-Z, Kim W-K, Yaremchuk MJ (Massachusetts Gen Hosp, Boston; Brigham and Women's Hosp, Boston; Harvard Med School, Boston)
Plast Reconstr Surg 93:714–722, 1994   130-95-7–23

Introduction.—Although onlay bone grafts are commonly used to recontour craniofacial bones, graft resorption sometimes occurs with time. The resorptive behavior of calvarial and iliac crest bone grafts were evaluated in the rabbit.

Methods.—A total of 32 white New Zealand rabbits received autologous anterior iliac crest and calvarium bone grafts to the snout. Animals were killed and specimens were studied on days 3, 10, and 70.

Results.—The calvarial graft contained significantly more area and volume than the iliac crest graft. By day 10, there was significantly more revascularization of the cancellous region than of the cortical region in both grafts. The cross-section area and the mean cortical thickness of the calvarian grafts were significantly bigger than those of the iliac crest grafts. The osteoclastic indices for the cancellous areas were significantly larger than for the cortex for both grafts. At 70 days all grafts demonstrated good bony union with their snout.

Conclusion.—Bone growth is related to revascularization. Calvarian grafts maintain more volume because they contain more cortical bone.

▶ In certain defects (e.g., mandibular defects), it is desirable to use cancellous bone because of the potential for revascularization and remodeling. However, for onlay requirements, the cortical bone graft appears to be better.—G.R. Holt, M.D., F.A.C.S.

Comparison of the Chondrogenic Potential of Free and Vascularized Perichondrium in the Airway
Hartig GK, Esclamado RM, Telian SA (Univ of Michigan, Ann Arbor)
Ann Otol Rhinol Laryngol 103:9–15, 1994   130-95-7–24

Introduction.—Some patients with severe laryngotracheal stenosis resulting from airway trauma fail multiple procedures designed to repair the stenosis. When the usual grafting materials are unsuccessful, further options must be developed. Cartilage formation in free and vascularized perichondrium placed in the airway was compared in an experimentally designed study. Once a significant advantage to vascularized grafts was confirmed, the effect of an intraoperative ischemic insult on cartilage formation in these grafts was evaluated.

Methods.—Vascularized perichondrium was chosen for its pliability, potential for bone or cartilage formation, resistance to infection, and rapid mucosalization. The rabbit model used offers an auricular perichondral graft that can be obtained in both free and vascularized forms. Airway defects were created in 38 New Zealand white rabbits. Sixteen received a free perichondral graft across the defect (group A), and 18 had defects covered with vascularized perichondrium (group B). Four animals (group C) received the same treatment as group B but had the central auricular artery and vein clamped for 2 hours to simulate conditions of a revascularization procedure. The animals were sacrificed at 8 weeks, and the airways were harvested for analysis.

Results.—The mean cartilage thickness was .15 mm in group A and .45 mm in group B. Both groups showed a bimodal distribution of cartilage thickness, with only 25% of group A grafts producing an average thickness of more than .3 mm vs. 78% of those in group B. The difference in cartilage thickness between the 2 groups was highly statistically significant. The 4 grafts in group C produced a mean cartilage thickness of .50 mm.

Conclusion.—In this rabbit model of airway defect, vascularized perichondrium provided significantly more cartilage than free perichondrium grafts. The vascularized perichondrium did not appear to be damaged by a 2-hour intraoperative ischemic insult. These grafts may be useful in laryngotracheal reconstruction, but they have yet to be evaluated in humans who have other factors that may influence the chondrogenic or osteogenic capacity of the grafts.

▶ This study showed promising results with use of a vascularized perichondral graft. Certainly, we need additional methods of treating tracheal stenosis. In humans, sites for such pedicled grafts might include thyroid cartilage alae with attached strap muscles and auricular conchal cartilage on a sternocleidomastoid muscle fascial pedicle.—G.R. Holt, M.D., F.A.C.S.

Applications of Image-Directed Robotics in Otolaryngologic Surgery
Kavanagh KT (Lake Cumberland Regional Hosp, Somerset, Ky)
Laryngoscope 104:283–293, 1994   130-95-7–25

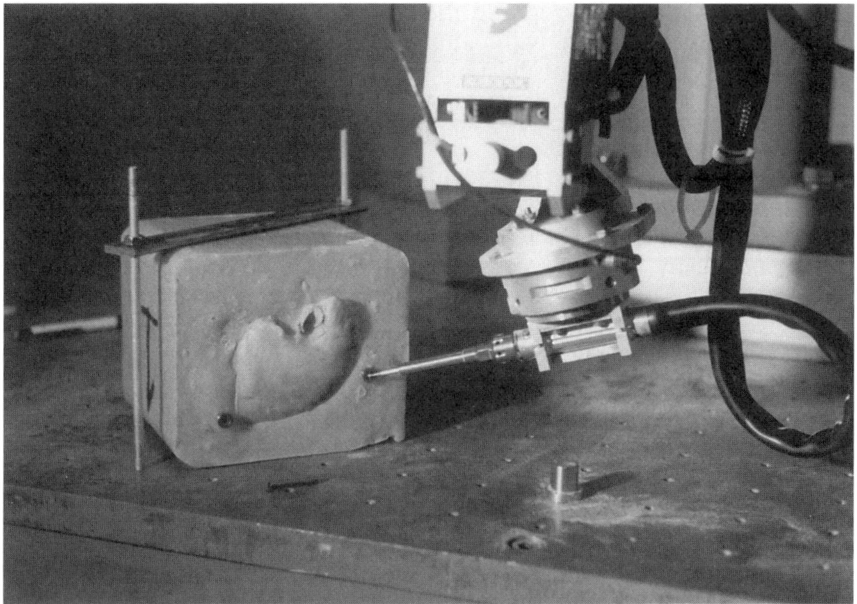

Fig 7–11.—Surgical block and robotic drill. (Courtesy of Kavanagh KT: *Laryngoscope* 104:283–293, 1994.)

Background.—Image-directed robotic surgery uses a three-dimensional image to assist a robot in tissue removal. Future use of robotics in otolaryngologic surgery was investigated.

Methods.—Five temporal bones were fixated in a block. Three orientation pins were then placed in the block. A three-dimensional reconstruction of the bone and pins was created and was then rotated, magnified, and sliced as needed. The surgical tool was then linked to the CT scannable orientation device. The robot's arm was manually moved so that the drilling tip in its arm touched the pins (Fig 7–11). The robot then oriented the pins to the CT scan. Five antrostomies were performed on the temporal bones. Measurements were then done of the planned removal area and the area of bone actually removed.

Results.—The average absolute error of drilling was .88 mm. As a result of an operator calibration error, 1 specimen had a .5-mm larger area of bone removed than had been planned. For another specimen, there was a sizable difference between the planned removal area and the bone removal defect. On average, the planned removal area was .66 mm larger than the bone-removal defect. The preoperative planned distance was shorter than the postoperative distance in 37 of the 50 measurements between the surgical site and the measured structure.

Conclusions.—Otorhinolaryngology is ideally suited for image-directed robotic surgery because the operation field can be readily fixed, and the abundant bony septa in the ear and sinuses decrease the likelihood that the soft tissue will shift. Antrostomies were performed on 5 human temporal bones using image-directed robotics. In none of the procedures was an adjacent structure violated. Future robotics improvements should result in greater drilling accuracy.

▶ This paper really caught my interest. Computer-assisted design/computer-assisted manufacturing (CAD/CAM) is routinely used when working with metals in industry, and the same engineering principles should be applicable to surgery that is guided by three-dimensional CT-coded boundaries. The major drawback of this approach is the lack of decision-making capacity that the human surgeon exhibits when the clinical situation is not the same as the scans had indicated.—G.R. Holt, M.D., F.A.C.S.

Vascularized Fascia as a Transferable Bed for Experimental Laryngeal Reconstruction
Delaere PR, Van Damme B, Feenstra L (Univ Hosp St Rafaël, Leuven, Belgium)
Ann Otol Rhinol Laryngol 103:215–221, 1994   130-95-7–26

Introduction.—The vascular fascial flaps have unique characteristics that might be useful in bringing a mucosal lining to the inner surface of a laryngeal defect. An experimental model was designed to examine the feasibility of a transferable vascular bed in laryngeal reconstruction after tumor removal.

Methods.—Thirty New Zealand white rabbits were divided into 3 groups of 10 animals each. No operative procedure was performed in group 1 (controls). Rabbits in group 2 had a hemilaryngeal defect reconstructed with vascularized fascia, autogenous cartilage, and an oral mucosal lining. In group 3, the vascularized fascia served as an internal lining with autogenous cartilage for support (Fig 7–12). Operative technique was identical for groups 2 and 3, except that the mucosal graft was not used in group 3. Six weeks after the operation, the vascular pedicle of the flap was dissected free, and the lateral thoracic artery was injected with blue Microfil so that the vascular pattern of the inner and outer fascial layers might be observed. The animals were then sacrificed and the larynges harvested. In a separate experiment, 15 rabbits were used to study reconstruction of the posterior glottis by introducing additional supporting cartilage strips within the vascular bed.

Results.—The mean laryngeal area measurements were 151.9 mm² for controls, 135.5 mm² for group 2, and 57.49 mm² for group 3. The fascia-lined group was significantly different than the control group. In group 2, a hydropic swelling of the superficial cells was visible over the oral mucosal graft in the subglottic area. Respiratory epithelium was the

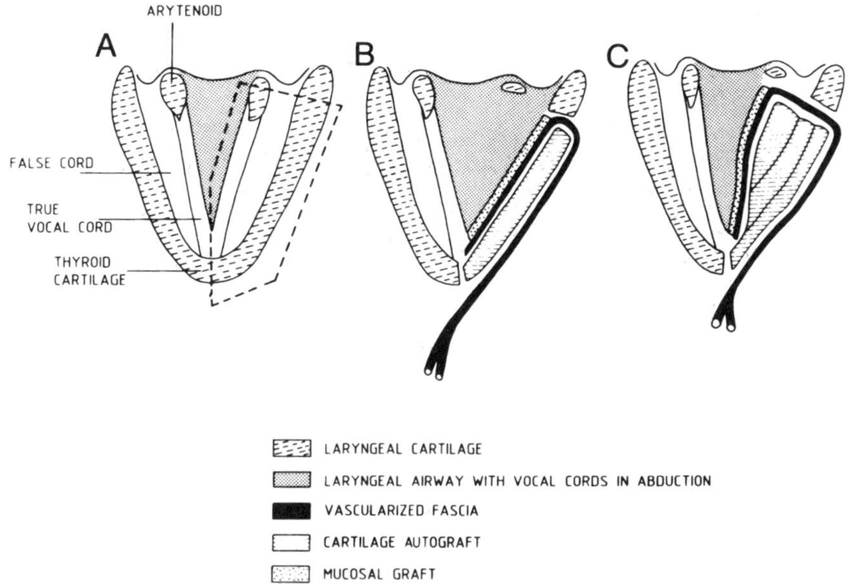

Fig 7–12.—Laryngeal reconstruction with vascularized fascia. **A,** outlining of resection, including vocal process of arytenoid cartilage. **B,** reconstruction with vascularized fascia rotated 180 degrees to bring mucosal lining inside and to protect cartilage autograft circumferentially in vascularized bed. **C,** reconstruction of posterior glottis by introduction of additional cartilage. (Courtesy of Delaere PR, Van Damme B, Feenstra L: *Ann Otol Rhinol Laryngol* 103:215-221, 1994.)

primary component of the epithelial lining in group 3. In animals undergoing reconstruction of posterior glottic bulk, those with 2 or 3 additional cartilage strips showed viable cartilage only in close contact with the vascularized layer.

Conclusion.—Reconstruction the larynx after removal of a transglottic tumor remains a challenge to the surgeon. The 3 laryngeal functions—maintenance of a sufficient airway lumen, prevention of aspiration, and production of sound—must be preserved. In the rabbit, a vascularized fascial flap was developed that is both consistently present and easy to isolate. The flap successfully brings mucosal and cartilage grafts into a laryngeal defect and suggests the possibility of a composite reconstruction for laryngeal repair.

▶ I was encouraged by the possibility of reconstructing laryngeal defects with the vascularized fascial flap. We use autogenous grafts routinely, sometimes in the larynx, and thereby understand their fate. Could this technique also be applied to the trachea?—G.R. Holt, M.D., F.A.C.S.

Moving?

I'd like to receive my *Year Book of Otolaryngology-Head & Neck Surgery* without interruption.
Please note the following change of address, effective:

Name: ____

New Address: ____

____

City: ________________________________ State: ________ Zip: ________

Old Address: ____

____

City: ________________________________ State: ________ Zip: ________

Reservation Card

Yes, I would like my own copy of *Year Book of Otolaryngology-Head & Neck Surgery*. Please begin my subscription with the current edition according to the terms described below.* I understand that I will have 30 days to examine each annual edition. If satisfied, I will pay just $72.95 plus sales tax, postage and handling (price subject to change without notice).

Name: ____

Address: ____

City: ________________________________ State: ________ Zip: ________

Method of Payment
○ Visa   ○ Mastercard   ○ AmEx   ○ Bill me   ○ Check (in US dollars, payable to Mosby, Inc.)

Card number: ____________________________ Exp date: ____________

Signature: ____

LS-0909

Your Year Book Service Guarantee:

When you subscribe to the *Year Book*, we'll send you an advance notice of future volumes about two months before they publish. This automatic notice system is designed to take up as little of your time as possible. If you do not want the *Year Book*, the advance notice makes it quick and easy for you to let us know your decision, and you will always have at least 20 days to decide. If we don't hear from you, we'll send you the new volume as soon as it's available. And, of course, the *Year Book* is yours to examine free of charge for 30 days (postage, handling and applicable sales tax are added to each shipment.).

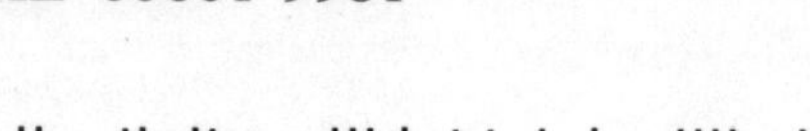

BUSINESS REPLY MAIL

FIRST CLASS MAIL   PERMIT No. 762   CHICAGO, IL

POSTAGE WILL BE PAID BY ADDRESSEE

Chris Hughes
Mosby-Year Book, Inc.
200 N. LaSalle Street
Suite 2600
Chicago, IL 60601-9981

BUSINESS REPLY MAIL

FIRST CLASS MAIL   PERMIT No. 762   CHICAGO, IL

POSTAGE WILL BE PAID BY ADDRESSEE

Chris Hughes
Mosby-Year Book, Inc.
200 N. LaSalle Street
Suite 2600
Chicago, IL 60601-9981

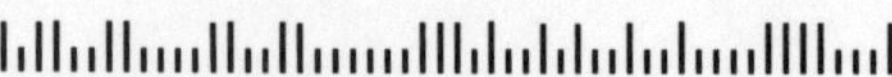

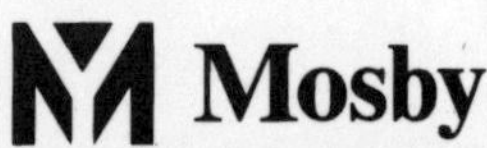

Dedicated to publishing excellence

8 Rhinology and Paranasal Sinuses

Response of the Nose to Exercise in Healthy Subjects and in Patients With Rhinitis and Asthma
Serra-Batlles J, Montserrat JM, Mullol J, Ballester E, Xaubet A, Picado C
(Hosp Clínic, Facultat de Medicina, Barcelona)
Thorax 49:128–132, 1994   130-95-8–1

Background.—Both the nose and the bronchi take part in regulating respiratory heat exchange. However, whereas thermal changes may lead to airway obstruction during exercise, they rarely lead to nasal obstruction in patients with rhinitis. Very little research has addressed the reasons for the differing exercise responses of the nose and bronchial tree. This issue was addressed in a study of patients with asthma, rhinitis, or both.

Methods.—Four groups of nonsmoking subjects were studied: 10 healthy controls, 15 patients with asthma and rhinitis, 10 patients with rhinitis only, and 11 patients with asthma only. All were studied during 6 minutes of bicycle ergometry, to reach a maximal heart rate of 80% of predicted. Forced expiratory volume in 1 second (FEV_1) was used to assess the bronchial response, and posterior rhinomanometry was used to assess the nasal response to exercise. Exercise-induced asthma was considered present in a decrease of 20% or more in FEV_1.

Results.—There were no significant differences in the degree of exercise-induced increase in heart rate and ventilation. The 2 groups of patients with asthma showed a significant decrease in FEV_1; the rhinitis-only group and the controls showed no change in this measure. Exercise-induced asthma developed in 50% of the patients with asthma. All 4 groups showed a similar degree of increase in nasal patency, with no difference between those with and without rhinitis. By 25 minutes after exercise, nasal patency returned to baseline. However, in the 13 patients with exercise-induced asthma, the nose remained significantly more patent between 10 and 30 minutes after exercise than in those without exercise-induced asthma.

Conclusions.—The nose and bronchi show different responses during exercise-induced airway obstruction. The bronchial response consists of narrowing, whereas the nasal response is increased patency. This difference suggests that different mechanisms govern the exercise responses of the upper airway vs. the central and peripheral airways.

▶ This article makes sense for those of us who run, particularly those who run with a head cold or allergic rhinitis exacerbation. The only problem is finding a way to run and carry Kleenex™ for the rhinorrhea.—G.R. Holt, M.D., F.A.C.S.

A Review of Revision Functional Endoscopic Sinus Surgery

King JM, Caldarelli DD, Pigato JB (Rush-Presbyterian-St Luke's Med Ctr, Chicago)
Laryngoscope 104:404–408, 1994   130-95-8–2

Objective.—Functional endoscopic sinus surgery (FESS) is a procedure of documented effectiveness, with up to 98% of patients achieving symptomatic improvements. However, for patients in whom FESS does not relieve persistent or recurrent sinus disease, revision surgery may be needed. The characteristics and results of a group of patients undergoing revision FESS after previous FESS or traditional sinus surgery were reviewed.

Methods.—Of 295 consecutive patients undergoing FESS during a 1-year period, 43 had a history of previous sinus surgery. There were 27 females and 16 males (mean age, 43 years). Thirty-three had had traditional surgery, and 10 had undergone a previous FESS procedure. In each case, recurrent sinusitis had failed to respond to antibiotics and other medical treatments. The main preoperative symptoms were facial pain, purulent rhinorrhea or postnasal drainage, and nasal obstruction. The patients were followed up for a mean of 14 months after undergoing revision FESS.

Results.—All patients underwent surgery on the maxillary ostia or sinus; 88% had surgical manipulation of the ethmoid sinuses and 49% of the sphenoid sinuses. There were no surgical complications. Thirteen patients had persistent disease after the revision FESS procedure and so were considered to be treatment failures. All but 2 of the patients in this group had had previous nonendoscopic sinus surgery; most had a history of oral steroid use and asthma. Three of the 4 patients with a history of aspergillosis failed revision FESS.

Conclusions.—Revision FESS has a success rate of 70% in this review. The procedure is safe, with no major complications. A number of factors associated with failed revision FESS are identified, but these need not be viewed as contraindications; treatment decisions should be individualized. The success of FESS might be enhanced by appropriate standardization and staging of sinus disease.

▶ Endoscopic sinus surgery is generally accepted as being efficacious for a well-defined group of indications. Old-fashioned exenterative surgery is *not* completely passé, however. This study nicely shows that the endoscope can be repeatedly used to identify recurrent disease and improve sinus physiology.—G.R. Holt, M.D., F.A.C.S.

A Comparison of Cocaine vs. Lidocaine With Oxymetazoline for Use in Nasal Procedures

Tarver CP, Noorily AD, Sakai CS (Univ of Texas Health Sciences Ctr, San Antonio)
Otolaryngol Head Neck Surg 109:653–659, 1993   130-95-8-3

Purpose.—Cocaine is still commonly used for anesthesia and vasoconstriction in patients undergoing nasal procedures. Some substance that offers the vasoconstrictive and anesthetic properties of cocaine without its disadvantages—including its controlled status, cardiac events, and expense—would be desirable. No single agent meets these criteria, but a combination of 2 agents, each with 1 of the desirable properties of cocaine, might do so. Cocaine was compared with a mixture of lidocaine and oxymetazoline (lido/oxy) to assess the degree of vasoconstriction and anesthesia.

Methods.—Twenty-two healthy young men were studied. All subjects were studied twice, once after receiving cocaine and again after receiving the lido/oxy combination. The medications were administered to the nasal cavity with a cottonoid pledget soaked with either 1 cc of 4% cocaine or .5 cc of 4% lidocaine mixed with .5 cc of .05% oxymetazoline. Laser Doppler flowmetry was used to evaluate blood flow. Semmes-Weinstein monofilaments were used to measure anesthesia, including both sensation threshold and pain perception.

Results.—Blood flow decreased to a greater extent after administration of lido/oxy than after administration of cocaine. Ten minutes after removal of the pledget, there were no differences between the 2 treatments in terms of pain perception change. However, after 50 minutes, lido/oxy was associated with a greater decrease in pain perception than cocaine. The 2 treatments were not significantly different in sensation threshold change.

Conclusions.—The lido/oxy combination appears to be an effective alternative to cocaine for patients undergoing nasal procedures. Further studies are needed to determine if the study methods predict the desired clinical responses and whether there might be some better combination than lido/oxy.

▶ A study such as this one gives us some evidence that a drug combination, rather than cocaine, may be efficacious in intranasal surgery. If the combination is shorter-acting, then a second application may be required before the end of the procedure.—G.R. Holt, M.D., F.A.C.S.

Nasal Packing After Routine Nasal Surgery: Is It Justified?
Von Schoenberg M, Robinson P, Ryan R (Middlesex Hosp, London)
J Laryngol Otol 107:902–905, 1993   130-95-8-4

Introduction.—The efficacy of nasal packing vs. no packing after nasal surgery has not been established. Previous studies have had design problems, have not reached significance because of small sample size, or have not adequately addressed the relationship between pain and nasal packing. Whether the routine use of nasal packing was advantageous vs. no packing was evaluated in terms of pain and complications.

Methods.—During an 18-month period, 95 adult patients undergoing routine nasal surgery were evaluated prospectively. Patients received either no packs, bismuth iodoform paraffin paste ([BIPP] an antiseptic dressing), or Telfa (a sterile, nonadherent absorbent pack). Only patients receiving packs were randomized. They were also randomized regarding whether they received a Silastic nasal splint for 1 week postoperatively. At 1 week and 3 months, patients were reviewed for: (1) postoperative pain scores using a visual analogue scale; (2) significant reactionary hem-

Pain Scores and Complications

Group number (*n*)	Without packs 24	With packs (all) 71	BIPP 27	Telfa 44
Mean pain scores				
First 24 hours	2.8	4.2	3.8	4.5
Pack removal	–	5.7	7	5
Seven days	2.8	4.3	3.9	4.5
Splint removal	1.4	5.4	6	5.1
Complications				
Haemorrhage				
Number	–	2	1	1
Percentage	–	2.8%	3.7%	2.2%
Vestibulitis				
Number	–	3	3	–
Percentage	–	4.2%	11.1%	–
Septal perforation				
Number	–	2	2	–
Percentage	–	2.8%	7.4%	–
Early adhesions				
Number	2	6	3	3
Percentage	8.3%	8.45%	11.1%	6.8%

(Courtesy of Von Schoenberg M, Robinson P, Ryan R: *J Laryngol Otol* 107:902–905, 1993.)

orrhage requiring intervention; (3) accidental pack displacement; (4) adhesions; or (5) development of vestibulitis and septal perforations.

Results.—Seventy-one patients received packs; 27 had BIPP, 44 had Telfa, and 24 had no packs. Patients receiving nasal packs experienced significantly more pain postoperatively and at pack removal, regardless of whether splints were used (table). The BIPP packs, with or without splints, were associated with more pain and complications than the Telfa or no pack.

Conclusion.—The routine use of nasal packing after nasal surgery is not justified, particularly with BIPP, because of the increased incidence of pain and complications. Nasal packing should be reserved for patients in whom reactionary hemorrhage is a concern. Preference should be given to Telfa packing.

▶ I have used ointment-coated Telfa packs since 1977, when I was introduced to their use by Dr. Milton Yoder. Since then, I have sworn by them, and I probably always will. However, I am still open to other views, such as those presented in this paper.—G.R. Holt, M.D., F.A.C.S.

Humoral Response to Subcutaneous, Oral, and Nasal Immunotherapy for Allergic Rhinitis Due to *Dermatophagoides pteronyssinus*

Piazza I, Bizzaro N (Hosp of San Doná di Piave, Venice, Italy)
Ann Allergy 71:461–469, 1993   130-95-8–5

Background.—Subcutaneous immunotherapy, which is widely used to treat patients with allergic respiratory diseases, reduces polyclonal and specific IgE and increases specific IgG. The efficacy of alternative forms of immunotherapy and the importance of IgG4 as a measurement of clinical improvement were investigated.

Methods.—Variations in total IgE and specific IgE, IgG, and IgG4 for *Dermatophagoides pteronyssinus* were studied in an open controlled trial of 57 patients. All patients were found to have perennial rhinitis from an allergy to house dust mites. Forty-three patients were given immunotherapy, and 14 served as controls. Seventeen patients received subcutaneous therapy, 14 received sublingual therapy, and 12 received local therapy. The findings were compared with the clinical course to uncover possible relations between serum and clinical changes.

Findings.—Subcutaneous immunotherapy had a significant clinical effect, but sublingual and nasal treatment did not. Specific antibody behavior in patients receiving subcutaneous immunotherapy was consistent with that which had been reported previously. In the sixth month of therapy, specific IgE levels began to decrease and specific IgG and IgG4 concentrations increased significantly. However, the changes were not associated with the clinical course. No significant specific antibody modifications resulted from the other 2 forms of therapy.

Conclusions.—The increase in specific IgG4 induced by subcutaneous immunotherapy was the most important finding. However, the change in specific IgG4 was not associated with clinical outcomes.

▶ Research in allergic disorders of the upper aerodigestive tract has become so much more sophisticated than when, as a resident, I was pulled, kicking and screaming, into seeing patients in the allergy clinic. I now have a greater appreciation of the science and clinical application.—G.R. Holt, M.D., F.A.C.S.

The Biochemistry of Neutralization

Trevino RJ (Louisiana State Univ, Shreveport)
Otolaryngol Head Neck Surg 109:844–846, 1993   130-95-8–6

Background.—Injections of low doses of common environmental antigens or irritants have been shown to result in reduced sensitivity during a subsequent exposure to the same antigens or irritants. The efficacy of this therapy was demonstrated, and its mechanism was explained.

Method.—In part I of the experiment, 20 patients who were undergoing skin end point titration (SET) in allergy testing for hay fever were observed. The SET comprised intradermal injection of fivefold dilutions of the allergenic extracts. The end point was designated as the dilution that initiated progressive positive whealing. Part II of the study was a double-blind, placebo-controlled test in which 40 patients were injected with the dose of antigen that was established as the end point during SET one week after the testing to determine whether this caused relief of symptoms. Ten additional patients were injected with placebo under the same conditions.

Results.—Although none of the patients was asked to give any response to part I of the study, 12 (60%) reported complete relief of symptoms during the test procedure or shortly thereafter. The other 40% reported some symptom relief. None indicated an increase in severity of symptoms after testing. In part II, none of the patients who received placebo reported relief of symptoms after the test injection. Of the 40 patients who received active ingredients, 27 (67.5%) reported relief of symptoms within 5 to 10 minutes of the injection.

Conclusion.—Administration of the end point dose of an antigen appears to bring relief of allergic symptoms in patients. It also protects the patient from anaphylactic reactions during the testing process. The biochemical mechanism of this protection is thought to include the production of intracellular prostaglandin E, which brings an increase in cyclic adenosine monophosphate and a decrease in cyclic guanosine monophosphate.

▶ This discussion helps explain the practical theory of SET. Although we are not always happy to see the prostaglandins at work, we are told that one type, prostaglandin E, may be protective against anaphylaxis.—G.R. Holt, M.D., F.A.C.S.

Anatomic Considerations in Complications of Endoscopic and Intranasal Sinus Surgery
Streitmann MJ, Otto RA, Sakai CS (Univ of Texas Health Science Ctr, San Antonio)
Ann Otol Rhinol Laryngol 103:105–109, 1994   130-95-8-7

Objective.—Although most complications of endoscopic and intranasal sinus surgery are minor, some are serious or even devastating, especially when the orbit or CNS sustains surgical injury. In a cadaver study, anatomical landmarks were located to guide surgeons performing sinus surgery.

Methods.—Distances and angular measurements of anatomical areas around the nasal sinuses were determined using 50 embalmed half-heads.

Results.—There were significant differences between males and females for distances from the anterior ethmoid artery to the ethmoid dome, posterior ethmoid artery, optic nerve, and basal lamella.

Conclusion.—To avoid serious injury when performing intranasal and endoscopic surgery, the surgeon must understand the anatomy of the area, and when possible, endoscopes and other surgical instruments should be calibrated.

▶ Every budding endoscopic sinus surgeon should memorize the data given in this paper. It will serve the surgeon well to know the ranges of distances found in the sinus three-dimensional anatomical relationships. These authors have done us a great service. Take advantage of their work. It will help you stay out of trouble.—G.R. Holt, M.D., F.A.C.S.

Possible Interactions With Terfenadine or Astemizole
Zechnich AD, Hedges JR, Eiselt-Proteau D, Haxby D (Oregon Health Sciences Univ, Portland Drug Use Review of Oregon, Salem)
West J Med 160:321–325, 1994   130-95-8-8

Background.—The use of terfenadine or astemizole with erythromycin or ketoconazole can prolong the QT interval and result in potentially fatal ventricular arrhythmias. The frequency and patterns of concurrent prescribing were investigated.

Methods and Findings.—The Oregon Medicaid prescription claims data for 22 months were reviewed. Between 1991 and 1992, use of terfenadine increased by 29% and peaked in June of each year. Terfenadine was among the most prescribed medications from March through July 1992. One hundred twenty-two episodes of concurrent terfenadine or astemizole use with macrolide antibiotic agents or ketoconazole were noted. Ninety-four percent of these episodes involved terfenadine. From 1991 to 1992, the frequency of concurrent use increased more than threefold. Patients received prescriptions from different physicians in 48% of these episodes but used different pharmacies in only 3%.

Conclusions.—The extensive, increasing use of terfenadine increases the possibility of serious interactions. Many physicians may be unaware of this. Good prospective screening by pharmacists may greatly decrease the incidence of concurrent prescribing.

▶ I think by now the otolaryngology community knows of this problem. However, we should make sure our primary care colleagues are also aware of it, because they may actually prescribe more than we do.—G.R. Holt, M.D., F.A.C.S.

Major Complications of Sinus Surgery: A Review of 1192 Procedures
Dessi P, Castro F, Triglia JM, Zanaret M, Cannoni M (Timone Univ, France)
J Laryngol Otol 108:212–215, 1994   130-95-8–9

Background.—Major complications remain a concern during sinus surgery. To evaluate the incidence, prevention, and management of these complications, the experience of an ear, nose, and throat surgeon at the Timone University Medical Center in France was reviewed.

Methods.—A retrospective review was done of 1,192 endoscopic sinus surgical procedures, involving 386 patients, performed from May 1987 to December 1991. The ratio of males to females was 2:1, with a mean patient age of 40 years. The same right-handed surgeon performed all procedures using endoscopic guidance. The indications for endonasal surgery were mainly polyposis (62%) and chronic sinusitis (31%). The procedures included 501 middle meatal antrostomies, 391 total ethmoidectomies, 191 sphenoidotomies, 61 anterior ethmoidectomies, and 48 inferior meatal antrostomies. Previous surgery had been done on 109 patients in the group.

Findings.—Five serious complications occurred in the group, including 3 orbitopalpebral hematomas and 2 CSF leaks. No deaths were reported. These complications occurred in 1% of all patients and in less than 1% of the procedures surveyed. All complications occurred in patients undergoing anterior ethmoidal surgery for polyposis. In light of this, complications occurred in 2% of patients undergoing this procedure. All complications were seen on the right side of the patient. Three of the 5 patients with complications had undergone previous surgery.

Conclusions.—These results call attention to several areas requiring caution. Right-handed surgeons may have difficulty performing procedures on the right side of the patient. Previous surgery may interfere with significant landmarks, which may increase the risk of complications. Intraoperative caution is urged to detect damage to the lamina papyracea by applying pressure to the eyeball. Similarly, CSF leaks can be detected intraoperatively by compression of the jugular vein. The experience and skill level of the surgeon are also key variables in accounting for complication rates.

▶ This is not the first report to implicate right- or left-handedness as a factor in surgical complications. We know that 1 tonsil is usually easier to remove than another, that a certain side may be easier for mastoidectomies, and that we tend to favor elevating 1 side during a septoplasty. Just be aware of this potential.—G.R. Holt, M.D., F.A.C.S.

The Effect of Terfenadine on Unilateral Nasal Challenge With Allergen

Wagenmann M, Baroody FM, Kagey-Sobotka A, Lichtenstein LM, Naclerio RM (Johns Hopkins Univ, Baltimore, Md)
J Allergy Clin Immunol 93:594–605, 1994   130-95-8–10

Background.—The H_1 receptor antagonists are the most popular drugs used in the treatment of allergic rhinitis. The effect of the H_1 receptor antagonist, terfenadine, on nasal reflexes after antigen challenge was investigated to distinguish H_1-mediated events from other contributing factors.

Method.—In this double-blind, randomized trial, 12 patients with seasonal allergic rhinitis were given either placebo or 60 mg of terfenadine. Filter paper disks were used for the unilateral administration of allergen and the collection of nasal secretions. Secretion weights, histamine content of recovered nasal secretions, and nasal airway resistance (NAR) were examined for each nostril, and sneezes were counted.

Results.—Placebo treatment led to significant changes in ipsilateral and contralateral secretion weights, ipsilateral histamine levels, ipsilateral NAR, and sneezing. No elevation was seen in contralateral histamine levels. Patients treated with terfenadine had a marked reduction in the number of sneezes and a decrease in ipsilateral and contralateral secretion weights, without affecting the increase in NAR. Terfenadine was also seen to lower histamine concentrations in ipsilateral secretions after allergen challenge. Similar results were achieved when identical nasal challenges were carried out with a tenfold lower dose of antigen.

Conclusion.—Although past studies have indicated that terfenadine had no effect on methacholine provocation and abolished ipsilateral and contralateral secretion weights after histamine challenge, this study demonstrates that sneezing after allergen challenge is brought almost exclusively by a reflex initiated through H_1 receptors. Thus, it appears that H_1 antagonism does not influence allergen-induced increases in NAR. Unilateral allergen challenge leads to bilateral increases in secretion weights, which are only partially inhibited by terfenadine. Therefore, mediators other than histamine appear to be implicated in the nasonasal reflex. Finally, as has been seen previously, terfenadine also reduces allergen-induced histamine release after challenge with the highest dose of antigen.

▶ This article is informative because of its review of the complex interactions of neuronal reflexes, cellular responses, and transmembrane vascular and intracellular fluid movement in the allergic nasal response.—G.R. Holt, M.D., F.A.C.S.

Intranasal Flunisolide Spray as an Adjunct to Oral Antibiotic Therapy for Sinusitis

Meltzer EO, Orgel HA, Backhaus JW, Busse WW, Druce HM, Metzger WJ, Mitchell DQ, Selner JC, Shapiro GG, Van Bavel JH, Basch C (Univ of California, San Diego; San Diego Diagnostic Radiology Med Group, Calif; Univ of Wisconsin, Madison; et al)

J Allergy Clin Immunol 92:812–823, 1993   130-95-8–11

Background.—Sinusitis is a common medical condition and a significant cause of morbidity. Because inflammation and edema of the mucosa of the nasal turbinates and sinus ostia cause drainage obstruction, a topical intranasal steroid may promote drainage and increase aeration of the sinuses. The efficacy of intranasal flunisolide, used as an adjunct to antibiotic therapy in decreasing the symptoms caused by the inflammation of allergic rhinitis, was studied.

Method.—On entry into the study, patients with symptoms and signs of acute or chronic sinusitis underwent a physical examination, provided a mucosal specimen for cytologic examination, and had a positive Waters' view radiograph. They were then randomly assigned to receive 7 weeks of amoxicillin/clavulanate potassium, 500 mg, with either a flunisolide .025% nasal solution, 2 sprays in each nostril 3 times a day, or placebo spray 3 times a day (phase I), followed by administration of flunisolide or placebo nasal spray alone 3 times a day for 4 weeks (phase II). At the end of phase I and at end point, patients underwent clinical assessments, sinus radiographs, nasal cytologic studies, and laboratory tests.

Results.—A total of 175 patients were randomized to groups: 89 received flunisolide and 86 received placebo. At the end of phase I, significant decreases in all clinical parameters as compared with baseline were seen in both flunisolide and placebo treatment groups. There was a trend toward greater improvement in the flunisolide-treated patients, but only the decrease in turbinate swelling/obstruction was statistically significant at the end of phase I compared with the placebo. Overall, global assessment by patients of the efficacy of treatment was significantly higher in the group treated with flunisolide at the end of phase I ($P =$ .007) and after phase II (.08). Improvement was seen in maxillary sinus radiographs in both treatment groups during phase I, with a slightly greater regression of abnormal findings in the flunisolide group after phase II. However, 80% of the radiographs were still abnormal at the end of phase I. Patients treated with flunisolide had a significant decrease in nasal cytogram compared with the placebo group. Flare-up during phase II occurred in 26% of the patients treated with flunisolide and in 35% of the placebo group. No significant adverse effects were seen in either group.

Conclusion.—Treatment with flunisolide topical nasal spray as an adjunct to antibiotic therapy was seen to be the most effective treatment in global evaluation and tended to improve symptoms, decrease inflammatory cells in nasal cytograms, normalize ultrasound scans, and assist regression of radiographic abnormalities compared with placebo spray. This modality may be a useful adjunct to antibiotic therapy in some patients.

▶ I can understand the concomitant use of topical steroid spray and antibiotics in acute sinusitis associated with allergic rhinitis. However, I am not certain whether this combination should be used in all cases of acute sinusitis. Remember, too, that topical nasal steroids may decrease the local (and desirable) tissue response to the infection.—G.R. Holt, M.D., F.A.C.S.

Use of Sinus X Ray Films by General Practitioners
Houghton DJ, Aitchison FA, Wilkinson L, Wilson JA (Royal Infirmary, Glasgow, Scotland)
BMJ 308:1608–1609, 1994   130-95-8–12

Background.—Plain sinus radiography is not generally indicated in the routine management of sinusitis. This may be justified by the large radiation exposure involved and the presence of radiologic abnormalities of the sinus in up to half of the population. The prevailing use of x-ray film by general practitioners was assessed, and current practice in sinus examination in radiology departments in Scotland was analyzed.

Method.—A total of 694 general practitioners in Greater Glasgow were asked to respond to a questionnaire about their use and interpretation of sinus x-ray films. A survey was also made of the routine sinus x-ray views used in 50 hospitals throughout the United Kingdom.

Results.—Responses were received from 584 general practitioners. Of these, 136 (23%) claimed to never request sinus x-ray films. Most of the others requested an estimated 1–3 or 3–5 per year. The indications selected by the 448 regular users of x-ray films included persistent facial pain, frequent attacks of acute sinusitis, requests from patient, to exclude neoplasm, chronic postnasal drip, prolonged absence from work and chronic nasal problems in childhood. Most of the regular users of x-ray films believed that sinus radiography was occasionally (269) or always (116) indicated when a patient was referred to an otorhinolaryngology specialist. The 4 findings most likely to influence management were antral opacity, deviated nasal septum, frontal opacity, and nasal polyps. Half of the 50 radiology departments provided general practitioners with 1 occipitometrial view; the others used this with occipitofrontal, lateral, or both views. Eight departments provided more views for otolaryngologists than for general practitioners.

Conclusion.—The response to this survey indicates that more than three quarters of general practitioners use sinus radiography, with the most common indication being facial pain. However, the single view provided by 50% of the radiology departments adequately shows only 1 of the 4 main paranasal sinuses. The survey showed that most general practitioners are aware of the significance of hard findings, (e.g., deviated nasal septum and nasal polyps). Such symptoms are appropriately shown by anterior rhinoscopy, easily performed with an auroscope. Sinus radiology is of little benefit, and general practitioners should be advised to give a full trial of topical steroid treatment to patients with chronic, nonspecific rhinosinusitis. Those patients who fail to respond to this treatment or who are suspected of having a neoplasm, polyp, or other structural nasal abnormality should be referred for assessment by a specialist.

▶ Specialists have often been misrepresented as ordering too many unnecessary and expensive tests. However, primary care physicians may, in fact, order more tests for ear, nose, and throat disorders than we otolaryngologists might, given our knowledge and experience in history-taking and our physical examination capabilities.—G.R. Holt, M.D., F.A.C.S.

Impairment of Nasal Mucociliary Clearance During Bone Marrow Transplantation
Sisson JH, Reed EC, Robbins RA, Anderson JR, Ogren FP, Diamond JS, Rennard SI, and the University of Nebraska Medical Center Bone Marrow Transplantation Pulmonary Study Group (Univ of Nebraska, Omaha; Omaha Veterans Affairs Med Ctr, Nebraska)
Bone Marrow Transplant 13:631–633, 1994   130-95-8-13

Purpose.—Mucositis is a well-known complication of chemotherapy and ionizing radiation administered before bone marrow transplantation (BMT). It is not known whether nasal mucociliary function is also impaired during BMT. Nasal mucociliary clearance before, during, and after BMT was examined.

Patients.—Nasal mucociliary clearance was assessed by measuring the saccharin transit time (STT) 10 days before BMT through 30 days after BMT, or until the STT returned to baseline. Ten men and 3 women aged 30–56 years completed the study.

Results.—Twelve of the 13 patients (92%) had a prolonged nasal STT at some time during the peritransplant period. The number of patients with ineffective nasal clearance was largest during the 5-day period immediately after bone marrow infusion. The STT remained prolonged during the 2 weeks after marrow infusion and returned to baseline within 30 days after marrow infusion. Prolonged STT values correlated with the appearance of mucositis.

Conclusions.—Nasal mucociliary clearance is significantly impaired during BMT in the majority of patients. Impairment of nasal mucociliary function may well have a role in the increased risk of upper respiratory tract infections reported for patients who have undergone BMT.

▶ This study gives us a better understanding of another factor in the development of sinusitis and other infections in patients who have undergone BMT. We must be vigilant and vigorous in the prevention and treatment of infections.—G.R. Holt, M.D., F.A.C.S.

A Comparison of Packing Materials Used in Nasal Surgery

Garth RJN, Brightwell AP (Royal Devon and Exeter Hosp, England)
J Laryngol Otol 108:564–566, 1994   130-95-8–14

Background.—Nasal packing is commonly used after septal or turbinate nasal surgery. Although the choice of packing material available to the surgeon has widened in recent years, surgeons often use packing material based on habit or practice. Packing materials, their effectiveness, ease of use, and comfort were examined and compared.

Methods.—A randomized, prospective design was used. Eligible patients underwent elective septal and turbinate surgery. A total of 48 patients enrolled, 73% of whom were male and 27% of whom were female. Packing material was randomized, and each side of the nose was packed with a different material. Combinations of Telfa®, bismuth iodoform paraffin paste (BIPP), paraffin gauze, and Merocel® were used as nasal packs. Performance of each pack was assessed using 10-cm visual analogue scores. The patients assessed their level of discomfort while the pack was in situ and during removal. The staff assessed bleeding, both while the pack was in situ and upon removal; ease of removal was also assessed.

Findings.—There was no statistically significant difference in discomfort in situ. However, the difference was significant on removal, with a high discomfort score of 6.0 for Merocel. No significant difference was seen in bleeding in situ. However, a significant difference was seen during removal. Brisk bleeding was associated with Merocel. No statistical significance was found for difficulty of removal, but the Merocel tended to stick.

Conclusion.—When the packing material was removed from the nose, the difference in performance became apparent. The Telfa and paraffin gauze provided better patient comfort and less bleeding as well as greater ease of removal.

▶ Hooray again for Telfa® packs!—G.R. Holt, M.D., F.A.C.S.

Orbital Complications in Functional Endoscopic Sinus Surgery
Corey JP, Bumsted R, Panje W, Namon A (Univ of Chicago)
Otolaryngol Head Neck Surg 109:814–820, 1993   130-95-8–15

Background.—Functional endoscopic sinus surgery has become a popular part of otolaryngology head and neck surgery. The most feared complications of these procedures are retro-orbital hematoma and other orbital complications. A 3.5-year experience with orbital complications of endoscopic sinus procedures was presented.

Findings.—The analysis included 616 endoscopic sinus procedures performed by attending surgeons or senior residents. Seven patients experienced 8 orbital complications. There were 5 orbital hemorrhages, 2 medial rectus injuries, and 1 nasolacrimal duct injury. All but 1 patient apparently had important predisposing factors, including intraoperative or perioperative hypertension, extensive polypoid disease, previous surgery with scarring, dehiscences of the lamina papyracea, inability to visu-

1. The lamina papyracea lies superior to and not any more lateral to the natural ostia
2. Operate lateral to the middle turbinate, never medial
3. The antrostomy should be placed just above inferior turbinate, with the surgical instrument lying on top of the inferior turbinate
4. The antrostomy should not be made more anterior than the anterior end of the middle turbinate
5. The nasofrontal duct lies at 6.0 to 6.5 cm from the nasal opening
6. The anterior ethmoid artery and base of the skull (posterior-superior fovea ethmoidalis) is 7 cm from the nasal opening
7. The sphenoid sinus anterior wall is 7 cm from the nasal opening
8. The basal lamella of the middle turbinate is 6 cm from the nasal opening (posterior ethmoids lie behind this)
9. The nasopharyngeal wall approximates the posterior sphenoid wall to within 1 cm
10. Identify and cannulate the sphenoid ostia if possible. The posterior middle turbinate may need to be removed to do this because the ostia lies half way up the anterior wall from the choana, just next to the septum
11. The anterior wall of the sphenoid sinus lies at a plane between the superior inferior turbinate and the bottom of the middle turbinate
12. The antrostomy is at the level of the inferior orbital rim
13. If the middle turbinate has to be removed, remove only the inferior part of the turbinate using a scissors; preserve the superior part as an anatomic landmark

Fig 8–1.—Anatomy relationships to prevent complications. (Courtesy of Corey JP, Bumsted R, Panje W, et al: *Otolaryngol Head Neck Surg* 109:814–820, 1993.)

Orbital Complications

Mechanisms of injury

Direct:	"Biting" or directly pulling blood vessels, nerve tissue, periorbital fat, rectus or oblique muscles, or nasolacrimal duct through iotrogenic or disease-related dehiscences or holes with forceps, "backbiters," etc.
Indirect:	Pulling extensive amounts of diseased polyp tissue or thick, scarred tissue (such as in cases previously operated on)

(Courtesy of Corey JP, Bumsted R, Panje W, et al: *Otolaryngol Head Neck Surg* 109:814–820, 1993.)

alize the maxillary ostium, violent perioperative coughing or sneezing, and chronic steroid use.

Discussion.—Morbidity from endoscopic sinus surgery can be minimized by knowing the type and incidence of complications, recognizing their signs, and managing them when they occur. Knowing the normal anatomical relationships can help in avoiding nasolacrimal duct injury

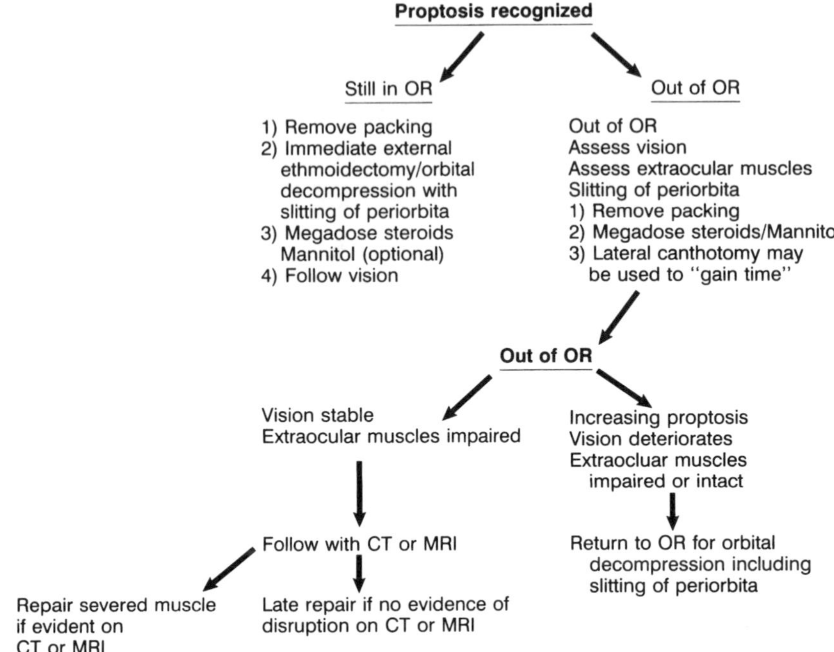

Fig 8–2.—Decision management tree for orbital proptosis, suspected retro-orbital hematoma, and suspected extraocular muscle damage. *Abbreviation:* OR, operating room. (Courtesy of Corey JP, Bumsted R, Panje W, et al: *Otolaryngol Head Neck Surg* 109:814–820, 1993.)

(Fig 8–1). Orbital complications can occur through both direct and indirect mechanisms (table), and may be noted during or after the operation. A decision-management tree for orbital proptosis, suspected retro-orbital hematoma, and suspected extraocular muscle damage (Fig 8–2) was developed.

▶ I encourage all endoscopic sinus surgeons, regardless of experience, to reread the important "predisposing factors" that these authors point out to us as warnings. No one can be too forewarned or fore-armed.—G.R. Holt, M.D., F.A.C.S.

Effect of Experimental Rhinovirus 39 Infection on the Nasal Response to Histamine and Cold Air Challenges in Allergic and Nonallergic Subjects

Doyle WJ, Skoner DP, Seroky JT, Fireman P, Gwaltney JM (Children's Hosp of Pittsburgh, Pa; Univ of Pittsburgh, Pa; Univ of Virginia, Charlottesville)
J Allergy Clin Immunol 93:534–542, 1994   130-95-8–16

Purpose.—Most studies suggest that individuals with allergic rhinitis (AR) have an increased magnitude of responses to intranasal histamine and methacholine challenge compared with nonallergic controls. These studies suggest that nasal responsiveness in subjects with seasonal AR varies over time, with greater responses occurring for challenges presented during and immediately after seasonal exposure to a relevant antigen. An attempt was made to clarify the altered responsiveness of the nose to intranasal challenge resulting from a rhinovirus-induced cold.

Methods.—The study sample comprised 20 subjects with seasonal AR and 18 nonallergic controls. All underwent paired intranasal histamine and cold air challenge sessions before and 8 to 13 days after experimental rhinovirus type 39 infection. Nasal responses were evaluated in terms of symptom scores for rhinorrhea and congestion, sneezing counts, weights of expelled secretions, and inspiratory conductance for nasal patency.

Results.—In both challenge sessions, the allergic subjects had a greater response than did the nonallergic subjects in terms of sneezing, symptoms of rhinorrhea and congestion, and secretion weights provoked by histamine. Secretion weights provoked by cold air challenge were also greater in the allergic group. On the paired challenge sessions performed after rhinovirus infection, the allergic subjects had greater sneezing, secretion weight, and rhinorrhea in response to histamine and greater secretion weight in response to cold air. The degree of enhanced responsiveness after viral infection was no different between the groups.

Conclusion.—Allergic and nonallergic individuals have increased nasal responsiveness to histamine and cold air challenge after rhinovirus infection. The increased responsiveness continues for a time even after subsistence of the priming stimulus, i.e., allergen exposure and rhinovirus infection in subjects with AR and rhinovirus infection in nonallergic subjects. The experimental model of inducing nasal hyperresponsiveness used in this study may be useful in evaluation of the various proposed mechanisms for modulation of nasal responsiveness.

▶ It was interesting to me that both allergic and nonallergic patients exhibited hyperresponsiveness of the nasal mucosa to histamine challenges after an upper respiratory tract infection (URI). Perhaps we should consider the use of a nonsedating antihistamine or a mast cell stabilizer for those patients with persistent nasal stuffiness after the other URI symptoms have abated.—G.R. Holt, M.D., F.A.C.S.

Bacteriology of Antrum in Adults With Chronic Maxillary Sinusitis

Erkan M, Aslan T, Özcan M, Koç N (Univ of Erciyes, Kayseri, Turkey)
Laryngoscope 104:321–324, 1994   130-95-8–17

Background.—A thorough understanding of the prevailing bacteriology is needed when treating patients with chronic maxillary sinusitis. The population of microorganisms in chronic maxillary sinusitis were identified when specimens were obtained, transported, and cultured by modern methods.

Patients and Findings.—A total of 126 patients aged 17–54 years were studied. Patients were seen over an 8-month period for complaints of chronic paranasal sinusitis. Swabs of the inflamed maxillary sinuses were obtained and processed for aerobic and anaerobic bacteria during endoscopy. Bacterial growth was noted in 113 of the 126 isolates. Anaerobic bacteria were isolated in 100 of the 113 cultures, accounting for the sole bacterial isolate in 59 instances. In the remaining 41 isolates, anaerobic bacteria were mixed with aerobic or facultative bacteria. Aerobic or facultative bacteria were present in 13 cases. A total of 323 bacterial isolates were recovered from the 113 culture-positive specimens. Of these, 228 isolates were anaerobes. In descending order of frequency, these included *Bacterioides* species, including *B. melaninogenicus* and *B. fragilis*, anaerobic cocci, *Propionibacterium acnes*, and *Fusobacterium* species. There were 95 aerobic or facultative anaerobic isolates. These included *Staphylococcus aureus*, group A β-hemolytic streptococci, α-hemolytic streptococci, and *Streptococcus pyogenes*, in descending order of frequency.

Conclusions.—Anaerobic organisms play an important role in chronic sinusitis. Successful treatment of maxillary sinusitis thus depends on the use of broad-spectrum antibiotics that include anaerobic bacteria. Persistent sinus inflammation and documented recurrent sinusitis with identifiable and related abnormalities in the osteomeatal complex may be considered indications for surgical intervention, the goal of which is to maintain physiologic function of the sinuses with as little destruction of normal sinus architecture and mucosa as possible.

▶ Sinus osteomeatal complex blockage leads to reduced oxygen tension in the sinuses and growth of anaerobic organisms. Effective drugs here might include Augmentin® (amoxicillin/clavulanate potassium), Flagyl® (metronidazole), and clindamycin, depending on your preference.—G.R. Holt, M.D., F.A.C.S.

9 Trauma and Reconstructive Surgery

A New Bilobed Design for the Sensate Radial Forearm Flap to Preserve Tongue Mobility Following Significant Glossectomy
Urken ML, Biller HF (The Mount Sinai Med Ctr, New York)
Arch Otolaryngol Head Neck Surg 120:26–31, 1994   130-95-9–1

Objective.—The preservation of tongue mobility and restoration of sensation are critical factors in oral rehabilitation. The radial forearm flap provides tissue that is thin, redundant, and pliable for reconstruction of the tongue. A new bilobed design of the sensate radial forearm flap is described that permits separation of the mobile tongue from the reconstructed floor of the mouth and the gingiva.

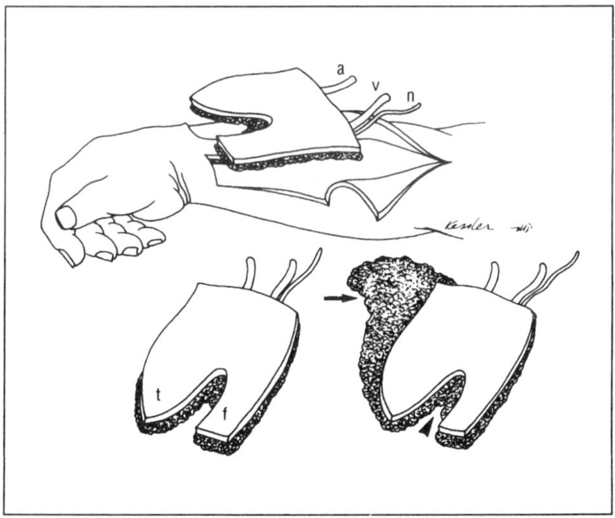

Fig 9–1.—Bilobed radial forearm free flap showing the radial artery (*a*), cephalic vein (*v*), and antebrachial cutaneous nerve (*n*). The proportions of the lobe used to reconstruct the tongue (*t*) and the lobe used for the floor of the mouth (*f*) will vary depending on the defect. Additional subcutaneous fat (*arrow*) may be harvested to provide bulk to the tongue base reconstruction. As the depth of the sulcus between the lobes is increased, a subcutaneous-fascial bridge may be preserved to enhance the vascularity to the lobe used to resurface the floor of the mouth (*arrowhead*). (Courtesy of Urken ML, Biller HF: *Arch Otolaryngol Head Neck Surg* 120:26–31, 1994.)

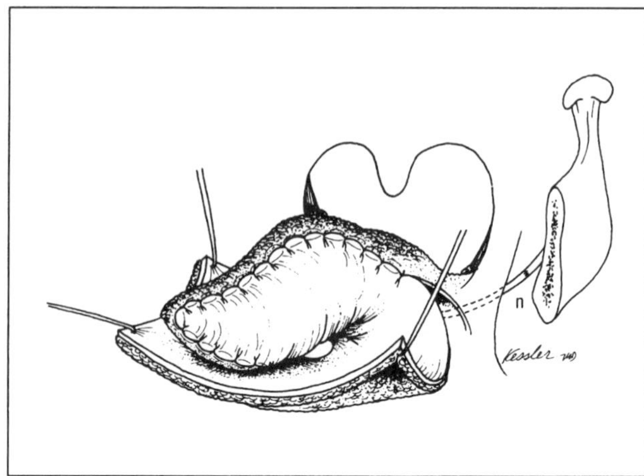

Fig 9–2.—Insetting of flap for reconstruction of the mobile tongue in a patient with a large defect of the floor of the mouth. The anastomosis of the antebrachial cutaneous nerve (*n*) to the lingual nerve is demonstrated. (Courtesy of Urken ML, Biller HF: *Arch Otolaryngol Head Neck Surg* 120:26–31, 1994.)

Technique.—The bilobed radial forearm free flap consists of 1 lobe used to restore the normal shape of the mobile tongue tip and a second lobe used to resurface the floor of the mouth and the gingiva (Fig 9–1). The depth of division between these 2 lobes varies with the defect. For longer separation between these lobes, a fascial subcutaneous bridge should be preserved to ensure adequate vascularity to both lobes. In defects that involve the tongue base, the length of the flap can be extended by raising skin flaps on the forearm in a subdermal plane, providing additional subcutaneous tissue to restore bulk to the neotongue. After insetting of the flap, microvascular anastomoses are performed, and the medial or lateral antebrachial cutaneous nerve is anastomosed to the lingual nerve (Fig 9–2). The lobe used to resurface the floor of the mouth and the gingiva should be fashioned with considerable redundancy to ensure that the mobile tongue is not tethered (Fig 9–3).

Outcome.—Ten patients who underwent significant glossectomy for squamous cell cancer underwent tongue reconstruction with the bilobed radial forearm free flap. All patients had at least one half of the mobile tongue resected, and a portion of the residual tongue had an intact motor supply. All 12 free flaps were successfully transferred without partial or total necrosis. All patients demonstrated mobile tongue tip, good articulation, and recovery of oral alimentation. The earliest recovery of sensation in the reinnervated forearm skin was 6 weeks. There were 2 donor site complications.

Conclusion.—For reconstruction of the oral cavity after significant glossectomy, the new bilobed radial forearm free flap provides a thin, pliable, and redundant tissue to preserve tongue mobility while prevent-

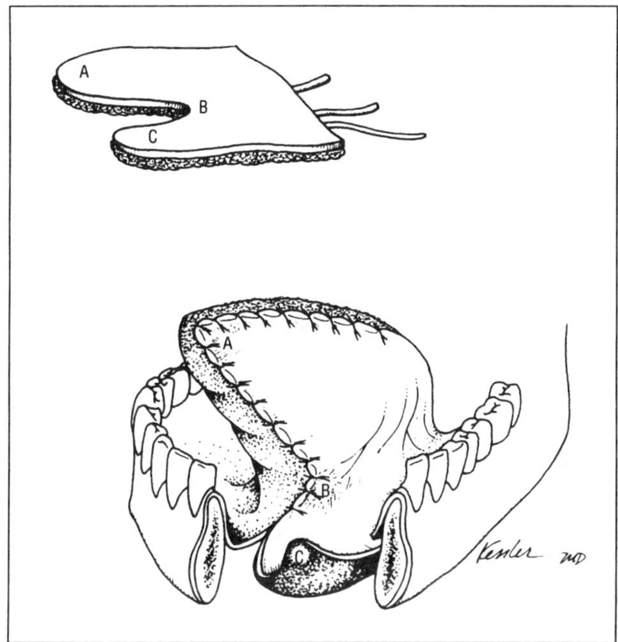

Fig 9–3.—Reconstruction of a hemiglossectomy defect with the bilobed flap. The separation of the floor of the mouth and the gingiva from the mobile tongue is reflected by the distance from points *B* to C. The redundancy of the lobe for the floor of the mouth enhances the tongue mobility and permits restoration of sulcular anatomy. (Courtesy of Urken ML, Biller HF: *Arch Otolaryngol Head Neck Surg* 120:26–31, 1994.)

ing tethering of the root of the tongue to the inner table of the mandible. Sensory re-education may improve functional sensation.

▶ These authors are leaders in oral reconstruction. They have devised what appears to be a very functional design for a free flap for tongue and floor-of-mouth reconstruction. Other flaps have not been tailored this nicely—excess bulk is designed "out" and "anatomical correctness" is designed "in."—G.R. Holt, M.D., F.A.C.S.

Use of Vicryl (Polyglactin–910) Mesh Implant for Repair of Orbital Floor Fracture Causing Diplopia: A Study of 28 Patients Over 5 Years

Mauriello JA Jr, Wasserman B, Kraut R (Univ of Medicine and Dentistry of New Jersey–New Jersey Med School, Newark)
Ophthal Plast Reconstr Surg 9:191–195, 1993   130-95-9–2

Introduction.—During a 5-year period, 28 patients underwent reconstruction of the orbital floor with Vicryl mesh (polyglactin-910) implants for significant preoperative diplopia resulting from entrapment of orbital tissues in the fracture site. Follow-up ranged from 1 month to 2 years.

Materials.—Vicryl mesh implants consist of 26.5- × 24-cm sheets, each of which is folded onto itself into 24 layers and packaged. The 24 layers are approximately 4 mm thick, and the sheet can be further folded onto itself to achieve greater thickness.

Methods.—The implant size and thickness is designed to prevent prolapse of tissue back into the fracture site and to avoid late enophthalmos. The implant is folded and cut to size depending on the depth of the defect and the surface area of orbital floor defect.

Outcome.—The implants varied in thickness from 5 to 56 layers. All but 1 patient showed objective and subjective improvement in motility, although 3 patients had only slight improvement in binocular field of vision. There were no late complications. Four patients had transient, low-grade eyelid inflammation, but none of the patients had acute infections that required implant removal.

Summary.—The layered Vicryl mesh is an excellent implant material for reconstruction of orbital floor fractures causing diplopia as a result of entrapment of orbital tissues in the fracture site. It is easily inserted and does not require fixation in the orbit. Vicryl mesh is soft and pliable and, therefore, is unlikely to compress orbital structures such as the optic nerve, extraocular muscles, and lacrimal sac. It is well tolerated by orbital tissues and absorbable; thus, it is unlikely to cause long-term complications such as infection, extrusion, or migration. Also, there is no risk of acquired infections associated with homologous tissue implants.

▶ We continue to seek the best implant material for orbital floor fractures. Silicone has been my personal choice over the years, but I have refrained from using that particular biomaterial recently. Gore-Tex® soft tissue sheeting is acceptable, and these authors tout the use of Vicryl® mesh, with good results reported.—G.R. Holt, M.D., F.A.C.S.

Preliminary Data on the Effect of Pharyngeal Flaps on the Upper Airway in Children With Velopharyngeal Inadequacy
Witsell DL, Drake AF, Warren DW (Univ of North Carolina, Chapel Hill)
Laryngoscope 104:12–15, 1994   130-95-9–3

Introduction.—The main surgical treatment for patients with velopharyngeal inadequacy caused by cleft palate, submucous cleft, or congenital velopharyngeal incompetence is the superiorly based pharyngeal flap. Although this procedure is generally safe and effective, some patients may have chronic nasal obstruction or obstructive sleep apnea develop. The changes in nasal airway size after the procedure were studied retrospectively.

Methods.—Pre- and postoperative data were analyzed for 7 children who underwent the superiorly based pharyngeal flap procedure. Measurements of the nasal airway size were obtained between 2 weeks and 5 months (average, 2.6 months) before the surgery and between 9 and 22 months (average, 13.5 months) after the surgery.

Results.—The cause of velopharyngeal inadequacy was unilateral complete cleft in 2 patients, occult submucous cleft in 2 patients, and bilateral complete cleft, unilateral incomplete cleft, and congenital velopharyngeal incompetence without cleft in 1 patient each. After adjusting the data for growth, 5 of the 7 patients had decreased nasal airway size after the surgery, which most affected the inspiratory phase of the breathing cycle. The nasal airway size increased in the other 2 patients.

Discussion.—These findings indicate that the effects of pharyngeal flaps on nasal airway size in children with velopharyngeal inadequacy are variable. Decreases are generally seen, but they are relatively slight and have a greater effect on inspiration than expiration, suggesting that the primary nasal deformities have already impaired the nasal airways. Some patients, however, may experience increased nasal airways. More long-term study of pre- and postoperative pressure-flow changes is necessary.

▶ Although this was a small series, the authors have gathered data that provide them with a sense of the complexity involved with the upper airway in patients with velopharyngeal insufficiency. Abnormal nasal airflow surely plays a role and must be adequately evaluated both pre- and postoperatively.—G.R. Holt, M.D., F.A.C.S.

Indications for the AO Plate With a Myocutaneous Flap Instead of Revascularized Tissue Transfer for Mandibular Reconstruction
Disher MJ, Esclamado RM, Sullivan MJ (Univ of Michigan, Ann Arbor; Ohio State Univ, Columbus)
Laryngoscope 103:1264–1268, 1993   130-95-9-4

Introduction.—For patients with full-thickness mandibular resection defects, the goals of reconstruction are to restore function and appearance while minimizing complications and morbidity. For this indication, reconstructing the mandible using a revascularized osseomyocutaneous flap is preferred. However, for dentulous patients with small lateral defects, they prefer the Arbeitsgemeinschaft furs Osteosynthesefragen (AO) mandibular reconstruction plate (MRP), which offers a quick, reliable replacement with no need for a donor site or advanced technical training. The results of primary AO MRP reconstruction in 16 patients were reported.

Patients.—All patients were dentulous and needed segment resection of the mandible for oncologic margins. The indications for AO MRP reconstruction included an expected lateral defect of less than 6 cm and the desire to maintain occlusion for functional reasons. Patients thought to be at especially poor risk for a lengthy reconstructive procedure were also considered for an AO MRP. The 16 patients were followed up for an average of 32 months after AO MRP reconstruction with no bone graft.

Outcomes.—The reconstruction was successful in 12 patients, who had long-term retention of the MRP. The overall complication rate was 38%, with 5 patients requiring a second or more operations. Four of the complications were serious and resulted in failure of the MRP reconstruction. The reasons for these failures involved exposure of the MRP in 3 cases and infection in 1. The mandibular defects ranged in size from 3 to 10 cm; this factor was not correlated with the type or rate of complications. For three fourths of the patients overall, rehabilitation was limited by disease progression.

Conclusions.—For certain patients requiring primary mandibular reconstruction, an AO MRP and a myocutaneous flap without a bone graft is a viable alternative. This procedure is appropriate in patients with small lateral mandibular defects, useful dentition, and advanced disease. It is also an alternative in patients who are judged too ill to withstand prolonged general anesthesia. Disease progression is the most important factor in the success of this technique.

▶ This seems to be a very reasonable approach to the small defect occurring in a dentulous mandible. However, bone graft reconstruction carries the potential for the subsequent implantation of osseointegrated teeth, which, in the long term, would be functionally superior than the use of an MRP.—G.R. Holt, M.D., F.A.C.S.

Endoscopic Laser Dacryocystorhinostomy
Metson R, Woog JJ, Puliafito CA (Massachusetts Eye & Ear Infirmary, Boston; Harvard Med School, Boston; Ctr for Eye Research, Boston; et al)
Laryngoscope 104:269–274, 1994   130-95-9–5

Introduction.—The surgical procedure of choice for opening obstructed lacrimal sacs has been external dacryocystorhinostomy (DCR) because of the difficulty visualizing and accessing the operative site using an intranasal approach. Forty-six endoscopic DCR procedures to relieve lacrimal obstruction were performed on 40 patients using a holmium:yttrium aluminum garnet (YAG) laser.

Technique.—A video camera attached to the endoscope is used throughout. A 20-gauge fiberoptic light probe is passed through a canaliculus into the lacrimal sac, transilluminating the lateral nasal wall to locate the lacrimal sac (Fig 9–4). The laser fiber is directed at the lateral nasal wall to vaporize approximately a 1-cm circle of mucosa, and the underlying bone is vaporized similarly. A suction-irrigation handpiece is used to maintain visualization. Penetration of the uncinate

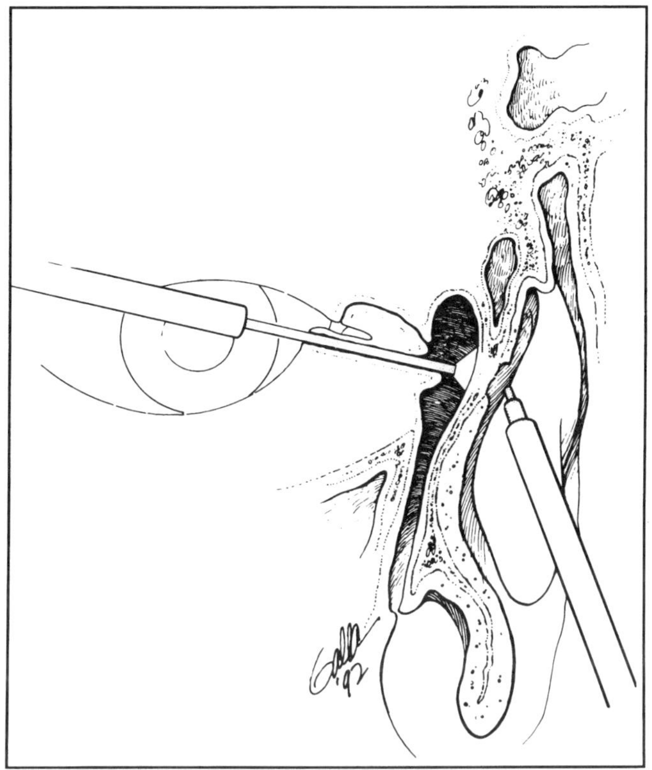

Fig 9–4.—The endoscopic approach to the lacrimal sac is shown in this frontal section through the right nasal cavity. A fiberoptic light probe is passed through a canaliculus into the lacrimal sac. Transillumination of the lateral nasal wall guides laser removal of mucosa and bone overlying the lacrimal sac. (Courtesy of Metson R, Woog JJ, Puliafito CA: *Laryngoscope* 104:269–274, 1994.)

process allows entry into an air space overlying the lacrimal sac. The lacrimal bone is opened and the medial wall of the lacrimal sac is exposed. Maxillary bone forming the anterior aspect of the lacrimal fossa is removed, exposing the medial sac wall so that the sac can be enlarged to a diameter of 5 to 10 cm. Stents attached to Silastic® tubing are passed through the superior and inferior canaliculi (Fig 9–5). Tubing ends are tied and left for 2 to 6 months during postoperative healing.

Results.—There were no complications. Lacrimal duct obstruction was successfully relieved in 34 of 40 patients (85%), with gradual closure of the surgical ostium in 5 of 6 patients with failed surgery. The revision procedure was unsuccessful for 4 of 5 patients in the failed group.

Conclusion.—The endoscopic laser DCR failure rate of 15%, compared with a 3% to 15% failure rate for external DCR, will probably decrease as practitioners become more experienced. The holmium:YAG laser is a likely choice for endoscopic laser DCR and has the potential to

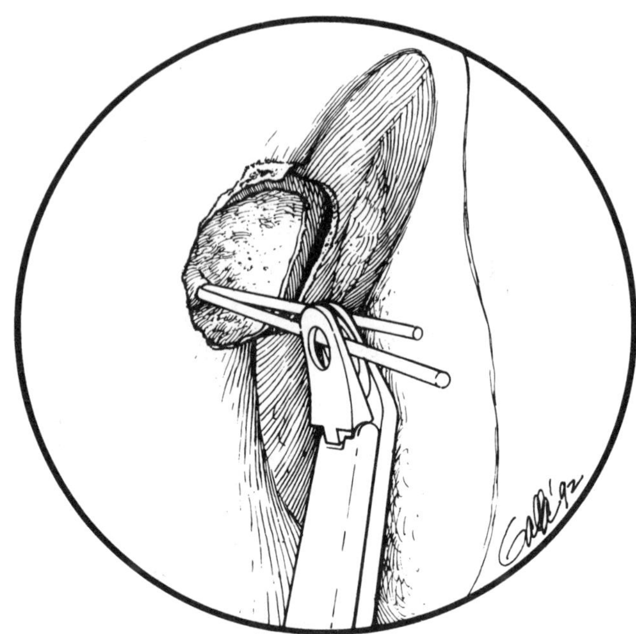

Fig 9–5.—Lacrimal probes threaded with Silastic® tubing are passed through the canaliculi, grasped with forceps, directed out of the nasal cavity, trimmed, and tied. Note the location of the internal common punctum where the catheters enter the sac interior. (Courtesy of Metson R, Woog JJ, Puliafito CA: *Laryngoscope* 104:269–274, 1994.)

decrease morbidity and eliminate the need for external incision. Further study is needed to establish the long-term efficacy of this method.

▶ Those of us who are not accomplished endoscopic sinus surgeons will have to use the proven external approach. For others, this will seem like an exciting technique that will clearly be helpful when other nasal and sinus diseases need attention.—G.R. Holt, M.D., F.A.C.S.

Expanded Unilateral Forehead Flap (Sail Flap) for Coverage of Opposite Forehead Defect

Iwahira Y, Maruyama Y (Toho Univ Hosp, Tokyo)
Plast Reconstr Surg 92:1052–1056, 1993   130-95-9–6

Background.—Simple coverage of facial skin defects is difficult from a cosmetic point of view. Tissue expansion combined with a unilateral forehead flap was used to reconstruct contralateral forehead defects.

Technique.—A skin expander with an exterior valve is implanted subcutaneously at the intact unilateral forehead area (Fig 9-6). The size of the expander should conform to the size of the forehead defect. The skin expander is filled

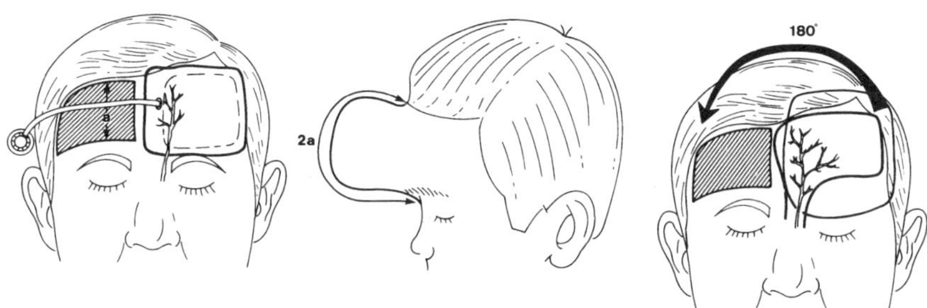

Fig 9–6.—**Left,** tissue expander is placed at unilateral forehead area subcutaneously. **Center,** expansion has been reached at twice the size of the forehead. **Right,** sail flap is elevated and rotated to the contralateral forehead defect with the pedicle, which includes the supratrochlear vessels. (Courtesy of Iwahira Y, Maruyama Y: *Plast Reconstr Surg* 92:1052–1056, 1993.)

with saline solution over time until the needed amount of skin becomes available. The expanded forehead flap is designed horizontally. After elevation, the flap is rotated 180 degrees with the pedicle, which includes the supratrochlear vessels, to cover the contralateral forehead defect. The donor site is closed primarily. The scar is hidden in the hairline.

Patients.—Five patients with unilateral forehead defects were treated according to the new technique. Total volume of the expanders ranged from 140 to 480 mL. The cosmetic outcome was excellent. Four patients had no complications. One patient had some superficial necrosis.

Conclusions.—The expanded unilateral forehead flap, also called a sail flap, gives excellent coverage of a contralateral defect of the forehead.

▶ What nice results were achieved in these forehead reconstructions! I especially liked the design that placed the donor suture line in the hairline.—G.R. Holt, M.D., F.A.C.S.

The Platysma Myocutaneous Flap: Indications and Caveats

Esclamado RM, Burkey BB, Carroll WR, Bradford CR (Univ of Michigan, Ann Arbor; Vanderbilt Univ, Nashville, Tenn)
Arch Otolaryngol Head Neck Surg 120:32–35, 1994   130-95-9–7

Background.—The use of the platysma myocutaneous flap to reconstruct defects of the floor of the mouth has seen limited popularity, despite its versatility, dependability, and ease of harvesting. Platysma flap reconstruction was studied in a group of 12 patients, and its role in the reconstructive armamentarium was defined.

Patients.—Twelve patients who were undergoing ablative resection of carcinoma of the oral cavity and oropharynx and reconstruction with a platysma myocutaneous flap participated in the study.

Technique.—To maximize flap viability, a U-shaped flap is designed as low in the neck as possible to increase the arc of flap rotation. The skin and platysma muscle are sharply elevated in the subplatysmal plane to allow for exposure to the neck. The ablation procedure is done, preserving the sternocleidomastoid muscle and facial artery when possible. The entire flap is turned into the defect. The neck flap is repositioned in the neck, and the skin island is designed to overlie the platysma muscle. The superior skin incision is then made through skin only and is elevated from the platysma muscle in the plane between the subcutaneous fat and the superficial cervical fascia to the level of the inferior border of the mandible. The flap is then rotated into the defect.

Results.—The overall flap survival was 92%. The common facial artery was lost in 3 patients, with flap survival occurring in each case. An exposed mandible was covered in 9 of the 12 patients, and the remaining 3 required thin soft tissue to close the surgical defect adequately. Three complications were directly related to the platysma myocutaneous flap: there was 1 skin paddle loss, but no pharyngocutaneous fistula as the underlying platysma muscle survived and granulated; 1 delayed pharyngocutaneous fistula presented 1 week after oral feeding but closed within 1 week; and 1 neck cellulitis developed that was resolved with antibiotic therapy.

Conclusion.—In this study, the platysma myocutaneous flap was shown to be highly reliable, with a 92% survival rate. For this level of success to be achieved, patients must be carefully evaluated and selected preoperatively. The method is ideal when reconstructive requirements demand soft tissue coverage of bare bone and restoration of the lingual and/or buccal sulcus to maintain full tongue mobility. The limitations of the platysma myocutaneous flap are its lack of bulk, limited skin availability, and lack of sensation. Therefore, it is less useful in cases where restoration of bulk is required, particularly in large tongue defects.

▶ Even though we are aware of the flap's limitations and its narrow range of indications, it is good to have it available for use in selected cases.—G.R. Holt, M.D., F.A.C.S.

Blindness After Maxillofacial Blunt Trauma: Evaluation of Candidates for Optic Nerve Decompression Surgery

Kallela I, Hyrkäs T, Paukku P, Iizuka T, Lindqvist C (Helsinki Univ Central Hosp, Finland)
J Craniomaxillofac Surg 22:220–225, 1994   130-95-9–8

Introduction.—Optic nerve blindness occurring in 1 or both eyes after severe midfacial trauma is difficult to diagnose and treat. Surgical decompression of the optic nerve is sometimes performed, but the results have been disappointing. Patients with post-traumatic loss of vision who could benefit from optic nerve decompression surgery were identified.

Patients.—Of 614 patients treated for midfacial fractures during a 5-year period, 10 (1.6%) had post-traumatic optic nerve blindness in 14 eyes. Four patients had loss of vision in both eyes. Four patients had isolated zygomatic fractures, and 6 had Le Fort fractures. Most patients had been involved in traffic accidents. All patients underwent plain radiography and CT before open reduction and miniplate fixation. Only 2 patients had optic nerve decompression.

Results.—All affected eyes had severe edema and ecchymosis of the periorbital region, with subconjunctival hemorrhage and chemosis. Computed tomographic scans showed involvement of the optic nerve in 11 eyes (80%). Three eyes with clinical evidence of optic nerve damage had normal CT scans. Swelling of the optic nerve was seen on the scans of 9 eyes. Only the 2 patients with gradual visual deterioration might have benefited from optic nerve decompression. The critical condition of 6 patients precluded immediate decompression surgery. However, even if the decompression surgery could have been done immediately after the accident, these patients would still have had a poor prognosis for a return of vision.

Conclusions.—Few patients with post-traumatic optic nerve blindness benefit from decompression surgery. Those with gradual loss of vision appear to be most likely to benefit from optic nerve decompression surgery.

▶ The National Eye Institute recently (and prematurely) closed out a study on optic nerve decompression because of poor results. It sounds as if we should be very careful about considering this therapy.—G.R. Holt, M.D., F.A.C.S.

The Self-Lined Superiorly Based Pull-Through Velopharyngoplasty: Plastic Surgery-Speech Pathology Interaction in the Management of Velopharyngeal Insufficiency

Johns DF, Cannito MP, Rohrich RJ, Tebbetts JB (Univ of Texas Southwestern, Dallas; Univ of Memphis, Tenn)
Plast Reconstr Surg 94:436–445, 1994   130-95-9–9

Background.—A newly developed surgical technique designed to overcome velopharyngeal insufficiency was described. Surgical intervention for this problem aims to provide a physiologic valving mechanism that yields a qualitative and quantifiable improvement in functional speech. A self-lined, superiorly based pull-through velopharyngoplasty was developed as a method for flap attachment that limits interpalatal dissection. The technique has been used in more than 150 patients during the past 12 years. Patients ranged in age from 3 to 56 years and had a variety of causes of velopharyngeal insufficiency.

Surgical Technique.—Preoperative videofluoroscopic views are obtained to determine the desired width of a superiorly based posterior pharyngeal flap. The flap is elevated using insulated-tip pinpoint electrocautery dissection in the prevertebral fascial plane. Blood loss is limited and visibility is enhanced by this method of dissection. A transverse full-thickness incision is made in the posterior aspect of the velum. The width of the slit is equal to that of the pharyngeal flap. The extreme distal portion of the uvula is transected, and the oral side of the velum is demucosalized posterior to the slit. Sutures are placed at the lateral aspect of the flap, and the proper level of attachment is determined by gently grasping the edge of the slit and moving the velum posteriorly and cephalad. The flap is folded on itself, providing full-thickness myomucosal lining. A superficial mucosal incision is made on the pharyngeal flap at the point where it passes through the palatal slit. To prevent fistula formation, the oral and nasal demucosalized raw surfaces of the flap and the velum are approximated with horizontal mattress sutures. Additional traction is placed on the flap during suturing to assure that it is under adequate tension.

Results and Conclusion.—Estimated blood loss averaged less than 10 mL, and the average operating time was 72 minutes. Fistula formation was reduced by superficial demucosalization of the flap at the site of the pull-through. Patients have scored well on measures of hypernasal resonance, nasal emission, and intelligibility. In general, the more severe the initial disorder, the greater the benefit of surgery. Postsurgical speech outcomes were better after the self-lined, pull-through procedure than after treatment with other types of pharyngeal flaps. In addition to significantly improving speech, the new technique has low complication and reoperation rates and maintains the anatomical integrity and physiologic function of the velar musculature.

▶ My only suggestion regarding surgical procedures for velopharyngeal insufficiency is that, during the procedure, it is helpful to look periodically at the nasopharynx from the nasal side using an endoscope to assess the closure from the perspective of our normal observation route.—G.R. Holt, M.D., F.A.C.S.

Mandibular Reconstruction With Osseointegrated Implants Into the Free Vascularized Radius
Mounsey RA, Boyd JB (The Toronto Hosp, Canada; Cleveland Clinic Florida, Ft Lauderdale)
Plast Reconstr Surg 94:457–464, 1994   130-95-9–10

Introduction.—It is often difficult to achieve complete oral rehabilitation after reconstruction of mandibular defects. Sixty-eight mandibular reconstructions were performed using the free vascularized radius during a 5-year period. The 4 patients described here underwent placement of

Patient	Reconstruction	Implants	Follow-up	Complications
1	6 × 4 cm skin 10-cm bone	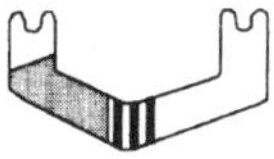	4 years	None
2	4 × 4 cm skin 12-cm bone (osteotomized to recreate contour)	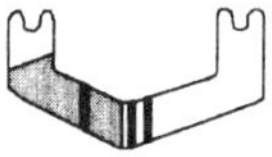	3 years	Hypertrophic granulations
3	5 × 4 cm skin 10-cm bone (osteotomized to recreate contour)	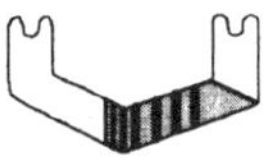	4 years	None
4	5 × 8 cm skin 9-cm bone	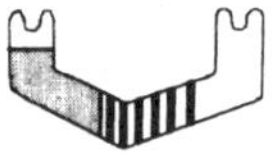	4 years	Loosening of implants; osteoradionecrosis of the mandible

Fig 9–7.—Details of reconstruction. (Courtesy of Mounsey RA, Boyd JB: *Plast Reconstr Surg* 94:457–464, 1994.)

osseointegrated implants after mandibular reconstruction with the free radial forearm flap.

Technique.—The radial forearm skin is transferred with or without bone, based upon the need for oral lining or skin replacement at the mandibular defect. The first phase of osseointegration is started 3 months after the initial defect is repaired and healing is complete. Titanium screw implants are placed into the bone using a low-speed drill. A cap is placed on the implant and the entire unit is covered with mucosa. Six to 12 months later, when bony ingrowth into the titanium screw is complete, the implant is uncovered for placement of an abutment that provides the link between the denture and the implant. Mucosal healing should occur by 4 weeks, when the denture is fitted by a prosthodontist.

Results.—The patient group included a 48-year-old woman and 3 men, ages 42, 29, and 48. Abnormalities resulted from recurrent ameloblastoma, gunshot blast (2 cases), and squamous cell carcinoma. The first patient has been followed up for 4 years and is satisfied with the procedure, both in terms of oral rehabilitation and cosmesis. She is able to chew and speak normally. Patients 2 and 3, both with gunshot wounds, have also had a satisfactory outcome; speech is normal or nearly normal and both can eat a regular diet. Hypertrophic granulation tissue complicated the second case, but the tissue was excised surgically and the procedure was completed. The fourth patient did well for a year, then experienced implant loosening and loss. Radiation damage to the mandible was thought to have made the bone susceptible to the microtrauma of mastication in this patient (Fig 9–7).

Conclusion.—The radius provides a good alternative to the free vascularized iliac crest for reconstruction of small-to-moderate lateral mandibular defects that require oral lining. Osseointegration can be performed successfully using the radial forearm flap, and implants can be placed directly into the free radius or into adjacent bone.

▶ Our own experience with osseointegrated implants in free and vascularized bone has been excellent. This technology has proved to be a winner!—G.R. Holt, M.D., F.A.C.S.

Surgical Treatment of Cleft Palate: 27 Years' Experience of the Wardill-Kilner Technique

Elander A, Lilja J, Friede H, Persson E-C, Lohmander-Agerskov A, Söderpalm E (Univ of Göteborg, Sweden)
Scand J Plast Reconstr Hand Surg 27:291–295, 1993   130-95-9–11

Purpose.—From 1958 to 1985, the Wardill-Kilner technique was used for the treatment of isolated cleft palate. In 1986, a new technique of soft palate closure at 6 months of age and residual cleft closure at 4 years of age was begun in an attempt to improve palatal growth and occlusion in patients with isolated cleft palate. To provide data for comparison with the new technique, the 27-year experience with the Wardill-Kilner technique was reviewed.

Patients.—The review included 230 patients with cleft palate who who underwent at a mean age of 13 months. In each case, the operation followed a modification of the push-back technique described by Wardill and Kilner (Fig 9–8). The cleft affected both the soft and hard palates in 47% of the patients and the soft palate only in 53%.

Outcomes.—Eight percent of the patients experienced postoperative dehiscences and fistulae. Dehiscence was more common in patients with clefts involving both the hard and soft palates than in those with soft palate cleft alone, 14% vs. 2%, respectively. Four percent of the patients required reoperation because of dehiscence, and 11 percent required palatopharyngeal flaps because of speech problems. Overall,15% of the patients underwent reoperation. The results improved in the latter part of the series.

Conclusions.—The Wardill-Kilner technique is a safe method of palatal closure that has comparatively low morbidity. Dehiscence is a more common complication when the cleft affects both the hard and soft palates, perhaps because of the difficulty of releasing tension in the border area between the hard and soft palates.

▶ In this technique, the Z-plasty of the nasal mucoperiosteum may help alleviate the discrepancy in tissue lengths with a push-back between the oral and nasal sides—perhaps improving high pharyngeal closure.—G.R. Holt, M.D., F.A.C.S.

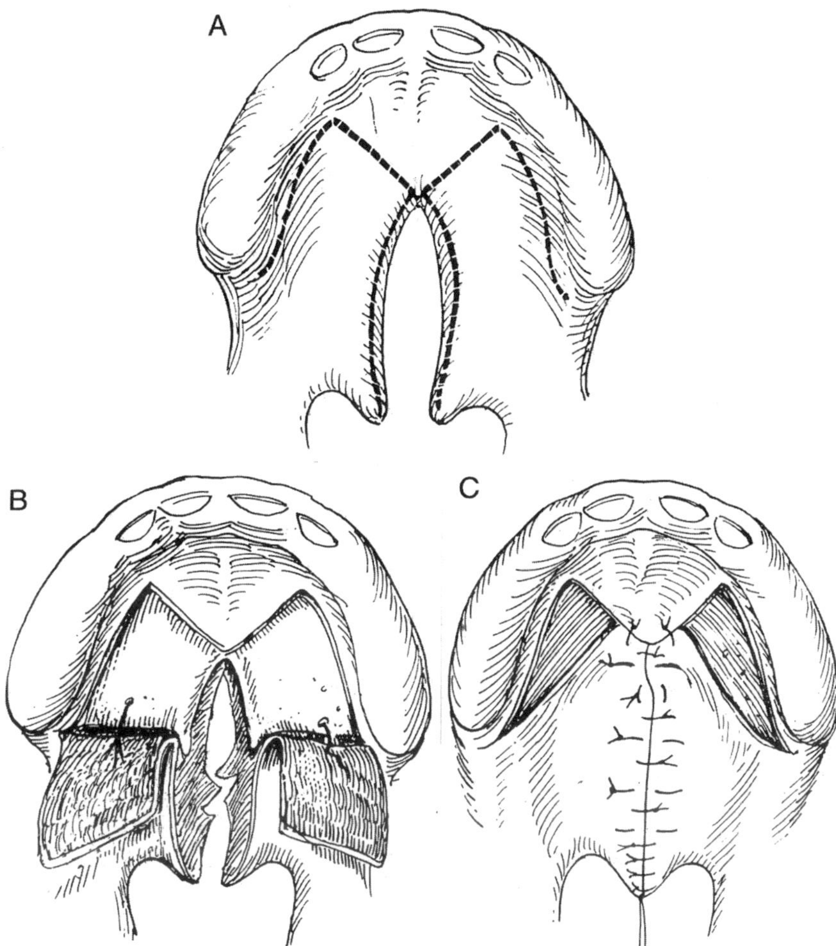

Fig 9–8.—Diagram of modification of the Wardill-Kilner technique for closure of palatal clefts. **A,** incision lines. **B,** mucoperiosteal flaps raised. Note lengthening of the nasal layer with a Z-plasty. **C,** oral layer closed. Lengthening of the oral layer is accomplished by a V–Y procedure in the anterior part. The bone is not covered by mucoperiosteum in the anterolateral part of the palate but is left to heal secondarily. (Courtesy of Elander A, Lilja J, Friede H, et al: *Scand J Plast Reconstr Hand Surg* 27:291–295, 1993.)

A Single Center's Experience With 308 Free Flaps for Repair of Head and Neck Cancer Defects

Schusterman MA, Miller MJ, Reece GP, Kroll SS, Marchi M, Goepfert H (Univ of Texas MD Anderson Cancer Ctr, Houston)
Plast Reconstr Surg 93:472–478, 1994

130-95-9–12

Introduction.—The aggressive nature of head and neck cancers often necessitates radical, and usually disfiguring, surgery. Simultaneous, reliable reconstructive surgery is important for restoring the patient's quality of life. The reliability of microvascular free flap transfer in reconstructive surgery of the head and neck was reported.

Methods.—The study prospectively examined 308 free flap procedures performed from May 1988 through February 1992 at the University of Texas M.D. Anderson Cancer Center.

Results.—A total of 86% of flap procedures were performed at the time of the original surgery. Most of the patients were white male smokers who consumed alcohol. Most resections were the result of squamous cell carcinoma; most tumors were T3, T4, or recurrent; and most flaps were from the radial forearm. The average patient was followed for 14 months, and 206 were alive at the last follow-up. The complication rate was 36%, with a venous thrombosis rate of 7%, a flap loss rate of 6%, and a flap salvage rate of 19%. Previous surgery and vein graft were significantly associated with flap loss.

Conclusion.—Microvascular surgery has improved the outcome of reconstructive surgery. Although the overall complication rate was 36%, only previous surgery and vein grafting increased the flap loss rate.

▶ A flap loss rate of 6% is very good. As more communities develop microvascular capabilities, microvascular flap use should increase. However, for the nonmicrovascular surgeon, this use of musculocutaneous flaps remains a viable alternative.—G.R. Holt, M.D., F.A.C.S.

Patient Fire Safety in the Operating Room

Chang BW, Petty P, Manson PN (Johns Hopkins School of Medicine, Baltimore, Md; Mayo Clinic and Found, Rochester, Minn)
Plast Reconstr Surg 93:519–521, 1994   130-95-9–13

Objective.—Each year in the United States, approximately 20–30 "patient fires" (fires erupting on a patient) occur during an operative procedure. Two cases were described.

Patients.—The first patient underwent excision of basal cell cancer of the left superior eyebrow under local anesthesia. A nasal cannula was placed, and towel drapes were placed over the nose and around the upper face and forehead. The second patient underwent a nasolabial flap for reconstruction of a defect resulting from excision of a basal cell carcinoma of the right alar region. A nasal cannula was placed in the mouth, but the drapes were placed beneath the chin. In both procedures, oxygen was used during the initial sedation and turned off. During cautery, a spark was produced and caused immediate flames. Both patients sustained first- or second-degree burns of the face. All burned areas healed uneventfully.

Discussion.—Patient fire occurs in the presence of 3 components: heat, fuel, and an oxidizer. Potential heat sources in the operating room include the electrocautery unit, lasers, overhead lights, fiberoptics, drills, and burrs. Fuel is abundant in the operating room, and includes drapes, hair, plastic oxygen tubing, aerosolized alcohol preparatory solutions, benzoin, Steri-Strips, and gastrointestinal tract gases. In any atmosphere oxygen-enriched above 21%, fuel sources will burn easily and will be harder to extinguish. Another source of oxygen is the thermal decomposition of nitrous oxide. Even cloth drapes can absorb and retain oxygen. The key to prevention of a patient fire is to disrupt any 1 of the 3 components.

▶ This has happened to me in the past. At first, I thought the electrocautery unit had shorted, but that was not the case. We now use only room air in any local surgical procedure in which electrocautery is necessary.—G.R. Holt, M.D., F.A.C.S.

10 Facial Plastic Surgery

Transconjunctival Approach to Lower Eyelid Blepharoplasty: Experience, Indications, and Technique in 300 Patients
Perkins SW, Dyer WK II, Simo F (Indiana Univ, Indianapolis; Emory Univ, Atlanta, Ga; St Louis Univ, Mo)
Arch Otolaryngol Head Neck Surg 120:172–177, 1994   130-95-10–1

Introduction.—The transconjunctival approach to lower lid blepharoplasty is not a new technique, but not much has been reported on this method. Transconjunctival blepharoplasty is ideal for young patients (15 to 30 years old) with familial pseudoherniation of orbital fat, as well as for older patients (30 to 50 years) with pseudoherniation of orbital fat but no true excess skin. The technique can be combined with a lower eyelid chemical peel to remove mild dermatochalasis and/or superficial rhytids. It is also very effective for revision or secondary blepharoplasty. Relative indications for transconjunctival blepharoplasty include patients

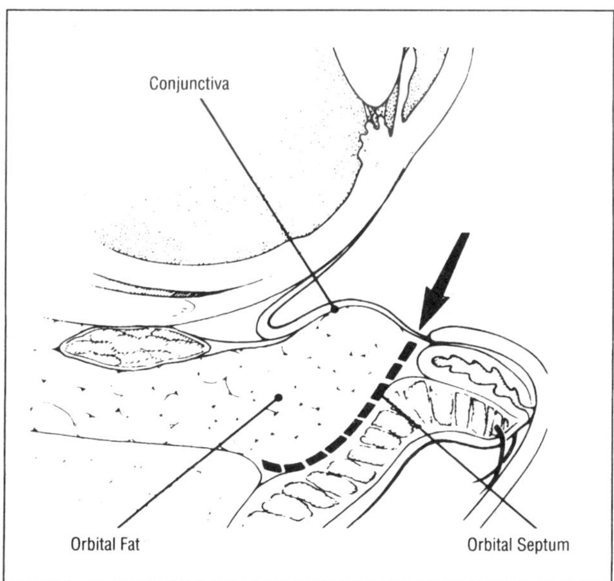

Fig 10–1.—Cross-sectional drawing of the anatomical structure of the orbit and lower eyelid, showing the conjunctival incision and approach to orbital fat between the orbital septum and orbicular muscle. (Courtesy of Perkins SW, Dyer WK, Simo F: *Arch Otolaryngol Head Neck Surg* 120:172–177, 1994.)

who specifically request no external scar, dark-skinned patients, and those with relative ptosis and scleral show or lateral rounding.

Technique.—The transconjunctival approach to lower lid blepharoplasty involves an incision through the conjunctiva and inferior retractor muscles, separation of the orbicularis muscle from the orbital septum, and anterior approach to the orbital septum (Fig 10–1). Closure is achieved by elevating the eyelid into position; no sutures are used. Associated adjunctive procedures include the "pinch technique" to remove redundant lower eyelid skin, and simultaneous chemical peeling for dermatochalasis, hyperpigmentation, and herniated orbital fat.

Outcome.—Results of 300 consecutive blepharoplasties performed with the transconjunctival approach were reviewed and all patients had satisfactory healing. Compared with 300 consecutive blepharoplasties performed with the standard skin-muscle flap transcutaneous approach, transconjunctival blepharoplasty was associated with significantly reduced short- and long-term complications. In the skin-muscle flap approach group, 32% had lower eyelid retraction that required massage or injection of an intralesional steroid, and 5% had lateral rounding. In contrast, none of the patients in the transconjunctival group required massage or intralesional steroids or had lateral rounding, and only 2% had friable granulation tissue at the conjunctival incision that required direct removal and superficial cauterization.

Conclusion.—For removal of the pseudoherniation of orbital fat of the lower eyelid, transconjunctival blepharoplasty should have a significant place in the surgical armamentarium of the facial plastic surgeon. The addition of the pinch technique and/or lower eyelid chemical peel provides complete results that patients desire.

▶ I believe this technique is indicated in the majority of patients with mild-to-moderate dermatochalasia and fat herniation. Some other technique must be used to remove excess skin. Watch the inferior rectus and inferior oblique muscles! For more senile eyelids, a lateral canthal resection and tightening can be performed on a lax lid.—G.R. Holt, M.D., F.A.C.S.

Vertical Dome Division in Open Rhinoplasty: An Update on Indications, Techniques, and Results

Adamson PA, McGraw-Wall BL, Morrow TA, Constantinides MS (Univ of Toronto)
Arch Otolaryngol Head Neck Surg 120:373–380, 1994   130-95-10–2

Objective.—Goldman's vertical dome division (VDD) is a useful adjunctive technique for refinement of the nasal tip. However, the procedure remains controversial because postoperative tip abnormalities have been reported. Experience with a modification of the VDD technique to

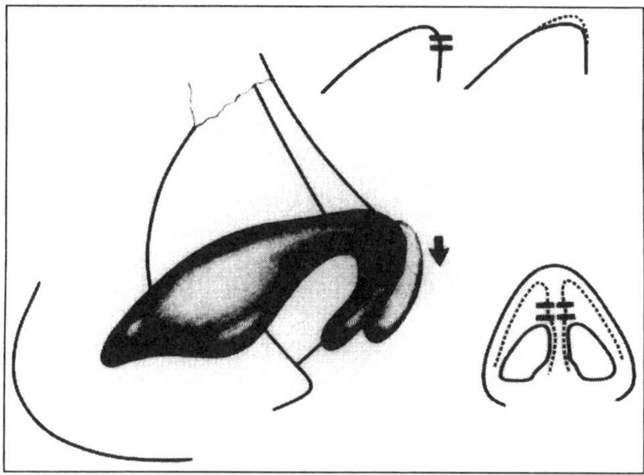

Fig 10–2.—Vertical dome division to the dome with overlap of the two segments. Reduction in tip projection as well as reduction in the infratip length is accomplished. (Courtesy of Adamson PA, McGraw-Wall BL, Morrow TA, et al: *Arch Otolaryngol Head Neck Surg* 120:373–380, 1994.)

reduce the incidence of the reported postoperative distortions and asymmetries was reviewed.

Technique.—The classic Goldman VDD involved dividing the alar cartilages; removing a portion of the alar cartilaginous lobule, as needed, to alter tip projection, rotation, or the width of the domal arch; and suturing the cartilages together again without overlap to recreate the alar margin. The modified technique

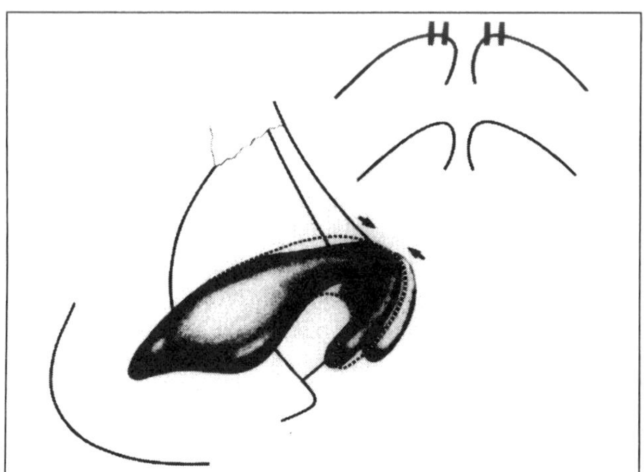

Fig 10–3.—A wide domal arch is corrected by dividing medial to the dome and overlapping to reduce the distance between the dome and the angle. Scoring of the cartilage to further refine the tip defining point is usually necessary. (Courtesy of Adamson PA, McGraw-Wall BL, Morrow TA, et al: *Arch Otolaryngol Head Neck Surg* 120:373–380, 1994.)

involves overlapping those portions of cartilage that would have been resected and suturing the overlapping portions to recreate the alar margin (Figs 10–2 and 10–3).

Patients.—Of 116 patients who underwent open rhinoplasty with VDD, 75 had VDD with cartilage resection and suturing, and 41 had VDD with cartilage overlap and suturing. Primary indications for VDD were lobule asymmetry, tip overprojection, a wide domal arch, a hanging or elongated infratip lobule, and the need for tip rotation.

Outcome.—Four patients (3.4%), including 3 who had the excisional procedure and 1 who had the overlap procedures, required revision of postoperative tip abnormalities. Two other patients had minor tip abnormalities not requiring surgical revision. Of the 6 postoperative tip abnormalities, 4 were caused by nasal bossae and 2 by lobule asymmetries. None of the patients sustained alar notching or lower nasal third pinching.

Conclusions.—Overlap/suture VDD for patients with complex tip abnormalities allows for more accurate anatomical reconstruction of the nasal lobule and avoids the postoperative cartilage displacement that often causes tip irregularities and asymmetries.

▶ This is a nice technique for our consideration. It probably is a more secure method than dividing and not suturing the cartilage together. I wonder whether the authors considered "beveling" the overlapping cartilage piece to smooth the contour less abruptly?—G.R. Holt, M.D., F.A.C.S.

Clinical Experience With the Tunable Pulsed-Dye Laser (585 nm) in the Treatment of Capillary Vascular Malformations
Achauer BM, Vander Kam VM, Padilla JF III (Univ of California Irvine Med Ctr, Orange)
Plast Reconstr Surg 92:1233–1241, 1993   130-95-10–3

Background.—A number of different lasers have been used for the treatment of the birthmark known as nevus flammeus or port-wine stain, which the authors designate capillary vascular malformation (CVM). Recent reports have suggested that the pulsed-dye laser, tuned to 585 rather than 577 nm, is the treatment of choice for CVMs. The 585-nm wavelength has been used in a wide range of anatomical areas; it permits treatment without local anesthesia and is associated with decreased healing time. The results of pulsed-dye laser treatment at 585 nm for CVM are reviewed.

Methods.—The investigators treated 134 such patients over a 5-year period; all were followed up for at least 2 years. Patient age range was 2 months to 66 years. Of these patients, 95 were available for evaluation of the results. The investigators' own classification system was used to describe each birthmark before and after laser treatment.

Results.—The results were classified as good or excellent in 74 of the 95 cases. Most patients in all classifications of preoperative severity showed improvement. The results were equally favorable for most patients in all age groups and with all birthmark colors; varying degrees of success were achieved in all anatomical areas and all ethnic groups. Up to 8 treatments were required to achieve maximum improvement. Only 1% of the patients experienced scarring; 3% had hypopigmentation.

Conclusions.—The pulsed-dye laser tuned to 585 nm is a useful treatment for CVM. It is effective in all age groups and can be used in some patients who previously were not candidates for laser surgery. Good-to-excellent aesthetic results can be achieved, with a minimal risk of complications, if the treatment is pursued to its completion. This article also includes a new system for the classification of CVMs.

▶ This modality seems to be excellent for CVMs. Not many specialists have training in and accessibility to this tunable pulsed-dye laser, so identify one in your area for potential referrals.—G.R. Holt, M.D., F.A.C.S.

Risk of Blood Contact Through Surgical Gloves in Aesthetic Procedures

Greco RJ, Wheatley M, McKenna P (Univ of Pittsburgh, Pa)
Aesthetic Plast Surg 17:167–168, 1993   130-95-10-4

Introduction.—Operating room personnel are at a particularly high risk of exposure to blood-borne pathogens such as hepatitis B virus (HBV) and HIV. Surgical gloves often have nonapparent perforations that can result in blood contact during operative procedures. The risk of exposure to blood during esthetic surgery was investigated.

Methods.—One hundred pairs of latex gloves used in consecutive esthetic surgical operations were collected and tested for holes. Sixty pairs had been used by 1 attending surgeon and 40 pairs by resident assistants. After each procedure, the type and duration of operation were recorded as well as any suspicion of blood contact and the maneuver that resulted in the contact. The gloves were overfilled with water to reveal a break, a method shown to be 100% effective in finding holes made with a 26-gauge or larger needle.

Results.—Perforations were detected in 32 (16%) gloves. In only 15 of those 32 operations were the surgeons aware of the perforations. The most common location of exposure (44%) was the left index finger. Perforations were more common in the surgeon's gloves (38.3%) than in the assistant's gloves (22.5%). Nearly all (90.6%) the holes were found after operations lasting more than 2 hours.

Conclusion.—Despite the use of gloves, plastic surgeons are at risk for blood exposure during esthetic surgery. Possible protective measures include changing the gloves during longer operations and reinforcing the nondominant index finger. Double-gloving has been shown to decrease blood exposure during other types of surgery but may reduce the dexterity required to perform esthetic surgery.

▶ If this article fails to send a chill up your back, you need to reread it. One of my former Fellows *always* double-gloved. I should learn from her.—G.R. Holt, M.D., F.A.C.S.

Temporalis Fascia Grafts in Open Secondary Rhinoplasty
Baker TM, Courtiss EH (Newton-Wellesley Hosp, Boston; Harvard Med School, Boston)
Plast Reconstr Surg 93:802–810, 1994   130-95-10–5

Background.—A common problem resulting from secondary rhinoplasty is parchment thin skin. An onlay graft of temporalis fascia is very satisfactory for covering the underlying osseocartilaginous framework or cartilage grafts in such cases. In closed rhinoplasty, precise placement of temporalis fascia grafts is difficult because the graft rolls. In an open rhinoplasty, however, the graft may be placed accurately and secured under direct vision (Fig 10–4). One experience with temporalis fascia grafts in open secondary rhinoplasties was reported.

Methods and Outcomes.—Six women, aged 31 to 57 years, underwent open secondary rhinoplasty. Five also had autologous cartilage grafts. The mean follow-up was 2 years. All patients had excellent dorsal contours. No osseocartilaginous irregularities were observed. Nasal infection developed in 1 patient who responded to antibiotics without removal of the fascia or cartilage graft. In 1 patient, biopsy specimens of the temporalis fascia and cartilage grafts were obtained 1 year after placement. Microscopic assessment confirmed the long-term viability of grafted tissues.

Conclusions.—Temporalis fascia grafts are very satisfactory in the management of thin skin in open secondary rhinoplasty. Clinical and histologic assessment confirms the long-term viability of these grafts.

▶ I like using temporalis fascia for many procedures, including eyelid and facial support, septal perforation repair, auricular reconstruction, and soft tissue augmentation. This article will lead me to try using it when properly indicated.—G.R. Holt, M.D., F.A.C.S.

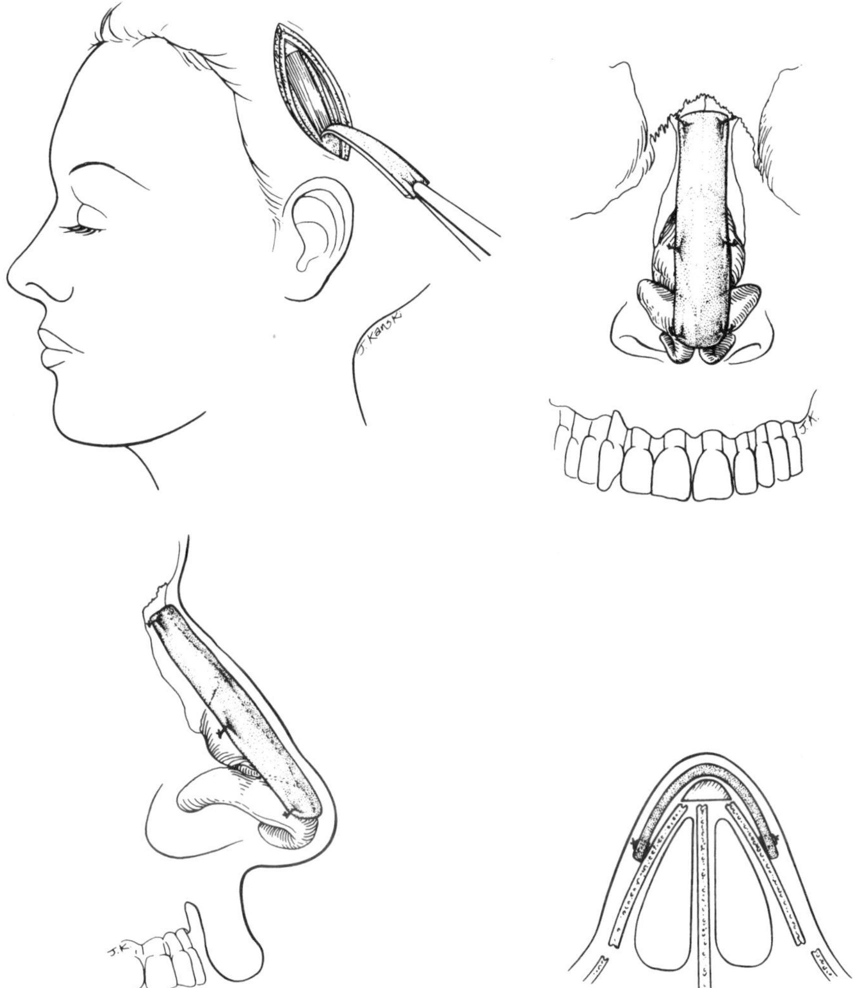

Fig 10–4.—Illustrations of technique. (Courtesy of Baker TM, Courtiss EH: *Plast Reconstr Surg* 93:802–810, 1994.)

Does Rhinoplasty Make the Nose More Susceptible to Fracture?

Guyuron B, Zarandy S (Mt Sinai Med Ctr, Cleveland, Ohio; Case Western Reserve Univ, Cleveland, Ohio)

Plast Reconstr Surg 93:313–317, 1994   130-95-10–6

Background.—Many patients who are considering undergoing rhinoplasty ask whether the operation will make the nose more susceptible to fracture. Insufficient data are available in the literature to answer this question. The vulnerability of the nose to fracture after rhinoplasty was investigated in a population-based study.

Methods.—Data on the incidence of nasal bone fracture in the general population were obtained from the National Center for Health Statistics. The investigators then studied 1,121 patients identified as having had routine elective rhinoplasty or septorhinoplasty for the occurrence of nasal fracture after their surgery.

Results.—The population statistics showed that an average of 51,200 nasal bone fractures occurred annually in the United States, with an average rate of .021% per year. Of the patients with a history of rhinoplasty, 24 had sustained 28 nasal bone fractures over a mean follow-up of 4 years. The 16 women and 8 men had a mean age of 27 years. The actual or crude rate of postrhinoplasty fracture was .624% per year compared with the age-standardized rate of .485%. Time from rhinoplasty to fracture ranged from 1 month to 6 years. For 16 patients, the average time from rhinoplasty to fracture was less than 1 year. More than 70% of patients were younger than 30 years at the time of postrhinoplasty fracture.

Conclusions.—Patients who have had rhinoplasty have an increased incidence of nasal fracture—perhaps 10 times higher than that of the general population. Fracture may be more common in the first year after rhinoplasty because the strength of the bone union has not reached its peak. As in the general population, postrhinoplasty nasal fracture is more common in individuals younger than 30 years.

▶ Of the estimated 51,200 nasal bone fractures occurring each year, I know that most of them have come in when I was on ER call. Seriously, my common sense tells me that after rhinoplasty, patients will always have a higher risk of refracture because of the manner in which bone healing occurs at the fracture sites.—G.R. Holt, M.D., F.A.C.S.

Bipedicled Axial Cross-Lip Flap for Correction of Major Vermilion Deficiency After Cleft Lip Repair
Wagner JD, Newman MH (Indiana Univ, Indianapolis; Univ of Michigan, Ann Arbor)
Cleft Palate Craniofac J 31:148–151, 1994   130-95-10–7

Introduction.—The most common secondary deformities after cleft lip repair are irregularities or deficiencies of the vermilion border. Vermilion deficiency is particularly severe in bilateral clefts (Fig 10–5). A technique was developed for correcting large vermilion deficits of the upper lip, using a bipedicled lower to upper cross-lip visor flap.

Operative Technique.—The procedure is performed with the patient under local or general anesthesia. An incision is made in the upper lip at the wet/dry vermilion border from commissure to commissure and is carried through the mucosa into the superficial layers of the obicularis muscle. The defect is mea-

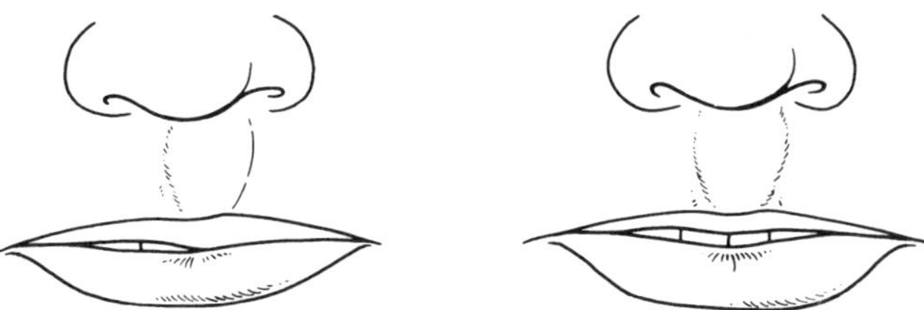

Fig 10–5.—Whistling deformity after unilateral cleft lip repair (**left**), and after bilateral lip repair (**right**). The bilateral deformity is characterized by diffuse lack of vermilion and is often associated with a deficient upper buccal sulcus. (Courtesy of Wagner JD, Newman MH: *Cleft Palate Craniofac J* 31:148–151, 1994.)

sured and the flap to be transferred is outlined on the lower lip. The anterior border of the flap is situated at the lower lip wet/dry vermilion border, extending posteriorly as required to fill the upper lip defect. After the flap is incised, it is rotated 180 degrees and inset into the transverse releasing incision of the upper lip. The pedicles are divided and inset after 10–14 days, when the flap is trimmed and inset into any remaining defect (Fig 10-6).

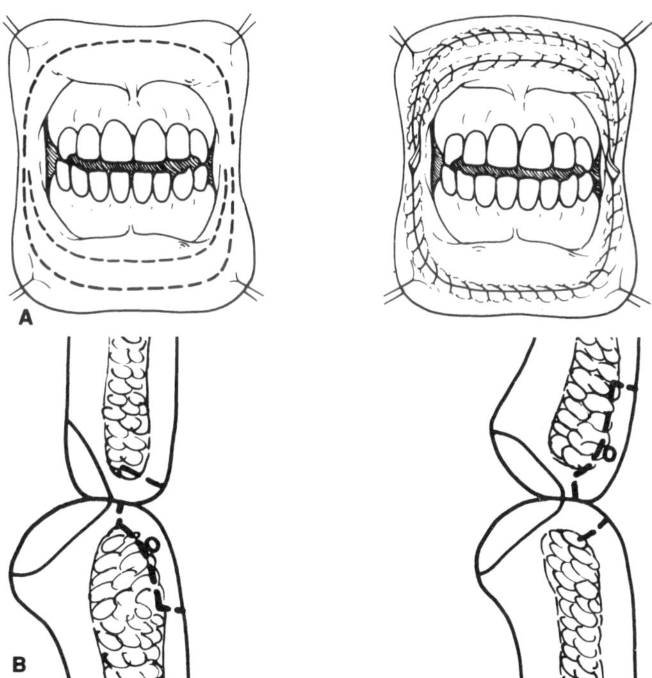

Fig 10–6.—**A,** flap planned on the lower lip to be transferred to the upper lip releasing incision (**left**), after transfer (**right**). Note bilateral axial pedicles at commissures, containing the labial coronary arteries, which are divided at the second stage 10-14 days later. **B,** sagittal view of flap, before transfer (**left**) and after transfer (**right**). (Courtesy of Wagner JD, Newman MH: *Cleft Palate Craniofac J* 31:148–151, 1994.)

Discussion.—In many cases of vermilion defect after bilateral cleft lip repair, there is an absolute shortage of vermilion and mucosa. This technique can manage sizable defects, however, providing ample bulk and lining without disturbing the obicularis oris muscular oral sphincter. The bipedicled axial cross-lip flap also balances the lips and does not complicate feeding.

▶ This technique struck me as being useful for vermilion deficiencies of any etiology. The flap is long and thin, so vascularity is certainly a concern, particularly in previously operated tissue.—G.R. Holt, M.D., F.A.C.S.

Modified Facelift Incision for Parotidectomy

Terris DJ, Tuffo KM, Fee WE Jr (Stanford Univ, Calif)
J Laryngol Otol 108:574–578, 1994   130-95-10–8

Objective.—The modified Blair incision is the standard technique for parotidectomies. A retrospective comparison of a modified facelift incision for parotid surgery with the standard modified Blair technique was made.

Methods.—The modified facelift incision follows the modified Blair procedure up to the point where the incision extends into the neck area. Then, instead of extending the incision down in front of the ear, the modified facelift incision extends down behind the ear for about 6 cm to expose the facial nerve and reveal the tumor of the parotid lobe (Fig 10–7). In group A, 18 patients, aged 21–61, had the modified facelift

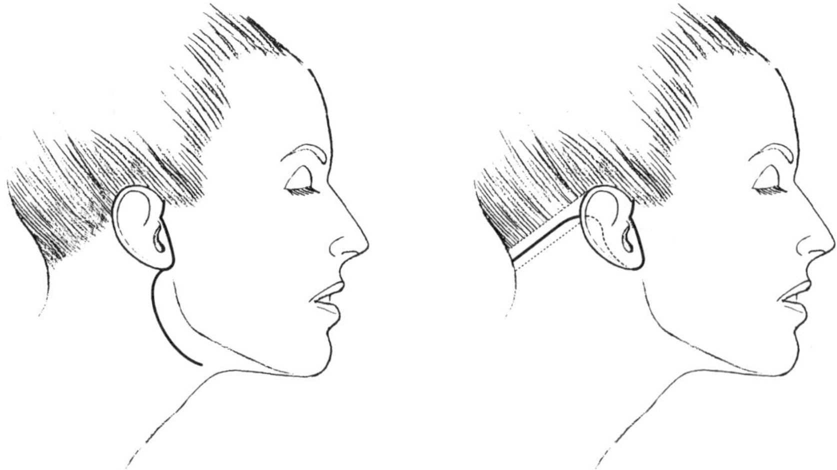

Fig 10–7.—The modified Blair incision is shown (**left**) and compared with the modified facelift incision (**right**). (Courtesy of Terris DJ, Tuffo KM, Fee WE Jr: *J Laryngol Otol* 108:574–578, 1994.)

procedure. In group B, 15 patients, aged 2–76 years, had the modified Blair incision. Patients were followed up for an average of 8 months.

Results.—Complications included 1 hematoma and 1 wound infection in each group, plus 1 salivary fistula and 1 facial nerve sacrifice and grafting in group A and 2 salivary fistulas in group B. The most common diagnosis was pleomorphic adenoma. There were 4 carcinomas. Surgeries lasted an average of 3 hours.

Conclusion.—The modified facelift procedure is safe, cosmetically desirable, yields satisfactory surgical exposure to the parotid and mastoid areas, and provides no additional risk of complications.

▶ The authors make a good case for this approach. I will try it next time. Just don't squeeze the flap.—G.R. Holt, M.D., F.A.C.S.

Early Excision of Nasal Hemangiomas: The L-Approach
van der Meulen JC, Gilbert PM, Roddi R (Academisch Ziekenhuis Rotterdam, The Netherlands)
Plast Reconstr Surg 94:465–473, 1994   130-95-10–9

Introduction.—Nasal hemangiomas tend to disappear with time, but their presence may cause severe psychological distress to the child. Although most physicians advocate postponing surgery until no further improvement is visible, the wisdom of this approach is debatable. Nine patients underwent early surgery in the involution phase with uniformly good results.

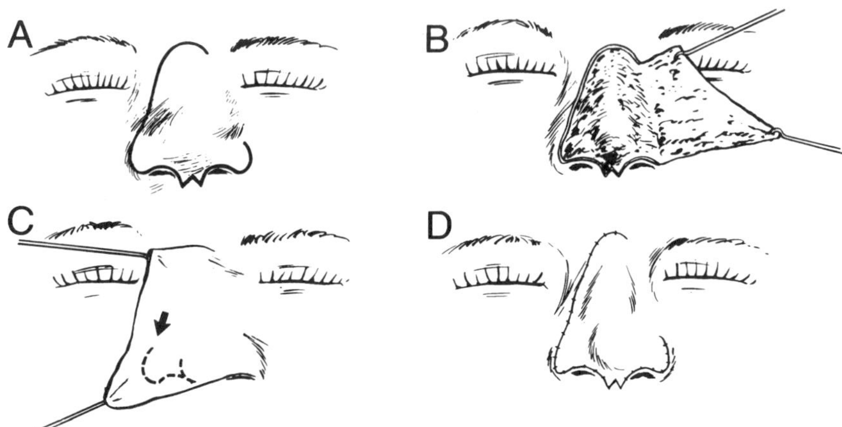

Fig 10–8.—The L-sign symbolizes different kinds of money (lira, lire, libra, livre). Livre also means book. The L-approach (**A**) permits opening of the nasal dorsum like a book (**B**). Any surplus can then be reduced (**C**), producing a more natural contour (**D**). (Courtesy of van der Meulen JC, Gilbert PM, Roddi R: *Plast Reconstr Surg* 94:465–473, 1994.)

Methods.—Nasal tip hemangiomas are relatively rare anomalies that may leave a mass of fibrofatty tissue and a sagging bag of atrophic non-elastic skin behind. All but one patient underwent surgery soon after first being seen for consultation. Two patients were 5 and 6 years of age at operation, but the others ranged in age from 8 months to 29 months. A low-flying bird incision (Rethi-incision) was used in 4 patients with a moderate hemangioma involving the nasal tip. In patients with a severe hemangioma involving the nasal tip and dorsum, an extended rhinotomy (L-approach, Fig 10–8) was used. The most difficult part of the operation involves redraping the skin over the denuded skeleton and restoring the nasal contours.

Results.—In 2 cases, the hemangioma could not be completely removed at the first operation. The results were good, however, in all 9 patients, with virtually normal nasal contours achieved. No skin was lost, and growth does not seem to be impaired. All parents expressed satisfaction with the results of surgery. The L-approach leaves no scar on the nasal dorsum or tip.

Conclusion.—Surgery before regression of the nasal hemangioma is more difficult, but a long wait may be required before the child enjoys a normal appearance. The L-approach allows for resection of excess skin resulting from the hemangioma's expanding effect on the nasal dorsum and tip. For selected patients and in experienced hands, this approach is preferable to the standard conservative treatment.

▶ Depending on the extent of involvement of the dorsal nasal skin that requires excision, this approach may not be possible. One can still include the midline forehead in the flap if needed.—G.R. Holt, M.D., F.A.C.S.

Intraoperative Custom Contouring of the Mandible
Glasgold AI, Glasgold MJ (Manhattan Eye, Ear, and Throat Hosp, New York)
Arch Otolaryngol Head Neck Surg 120:180–184, 1994   130-95-10–10

Objective.—Although their design reflects an increasingly sophisticated understanding of mandibular contouring, the chin implants that are currently available do not sufficiently meet the need for precise profile correction. The use of a newly developed extension wafer that allows custom mandibular contouring in patients undergoing augmentation mentoplasty was examined.

Methods.—The study included 100 consecutive patients who were undergoing elective augmentation mentoplasty. All operations were performed via a standard submental approach. Chin implants were sutured to the periosteum of the mandibular rim; when needed, Silastic extension wafers were inserted under the implant and fixed to it with sutures (Fig 10–9). The results were evaluated in terms of profile augmentation, the ideal for which was defined as projecting the most anterior point of

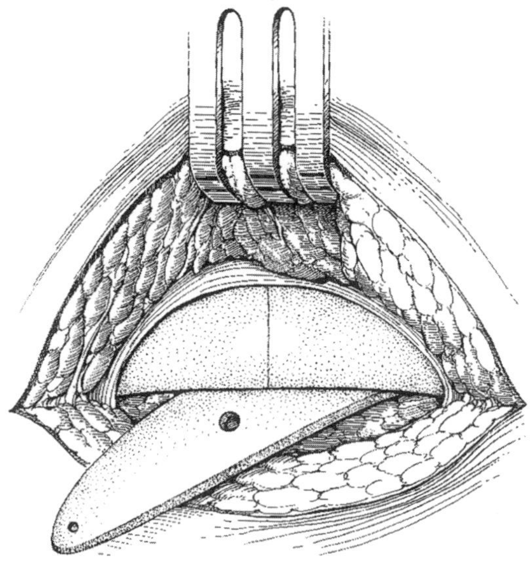

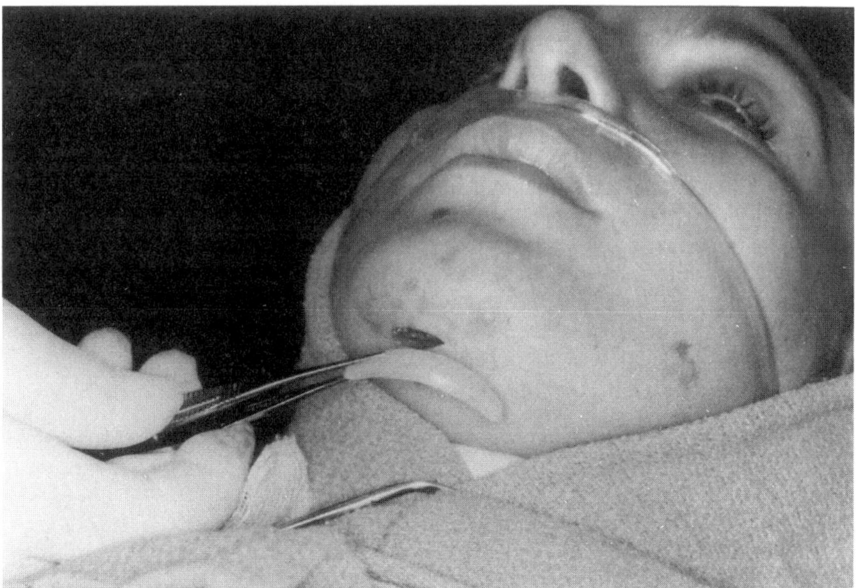

Fig 10–9.—Illustration and photograph of wafer being inserted under implant. (Courtesy of Glasgold AI, Glasgold MJ: *Arch Otolaryngol Head Neck Surg* 120:180–184, 1994.)

the patient's chin on profile to within 2 mm of a vertical line from the lower lip.

Results.—The mean amount of augmentation needed was measured preoperatively as 5.5 mm. A commercial implant did not provide the desired amount of profile augmentation in 20 patients, so a 2-mm extension wafer was used. At 6 months' follow-up, all patients were satisfied with their results. None has had any infection, implant rejection, or slippage. According to the stated criteria, 98% of the patients achieved ideal profile augmentation, the exceptions being 2 patients with fairly extreme micrognathia.

Conclusions.—The use of insertion wafers can improve the ability to perform custom contouring of the mandible in augmentation mentoplasty. By eliminating the need for sizers and reducing surgical manipulation, insertion wafers can markedly decrease surgical trauma in patients needing multiple insertion, with resulting reductions in discomfort and infection risk. The wafer can be added in a secondary office procedure if the original augmentation is deemed inadequate.

▶ The notion of "fine-tuning" the chin implant through the use of augmentation wafers is a good one. If the patient is concerned about having a silicone implant placed in the face, the surgeon must be familiar enough with biomaterials (as are these authors) to point out the differences between solid silicone and the gel-filled, polyurethane-covered breast implant.—G.R. Holt, M.D., F.A.C.S.

Infections Requiring Hospital Readmission Following Face Lift Surgery: Incidence, Treatment, and Sequelae
LeRoy JL Jr, Rees TD, Nolan WB III (Manhattan Eye, Ear, and Throat Hosp, New York)
Plast Reconstr Surg 93:533–536, 1994   130-95-10–11

Introduction.—As the dissection techniques used in facelift surgery go farther and deeper into the face and neck, the incidence or severity of postoperative infections might be expected to increase. The reported incidence of infection is less than 1%, with mainly minor, localized infections. However, more severe infectious complications, including severe cellulitis, abscess formation, sepsis, and flap necrosis, can occur. The perioperative factors, clinical findings, treatment, and outcome of major infections in a series of patients who had undergone facelift procedures were reviewed.

Patients.—Of 6,166 consecutive patients who underwent face lift operations over a 7-year period, 11 had infectious complications requiring hospital readmission, for a rate of .18%. There were 10 women and 1 man (average age, 62 years). Indications for readmission were abscess requiring surgical drainage in 7 patients and severe cellulitis in 4. All abscess cultures showed *Staphylococcus* species as the predominant organism. Culture in 2 of 3 patients admitted 3 weeks after surgery revealed gram-negative organisms as well as *Staphylococcus* organisms. No significant associations were noted with past medical history, perioperative antibiotic use, surgical equipment used, complexity of dissection, drain use, or hematoma formation. None of the patients had systemic signs or grossly abnormal laboratory findings at the time of readmission. Three patients were left with minor scarring as a result of their infection; the other 8 had no sequelae.

Conclusions.—Major infections are a rare complication of face lift surgery. Standard management approaches, if provided in a timely fashion, will usually yield a satisfactory outcome with little morbidity. The culture results in this study suggest that all face lift patients should receive initial *Staphylococcus* coverage. Those readmitted more than 1 week after surgery may be considered for gram-negative coverage, pending culture results.

▶ The authors remind us that although infections are unusual after a face lift, they can occur. Perioperative use of antibiotics seems prudent. As you dissect deeper into the face, remember that more anatomical spaces are opened to potential infection.—G.R. Holt, M.D., F.A.C.S.

Anesthetic Practices in Ambulatory Aesthetic Surgery
Courtiss EH, Goldwyn RM, Joffe JM, Hannenberg AA (Newton-Wellesley Hosp, Massachusetts; Beth Israel Hosp, Boston; Harvard Med School, Boston; et al)
Plast Reconstr Surg 93:792–801, 1994   130-95-10–12

Background.—Aesthetic surgery is widely practiced on an outpatient basis, and a number of anesthetic techniques are available. How often various anesthetic techniques are used and whether practice varies by surgery location were investigated.

Methods.—A carefully designed 16-page questionnaire was sent to the 805 actively practicing members of the American Society of Aesthetic Plastic Surgery. The response rate was 77%.

Findings.—More than 50% of the respondents performed aesthetic surgery in their offices at least half the time. About half never performed aesthetic surgery in the hospital, and most never used a free-standing ambulatory surgical center. A number of preoperative laboratory studies were routinely ordered, regardless of the location of the surgery or patient age. The most common of these studies were complete blood count, urinalysis, hematocrit/hemoglobin, coagulation studies, and bleeding time. In all settings, local anesthesia with intravenous sedation was widely used. The most commonly used agents were lidocaine, bupivacaine, and cocaine; 95% of respondents used epinephrine. In two thirds of office surgeries in which local anesthesia was used, neither a nurse anesthetist nor an anesthesiologist was present. About half of the office surgical units used general anesthesia, which was administered by anesthesia personnel. Anesthesiologists and nurse anesthetists performed this function with roughly equal frequency. Regardless of surgical location, similar intensity and methods of patient monitoring were used.

Conclusion.—In ambulatory esthetic surgery, similar laboratory evaluation, monitoring, and anesthesia practices are followed, regardless of the location of the surgery. Given the high response rate and target population of this study, the results are believed to give a reliable reflection of current practice.

▶ This is an interesting study of independent office surgical centers. It shows me that standards of care are essentially function-driven, and that practitioners do what is commonly considered necessary to provide safety for their patients.—G.R. Holt, M.D., F.A.C.S.

Silicone Facial Implants: Are They Safe?
Silver FH, Glasgold AI (Univ of Medicine and Dentistry of New Jersey–Robert Wood Johnson Med School, Piscataway, NJ; Robert Wood Johnson Univ Hosp, New Brunswick, NJ)
J Long-Term Effects Med Implants 3:313–320, 1993   130-95-10–13

Background.—The recent publicity surrounding the use of silicone gel-filled breast implants has affected the medical device industry. Tissue reactions are wide ranging and include lymphadenopathy, fever, joint pain, mixed connective tissue disease, scleroderma, Sjögren's syndrome, rheumatoid arthritis, arthralgias, systemic lupus erythematosus, and iritis. Although granuloma formation has been noted, reports of immunologic diseases are scarce. The focus has been on breast implants, but there are other permanent implants made from silicone. The adverse effects of facial implants in the form of fluid, particles, and solid implants were reviewed to evaluate the occurrence of similar reactions.

Types of Implants.—Silicone fluid is not approved by the Food and Drug Administration for any medical indication, and action has been taken against physicians who "promote" its use. The fluid has been shown to be safe when used to correct postrhinoplasty defects, age-related rhytides, and acne scars, among other conditions. Safeguards include using the microdroplet technique; undercorrection of the area; 6- to 12-week treatment intervals; use of pure, medical-grade silicone; and use of silicone for precision. Silicone powder has been used for filling tissue depressions that have rigid back support. Particles are injected and molded manually. Only 2 hematomas have been reported to result from 50 procedures. Solid implants have been used on the chin, orbital floor, and in various nasal augmentations. Complications after procedures on the chin were least with the silicone prostheses and most with acrylic and Proplast prostheses. Nasal implants are more troublesome because of slippage or extrusion.

Complications.—There are conflicting reports on tissue responses. Adverse reactions range from pain, swelling, ecchymosis, overcorrection, inflammation to embolism, granulomatous response, and connective tissue disease in spite of some reports citing no adverse effects. Solid implants show fewer adverse reactions such as asymmetry, extrusion, and foreign-body reactions.

Comment.—On the basis of the literature and federal regulator stances, the conflicting reports regarding the safety of liquid silicone and its link with autoimmune diseases argue against its use. Solid implants currently have the lowest complication rate of all implants studied, yet further long-term studies need to be conducted to improve our understanding of complication rates.

▶ If a facial surgeon continues to use silicone implants, he or she must be very familiar with the body of literature concerning silicone's biocompatibility, both to adequately inform the patient and to decide whether to use them. I have decided to substitute other biomaterials in instances where I had previously used silicone.—G.R. Holt, M.D., F.A.C.S.

11 Larynx and Airway

Determining the Site of Airway Collapse in Obstructive Sleep Apnea With Airway Pressure Monitoring
Katsantonis GP, Moss K, Miyazaki S, Walsh J (Park Central Inst, St Louis, Mo; Deaconess Hosp, St Louis, Mo; Mito Natl Hosp, Japan)
Laryngoscope 103:1126–1131, 1993   130-95-11–1

Background.—Identifying the collapsing or stenotic site of the pharyngeal lumen in patients with obstructive sleep apnea (OSA) is essential for selecting the appropriate surgical intervention. There are many available methods for determining the site of airway collapse in patients with OSA. However, their efficacy has been suboptimal, and the selection of surgical candidates remains difficult. The value of airway pressure monitoring in patients with OSA to determine the site of airway collapse was investigated.

Methods.—Twenty patients had complete polysomnography and simultaneous upper airway pressure monitoring with a custom-made, soft silicone-covered catheter with a diameter of 2.3 mm. The catheter had 4 solid-state microtip pressure sensors: 1 in the posterior nasopharynx, 1 just caudal to the tip of the uvula, 1 at the level of the hyoid bone, and 1 in the midesophagus. The levels of airway collapse were determined by pressure pattern changes between transducers.

Findings.—Airway collapse was limited to or began at the oropharyngeal region in 14 patients. In 7 patients, the obstruction extended to the base of the tongue, and in 2, to the entire collapsible upper airway. Four patients had collapse at the base of the tongue. Two additional patients had collapse at the hypopharynx. The airway collapse site remained fairly constant through the sleep stages and in different sleep positions. Of the 4 patients undergoing uvulopalatopharyngoplasty and postoperative polysomnography, responses were favorable in 2.

Conclusions.—Although airway pressure monitoring is an excellent way to study the dynamics of the airway in patients with OSA, its clinical usefulness and accuracy have yet to be established. However, newer instrumentation makes the procedure easy to do, with insignificant morbidity. Airway pressure monitoring should be done more often in medical centers with the appropriate equipment so that more data can be obtained.

▶ I predict that clinically significant technologic advances in airway monitoring for OSA will occur in this decade, perhaps enabling us to be more precise in determining the site of obstruction and to provide more focused therapy.—G.R. Holt, M.D., F.A.C.S.

Function of the Posterior Cricoarytenoid Muscle in Phonation: In Vivo Laryngeal Model
Choi H-S, Berke GS, Ye M, Kreiman J (Univ of California, Los Angeles)
Otolaryngol Head Neck Surg 109:1043–1051, 1993   130-95-11–2

Background.—Several electromyographic studies indicate that the posterior cricoarytenoid (PCA) muscle is not simply an abductor of the vocal folds but also has some function in phonation. However, researchers have not definitively established the function of the PCA muscle in phonation.

Methods.—An in vivo canine laryngeal model was used to study the function of the PCA model. Five adult mongrel dogs were studied under varying conditions of nerve stimulation. Subglottic pressure and electroglottographic, photoglottographic, and acoustic waveforms were documented.

Findings.—The fundamental frequency (F0), subglottic pressure, and open quotient (OQ) were significantly reduced with PCA muscle stimulation level in the dynamic study. Superior laryngeal nerve (SLN) stimulation condition also significantly influenced pressure and OQ, but not F0, independent of the effects of PCA muscle stimulation. Both pressure and OQ significantly decreased with SLN stimulation in all PCA muscle stimulation conditions. The level of PCA muscle stimulation significantly affected all dependent measures. Across SLN conditions, each level of PCA muscle stimulation significantly differed from all others for all dependent variables. In addition, vocal efficiency decreased as PCA muscle stimulation increased. The SLN stimulation condition significantly influenced F0, pressure, and OQ, but not intensity. There were also significant interactions between PCA muscle and SLN stimulation for F0, pressure, and OQ.

Conclusions.—In this canine model, subglottic pressure, F0, sound intensity, and vocal efficiency decreased as stimulation of the posterior branch of the recurrent laryngeal nerve was increased. Therefore, the PCA muscle acts to brace the larynx against the anterior pull of the adductor and cricothyroid muscles, as well as to control the phonatory glottal width.

▶ This interesting paper suggests that the PCA muscle is more involved in laryngeal dynamics than was previously thought. It is clear that in those patients who have abductor spasmodic laryngeal dysfunction, there is greater diminishment of vocal function than one would expect; therefore, perhaps the PCA is coming into play in the ways that this article suggests.—G.R. Holt, M.D., F.A.C.S.

A Comparison of the Efficacy of Unilateral Versus Bilateral Botulinum Toxin Injections in the Treatment of Adductor Spasmodic Dysphonia

Maloney AP, Morrison MD (Univ of British Columbia, Vancouver)
J Otolaryngol 23:160–164, 1994   130-95-11–3

Background.—Adductor spasmodic dysphonia caused by focal dystonia is treated by injection of the thyroarytenoid-vocalis complex with botulinum toxin type A (Botox). This treatment appears to work via presynaptic motor endplate blockade, irreversibly preventing the release of acetylcholine and thus causing muscle paresis. Some practitioners use unilateral and some bilateral Botox injection; unilateral injection may reduce the severity of the side effects of whisper voice and aspiration in the weeks after treatment. The efficacy of unilateral and bilateral injection were compared in terms of these side effects and of the duration of benefit in a retrospective/prospective study.

Methods.—The analysis included 24 patients who were treated with unilateral or bilateral Botox injection for adductor spasmodic dysphonia. A retrospective chart review was performed to collect patient data; the results were updated by a prospective telephone interview. All patients were initially treated with bilateral injection with electromyographic guidance. When they returned for repeat injection, the possible differences in voice recovery and side effects were explained and the patients were offered unilateral injection.

Results.—The average number of treatments per patient was 3.3 for bilateral injections and 1.5 for unilateral injections. Average Botox dosage was 2.5 mouse units (MU) for bilateral injections and 4.5 MU for unilateral therapy. The effect of the injections lasted for an average of 15 weeks for bilateral injections vs. 11 weeks for unilateral injection. The average duration of side effects was 3 vs. 2 weeks, respectively. Men had a significantly longer duration of benefit with bilateral injection, whereas women showed no such difference. Both sexes had significantly reduced aspiration and men had significantly reduced breathiness with unilateral injection. On subjective voice ratings, improvement was rated significantly superior with bilateral treatment: 88% of patients reported good to excellent results, compared with 46% of the unilateral group. Seventy-one percent of patients preferred bilateral injection.

Conclusions.—Bilateral injection of the thyroarytenoid-vocalis complex with Botox appears to yield longer-lasting results than unilateral injection for patients with adductor spasmodic dysphonia. If side effects are severe with bilateral injection, unilateral injection may be tried; however, the patient should understand that the vocal benefit and duration of effect will be lessened.

▶ This paper nicely reviews for us the dilemma of unilateral vs. bilateral injections. Because each patient has his or her own symptoms, needs, expectations, and responses, in the end I see it as a necessity to individualize the dosage and injection sites to better serve the patient.—G.R. Holt, M.D., F.A.C.S.

Configuration of the Glottis in Laryngeal Paralysis: I. Clinical Study
Woodson GE (Univ of California, San Diego)
Laryngoscope 103:1227–1234, 1993   130-95-11–4

Objective.—The cricothyroid muscle is generally believed to be responsible for the paramedian position of the vocal fold in patients with recurrent laryngeal nerve paralysis. However, the available evidence in support of this theory is inconclusive. The expected cadaveric vocal fold position after vagus nerve lesions has been reported in patients with an intact superior vocal nerve as well. The configuration of the glottis was compared in patients with unilateral paralysis caused by known lesions of the recurrent laryngeal or vagus nerve.

Methods.—Fourteen patients were referred for treatment of glottic insufficiency. In all cases, the site of the lesion could be established either electromyographically or anatomically. In 7 patients, the vagus nerve had been injured or sacrificed in the course of tumor resection; the other 7 patients had lesions of the recurrent laryngeal nerve. All patients, as well as a number of normal individuals examined for other reasons, underwent videolaryngoscopy. The images were objectively measured to determine whether the cricothyroid muscle had a significant effect on the position of the paralyzed vocal fold.

Results.—In the patients with laryngeal paralysis, the altered configuration of the glottis could not be adequately characterized by standard terms of vocal fold position. Shortening of the paralyzed fold and anterior rotation of the arytenoid were observed. There was a tendency toward a more lateral vocal fold position in patients with vagus nerve lesions; however, there was no significant difference in fold position between the 2 groups.

Conclusions.—In patients with laryngeal paralysis, the paralyzed vocal folds are not necessarily denervated. Many factors can influence the position of the glottis; the site of the nerve lesion cannot be diagnosed on the basis of fold position. The length of the vocal fold is affected as well as its rotational position; procedures to medialize the paralyzed fold address only its rotation in the axial plane without correcting its deficient length.

▶ This is an excellent paper from a fine laryngologist. The discussion helped me sort out the clinical problems of varied true vocal cord position in paralysis. Also, with anterior/posterior shortening in the bilateral paralyses, widening of the cross-section of the vocal fold can further reduce glottic opening.—G.R. Holt, M.D., F.A.C.S.

Airway Resistance and Work of Breathing in Tracheostomy Tubes
Mullins JB, Templer JW, Kong J, Davis WE, Hinson J Jr (Univ of Missouri, Columbia, Harry S Truman Mem Veterans Affairs Hosp, Columbia, Mo)
Laryngoscope 103:1367–1372, 1993   130-95-11–5

Background.—The variables of diameter and length change the airflow dynamics and work of breathing through tracheostomy tubes. The airflow dynamics of neonatal, pediatric, and adult tracheostomy tubes were evaluated.

Methods and Findings.—Flow rates were plotted against change in pressure for inspiratory and expiratory flow. Resistances for each tube were then determined. The expiratory resistances were greater for the neonatal tubes and for pediatric tubes 0 and 00. Inspiratory resistances were the limiting factor in the adult tubes and the larger pediatric tubes. Calculated resistances were compared with known physiologic airway resistances. The upper airway resistance of adults was most closely simulated by adult tubes 8 and 10. Neonatal tube 0 was apparently most appropriate for newborns. Increasing tube diameter and decreasing tidal volume and respiratory rate reduced the amount of work needed to maintain a given flow.

Conclusions.—In patients undergoing tracheotomy for long-term management, the best choice may be the tube with flow characteristics most closely resembling those of the upper respiratory system to maintain respiratory homeostasis. A tracheostomy tube with a larger inner diameter may be better for patients undergoing tracheotomy to facilitate weaning from a ventilator.

▶ This nice paper that encourages us to think in scientific and physiologic terms about the choice of tracheostomy tubes, particularly in the newborn and the ventilator-dependent patient.—G.R. Holt, M.D., F.A.C.S.

Teflon Granulomas and Overinjection of Teflon: A Therapeutic Challenge for the Otorhinolaryngologist
Kasperbauer JL, Slavit DH, Maragos NE (Mayo Clinic and Found, Rochester, Minn; VA Med Ctr, Brooklyn, NY)
Ann Otol Rhinol Laryngol 102:748–751, 1993   130-95-11–6

Background.—Teflon granulomas and overinjection of Teflon® with resulting laryngeal dysfunction are uncommon reactions that are difficult to manage, mostly because of inflammatory responses to the injected Teflon. The management of 16 patients with symptoms of dysphonia and/or airway obstruction secondary to Teflon granulomas or overinjection was reported.

Patients and Outcomes.—The patients were 12 women and 4 men who were undergoing surgery for symptoms secondary to Teflon granulomas or vocal folds overinjected with Teflon. Initial symptoms included airway obstruction, coughing, choking, swallowing problems, and dysphonia. All patients underwent granuloma and Teflon removal endoscopically through a lateral cordotomy. An additional procedure was needed to adequately remove Teflon and the associated inflammation in 5 patients (31%). In 2 patients, the Teflon granulomas were so large that a tracheotomy was needed in conjunction with Teflon removal. Selecting the appropriate second procedure and the time of intervention was challenging.

Conclusions.—Teflon removal from the vocal cords is possible, with a resultant improvement in dysphonia. After Teflon removal, a second procedure is often needed for dysphonia. Thyroplasty and/or arytenoid adduction can be successfully used to manage dysphonia after Teflon removal.

▶ Many of us see these patients now, after the "golden age of Teflon." You need to see only 1 or 2 such patients before you realize you no longer want to use Teflon. Large granulomata may even require laryngofissure with a tracheostomy and the choice of a primary or secondary thyroplasty.—G.R. Holt, M.D., F.A.C.S.

Hydroxylapatite Laryngeal Implants for Medialization: Preliminary Report
Cummings CW, Purcell LL, Flint PW (Johns Hopkins Univ, Baltimore, Md)
Ann Otol Rhinol Laryngol 102:843–851, 1993   130-95-11–7

Background.—Laryngeal implantation for medialization has led to improved management of patients with vocal fold motion impairment. Preliminary data assessing the use of preformed hydroxylapatite laryngeal implants and instrumentation for prompt determination of implant size and position were reported.

Patients and Methods.—Implantation with hydroxylapatite prostheses was performed in 39 patients for treatment of incomplete glottic closure. Of these patients, 35 had vocal fold paralysis, and 4 were given a diagnosis of soft tissue deficits or bowing. A window was created in the thyroid ala using a standard fenestra template. One of 5 prosthesis templates, ranging from 3 to 7 mm, were inserted through the window to determine correct size and position (Fig 11–1). The corresponding implant was then inserted and anchored with a hydroxylapatite shim.

Results.—The 35 patients treated for laryngeal paralysis were assessed for reporting purposes. Of them, 31 reported subjective improvement. Improvement was also observed in 13 of 15 patients with complete preoperative and postoperative objective voice function measurements. There was 1 instance of implant extrusion and 1 instance of airway obstruction secondary to edema. No other complications were noted.

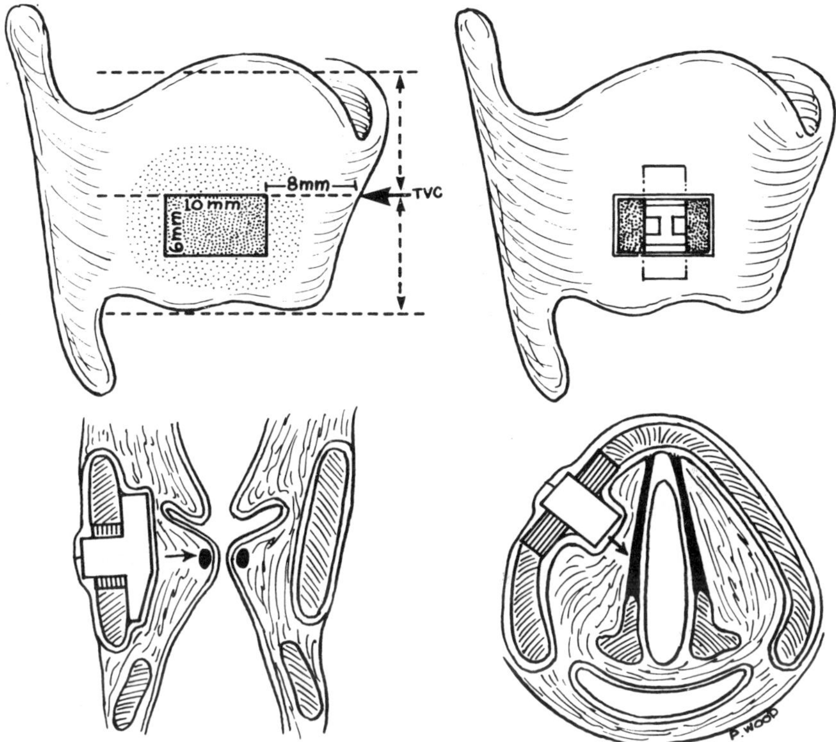

Fig 11–1.—Medialization thyroplasty. Horizontal fenestra with the implant in the vertical position and the beveled surface of the implant directed inferiorly to accommodate conus elasticus. (Courtesy of Cummings CW, Purcell LL, Flint PW: *Ann Otol Rhinol Laryngol* 102:843–851, 1993.)

Conclusions.—Based on preliminary data, the prefabricated hydroxylapatite implant appears to be effective for medialization thyroplasty. Associated benefits include readily available implant selection, prompt identification of size and position, and improved implant stabilization.

▶ I think we have to consider implant material other than silicone block for use as a thyroplasty "shim." Hydroxyapatite seems to be a possible candidate.—G.R. Holt, M.D., F.A.C.S.

Use of Laryngeal Muscular Tenotomy for Bilateral Midline Vocal Cord Fixation

Rontal M, Rontal E (Univ of Michigan, Ann Arbor)
Ann Otol Rhinol Laryngol 103:583–589, 1994   130-95-11–8

Objective.—Bilateral midline vocal cord fixation (BMVCF) can cause sudden or slow-onset airway obstruction, which can be life threatening.

Treatment tries to establish a laryngeal airway. The use of laryngeal tenotomy as an effective treatment for BMVCF was described.

Methods.—Six of 8 patients with BMVCF had this condition develop after endotracheal intubation. All patients had respiratory obstruction and received a tracheotomy. All patients had a tenotomy in which the intralaryngeal muscles were detached from the arytenoid, moving the vocal cords away from the midline and opening the glottis. After recovery, tracheotomies were plugged.

Results.—All 8 patients were decannulated, and none experienced aspiration. In 3 patients, medication was provided to inhibit gastrointestinal reflux. All voices were good. Only 1 patient required reoperation to enlarge his airway because of the energy requirements of his job.

Conclusion.—This procedure for treating vocal cord paralysis, which involves muscular release with no removal of cartilage, results in less damage to tissue and faster healing.

▶ I recently tried this technique after reviewing this article. The authors' experienced success in their 8 patients. If it works for me, I will be very pleased, because it is difficult to decannulate patients with BMVCF.—G.R. Holt, M.D., F.A.C.S.

Use of the Carden Anaesthetic Tube for Surgery Around a Tracheostome
Strachan DR, Grace ARG, Jackson IJB, Richardson GL (York District Hosp, England)
J Laryngol Otol 108:46–48, 1994   130-95-11–9

Background.—The Carden anesthetic tube is widely used to facilitate microlaryngeal surgery. This tube features a built-in jet tube through which the lungs are ventilated by jetting oxygen. This eliminates the Venturi effect in the operative field. Air blows out during both inhalation and exhalation, minimizing the risk of blowing blood and debris into the lungs. In microlaryngeal surgery with the Carden tube, the cuff inflating tube is only 1.5 mm and the jet tube is 3.5 mm in width, thus causing minimal obstruction of the surgical field of view. The use of the Carden anesthetic tube during surgical procedures in and around a tracheostomy was described.

Techniques.—General anesthetic is usually deemed preferable to local anesthetic for the creation of a tracheoesophageal fistula for insertion of an artificial voice prosthesis. The Groningen and Provox prostheses are generally replaced using local anesthesia, although in some situations (including patient preference, patients requiring pharyngoesophageal dilation, and those undergoing concomitant surgical procedures), a general anesthetic is preferred. In such cases, a Carden endotracheal tube can greatly facilitate access to the operative field while maintaining control of ventilation. The Carden tube is also a useful adjunct for patients who require refashioning of the tracheostomy and upper trachea. The use of this tube is contraindicated in certain situations, however, including severely narrowed trachea, severe chronic obstructive airways disease, and for obese patients.

The procedure begins by preoxygenating the patient for about 4 minutes with a face mask held against the tracheostomy, followed by induction of anesthesia and muscle paralysis. The surgeon then uses a Magills or other packing forceps to introduce the Carden tube into the trachea. The cuff is inflated, the jet tube is attached to the jetting apparatus, and ventilation is initiated. When a prosthetic valve for voice rehabilitation is placed after laryngectomy, the optimal site for creation of the tracheoesophageal fistula is about 10 mm from the mucocutaneous junction on the anterior margin of the trachea. This distance is slightly less with a Blom-Singer valve. This technique provides excellent access for the creation of a fistula or changing of a prosthetic valve.

Discussion.—The Carden anesthetic tube with jet ventilation can improve surgical access to the upper trachea and tracheostomy after laryngectomy. The Carden tube facilitates any surgical procedure in this area, including creation of a tracheoesophageal fistula, changing of prosthetic valves, and refashioning of a tracheostomy.

▶ For the patient requiring tracheostomal revisions or a secondary tracheoesophageal puncture, this method of anesthesia should be considered. Remember, however, that any obstruction to air egress from the trachea can lead to a tension pneumothorax.—G.R. Holt, M.D., F.A.C.S.

Intelligibility of Tracheoesophageal Speech Among Naive Listeners
Smith LF, Calhoun KH (Univ of Texas, Galveston)
South Med J 87:333–335, 1994   130-95-11–10

Introduction.—The most common method of speech rehabilitation for patients with total laryngectomy is tracheoesophageal (TE) speech. Expert listeners and only patients with excellent TE speech have been used in most previous studies to compare intelligibility of TE speech with esophageal, artificial larynx, and normal speech. Twenty nonexpert, or "naive," listeners were used to determine speech intelligibility in 8 patients with varying speech skills who used TE speech as a primary communication.

Method.—A closed list of phonetically balanced words and an open list of spondee words were used to determine speech intelligibility. In both tests, patients were assigned different word lists to eliminate word familiarity in listeners.

Results.—Intelligibility was 71% for phonetically balanced words, 82% for the open list of spondee words, and 76% overall. Intelligibility of TE speech among the 8 patients varied from 61% to 91%.

Conclusion.—The wide range of intelligibility in TE speech indicated that it is significantly less intelligible to naive listeners than laryngeal speech. Although TE speech is an excellent method, further research is needed to improve voice rehabilitation for patients with laryngectomy.

▶ Usually the best listeners for TE speech include the otolaryngologist and close members of the patient's family. Both of these groups have an interest in and a need to understand such speech, and they certainly have daily experience.—G.R. Holt, M.D., F.A.C.S.

Laryngeal Microsurgery Under General Anesthesia Using Small-Bore Endotracheal Tubes: Blood Gas Analysis

Altissimi G, Gallucci L, Prattichizzo L, Arcamone D, Monacelli C (Univ of Perugia, Italy)
Laryngoscope 104:325–328, 1994   130-95-11–11

Background.—Endotracheal intubation with small-bore tubes allows increased visualization of the operative field during direct microscopic suspension laryngoscopy. However, time under anesthesia becomes important when considering the effects of oxygen pressure (PO_2) carbon dioxide pressure (PCO_2), and the acid-base balance relative to the insufflation of the anesthetic at high levels of blood flow and pressure and the difficult elimination of PCO_2 through a small-bore nasotracheal tube.

Methods.—Variations in PO_2, PCO_2, bicarbonate (HCO_3), percentage saturation of O_2, and pH levels were examined during general anesthesia through small-bore endotracheal tubes in 39 patients undergoing laryngeal microsurgery. Duration of surgery ranged from 10 to 100 minutes.

Results.—Levels of PCO_2 above 50 mm Hg were observed only in the 100th minute, but the average PCO_2 value of 54.55 mm Hg fell within the normal limits of a permitted hypercapnia. The pH values tended to fall in correlation to the increase in PCO_2, but the drop was significant only at the 100th minute. However, pH levels of 7.22 at the 100th minute did not constitute a risk because they were above the > 7.00 safeguard level. There were no significant changes in PO_2 and percentage saturation of O_2. The HCO_3 levels fluctuated during surgery, but the variations were not statistically significant.

Conclusion.—General anesthesia with small-bore endotracheal tubes can be safely used for laryngeal microsurgery when operating times are shorter than 100 minutes. Hypercapnia tends to develop gradually as a result of the difficulty in expelling CO_2 through small-bore tubes, but the levels of PCO_2 do not reach dangerous levels. The acid-base balance is significantly modified only in the final stages of the operation.

▶ Copy this article and show it to your own anesthesiologist. A lot of them think a small tube is a #7 endotracheal tube. These 5-mm Coplans tubes could really help with visualization of the larynx, especially during vocal fold surgery.—G.R. Holt, M.D., F.A.C.S.

Long-Term Changes in Vocal Quality Following Isshiki Thyroplasty Type I

Leder SB, Sasaki CT (Yale Univ, New Haven, Conn)
Laryngoscope 104:275–277, 1994   130-95-11-12

Objective.—For correction of unilateral vocal-fold paralysis, thyroplasty type I uses a Silastic implant for external medialization of the abducted true vocal fold by lateral compression. Short-term results in 13 patients who underwent Isshiki thyroplasty type I for unilateral vocal-fold paralysis indicated significantly higher habitual vocal intensity and significantly longer maximum phonation time, both immediately after phonosurgery and up to 3 months post thyroplasty. The longitudinal changes of medialization thyroplasty in 5 of these patients was described.

Patients.—Five women with unilateral vocal-cord paralysis were followed up for as long as 4 years, 4 months after thyroplasty type I. None had any periphonosurgical or postphonosurgical complications.

Outcome.—During oral reading, patients exhibited significantly higher vocal fundamental frequency (191.4 Hz), significant moderation of habitual vocal intensity (43.6 dB), and significantly longer maximum phonation time (9.8 seconds) compared with prethyroplasty. The thyroplasty patients also exhibited significantly more breath groups both prethyroplasty and post thryoplasty compared with women without laryngeal pathology. In the thyroplasty group, there was a clinically but nonstatistically relevant reduction in the number of breath groups prethyroplasty compared with after thyroplasty.

Discussion.—Initially, improved vocal-fold adduction increases habitual voice intensity, most likely from continuation of increased breath support patterns necessary to compensate for inadequate glottic closure. With time, self-adjustment or relearning of the more natural breath support patterns, consistent with improved vocal-fold adduction and glottic closure, allows for reduced vocal effort and a corresponding decrease in overall habitual voice intensity. Improved glottic closure allows the maximum phonation time to increase more than 4 seconds, resulting in improved breath support for speech production and a concomitant reduction in breath groups during oral reading.

Conclusion.—The long-term success of Isshiki thyroplasty type I on both vocal quality and speech production skills is positive and lasting.

▶ The type I thyroplasty has become an important and welcome technique for aiding vocal cord paralysis. However, maximal improvement is not gained from the procedure alone but, also, from concomitant speech therapy in which vocal habits appropriate to the altered anatomy can be learned and practiced.—G.R. Holt, M.D., F.A.C.S.

Tracheostomy and Percutaneous Endoscopic Gastrostomy in the Management of the Head-Injured Trauma Patient

D'Amelio LF, Hammond JS, Spain DA, Sutyak JP (Univ of Medicine and Dentistry of New Jersey-Robert Wood Johnson Med School, New Brunswick)
Am Surg 60:180–185, 1994   130-95-11–13

Introduction.—The timing of tracheostomy (TRACH) and percutaneous endoscopic gastrostomy (PEG) in head-injured trauma patients was analyzed to determine how long they were in ICU, hospital length of stay, days of mechanical ventilation after TRACH/PEG, complications, and mortality. The timing of TRACH has been debated, particularly regarding its long-term incidence of subglottic stenosis, and it is often compared with tracheomalacia with endotracheal intubation. The safety of TRACH in the critically ill patient has been questioned, as long-term tracheal complications and perioperative morbidity were previously believed to be high. The role of PEG has also been debated with regard to the relative risk of gastric vs. jejunal feedings in terms of aspirations.

Methods.—During a period of 21 months, 31 head-injured trauma patients (mean age, 38 years) underwent TRACH and PEG. The patients were divided into early (less than or equal to 7 days) and late (greater than 7 days) groups, on the basis of the interval between injury and TRACH/PEG. Days to full enteral nutrition were also recorded in relation to esophagogastroduodenoscopy findings with PEG. Defined complications included aspiration, diarrhea, sinusitis, feeding intolerance, and new pneumonia.

Results.—Twenty-one head-injured patients underwent TRACH-PEG within 7 days of hospital admission, with a mean of 4.6 days. Ten other patients had TRACH/PEG at a mean of 13.2 days after being admitted to the hospital. Early TRACH/PEG resulted in shorter total ICU length of stay (12.6 vs. 26.2 days). Length of stay in the ICU after TRACH/ PEG was shortened (8 vs. 15.1 days), as were hospital stay (34 vs. 49 days) and course of mechanical ventilation (4.6 vs. 11.7 days). Full esophagogastroduodenoscopy at the time of PEG revealed pathologic diagnosis in 11 of 20 early patients and 4 of 8 late patients, but the esophagogastroduodenoscopy findings did not mandate specific therapy beyond routine prophylactic use of sucralfate. Full enteral nutritional support was accomplished earlier (5.4 vs. 7.6 days) in the early group; however, this was not statistically significant. No complications resulted. No unnecessary procedures were performed. All patients ventilated less than 48 hours after TRACH required long-term airway protection and suctioning access.

Conclusion.—Tracheostomy and percutaneous endoscopic gastrostomy performed within the first 7 days of head injury in the trauma patient is the procedure of choice for enteral nutrition, long-term airway protection, and mechanical ventilation. It shortens the ICU and hospital length of stay as well as the course of mechanical ventilation.

▶ This study reflects my own practice experience and preferences. On the whole, TRACH and PEG are positive interventions that help patients and also help health care professionals provide care for such patients. The risk/benefit ratio clearly is in the patient's favor.—G.R. Holt, M.D., F.A.C.S.

Airway Endoscopy in the Diagnosis and Treatment of Bacterial Tracheitis in Children

Eckel HE, Widemann B, Damm M, Roth B (Univ of Cologne, Germany)
Int J Pediatr Otorhinolaryngol 27:147–157, 1993   130-95-11–14

Background.—The initial symptoms of bacterial tracheitis (BT) in children are those of viral laryngotracheobronchitis or epiglottitis. However, such patients do not respond to appropriate treatment for these diseases, and acute respiratory decompensation often develops. Because the treatment and outcome of BT are so different from those of viral laryngotracheobronchitis and epiglottitis, the diagnosis must be prompt and accurate.

Methods.—The significance of different diagnostic features was studied in 11 patients, aged 8 months to 11.5 years. A chart review indicated that these patients met the criteria for BT.

Findings.—All had inspiratory stridor and respiratory distress, but the presence of cough, hoarseness, and fever were inconsistent. Duration of symptoms and length of prodromal period were also variable. Leukocyte counts ranged from 3.7 to 14.7 cells/nL. Differential blood counts demonstrated band cells in 1% to 41% of leukocytes. There was a marked left shift above 30% in 3 patients. In 2 patients, C-reactive protein was mildly increased and markedly increased in 1 patient. In 10 of the 11 children, chest radiographs led to diagnosis of pneumonia, bronchopneumonia, acute bronchitis, and lobar dystelektasia. In most patients, Gram stains of the purulent secretions showed polymorphonuclear leukocytes with gram-positive cocci. The most common bacterium cultured was *Staphyloccocus aureus*. All children had a normal supraglottic and glottic larynx on laryngoscopy. In 8 children, tracheobronchoscopy showed typical BT findings—membranous inflammation or copious mucopurulent secretions in the trachea with notable subglottic edema. This enabled a definitive diagnosis. The resolution of the inflammatory process typically required 1 to 2 weeks. None of the patients needed a tracheostomy. There were no instances of cardiopulmonary arrest or toxic shock syndrome, but severe adult respiratory distress syndrome developed in 1 child, necessitating prolonged assisted artificial ventilation. Length of hospitalization ranged from 1 to 3 weeks. None of the children died or had significant long-term morbidity.

Conclusions.—There is no single clinical, radiologic, or laboratory feature that reliably predicts BT. Airway endoscopy is the only diagnostic procedure able to distinguish BT from other forms of acute obstructive upper airway disease accurately and promptly. Endoscopy can be both diagnostic and therapeutic. Children with mild airway obstruction can be managed medically and observed.

▶ If the child's clinical condition warrants concern about BT, then endoscopy should be performed urgently. Endoscopy also provides a means of aspiration for cultures and cleaning of the exudate within the airway.—G.R. Holt, M.D., F.A.C.S.

12 Head and Neck Oncology

Professional Burnout Among Head and Neck Surgeons: Results of a Survey
Johnson JT, Wagner RL, Rueger RM, Goepfert H (Univ of Pittsburgh, Pa; MD Anderson Cancer Ctr, Houston)
Head Neck 15:557–560, 1993   130-95-12–1

Background.—Burnout can develop in any highly productive, hardworking individual. Burnout among physicians has not been studied extensively. A survey was done to document professional burnout among head and neck surgeons.

Methods.—Approximately 1,045 surveys were mailed to members of the American Society of Head and Neck Surgery and the Society of Head and Neck Surgeons. Questionnaires were received from 395 physicians, for a 39% return rate. The mean age of the respondents was 48 years.

Findings.—Physicians worked an average of 66 hours a week. More than 70% of their time was devoted to patient care; 30% to 50% of this time was spent managing head and neck cancer. Thirty-four percent of the physicians said they were burned out. However, only 27% were frustrated with disease, compared with 67% frustrated by government requirements and 58% frustrated with the economics of medical practice. Ninety-seven percent said they liked their work.

Conclusions.—Although most of the head and neck surgeons responding to this survey said they enjoyed their work, the stress of extending working hours to care for severely ill patients and the increased need to deal with government and economic demands were major concerns. These issues need to be discussed and confronted to enhance the ability of physicians to function productively.

▶ This excellent paper should raise the specter of concern in our profession for those of us who deal with head and neck cancers. The frustration that we feel probably comes from dealing with the bureaucracies of the government and insurance companies. I fear that, because of capitation and managed care, many will view cancer surgery as too costly and will recommend nonsurgical care on the basis of cost and time alone. Let's not let that happen.—G.R. Holt, M.D., F.A.C.S.

Microlaryngoscopic Surgery for T1 Glottic Lesions: A Cost-Effective Option

Myers EN, Wagner RL, Johnson JT (Univ of Pittsburgh, Pa)
Ann Otol Rhinol Laryngol 103:28–30, 1994   130-95-12-2

Objective.—For the treatment of T1 glottic lesions, microlaryngoscopy (ML) with excision of the lesion with or without laser use, vertical partial laryngeal surgery, and irradiation provide primary cure rates greater than 85%. In the present cost-conscious environment, there is a need to define treatment costs along with medical decision-making to provide cost-effective treatment.

Study Design.—The cost-effectiveness of ML with or without laser treatment was studied in a retrospective review of 50 patients with invasive and microinvasive squamous cell carcinoma who underwent treatment between 1978 and 1990. Cost analysis was performed for each treatment modality and hospitalization by averaging 10 hospital bills and related service bills and extrapolating 1992 health care costs into the treatment options for T1 glottic carcinoma. By using previous reports, analysis of cost-effectiveness was also performed for other treatment options for T1 glottic lesions, including hemilaryngectomy and radiotherapy.

Findings.—During an average follow-up of 48 months, 46 (92%) patients were cured by primary ML with excision, requiring an average of 2 procedures (range, 1 to 6). Four (8%) patients failed ML treatment, but all were successfully salvaged by hemilaryngectomy or irradiation. Similar cure rates had been reported after hemilaryngectomy or radiotherapy for T1 glottic lesions. The costs of treatment for T1 glottic cancer were $12,956 per patient for ML, $35,616 per patient with hemilaryngectomy,

TABLE 1.—Costs of Treatment for Glottic Carcinoma

Type of Treatment	Total Costs*
Microlaryngoscopy plus excision with or without laser (1 procedure)	$6,478
Microlaryngoscopy plus excision with or without laser (2 procedures)	$12,956
Radiotherapy	$27,000
Hemilaryngectomy	$35,616
Total laryngectomy	$25,649
Laryngoscopy	$5,588

* Costs include hospital, surgeon, radiology, radiation oncology, ancillary services, and technical and professional components, where applicable (1992 figures).

(Courtesy of Myers EN, Wagner RL, Johnson JT: *Ann Otol Rhinol Laryngol* 103:28–30, 1994.)

TABLE 2.—Costs for Theoretic Group of 100 Patients
Undergoing Microlaryngoscopy With Excision

ML (100 patients) = ($6,478 × 2) × 100 patients = $1.3 million.

Eight patients would fail this regimen and need further treatment.

Two patients would have HL for salvage and 6 patients would undergo XRT. Therefore,

HL (2 failures) = $35,616 × 2 patients = $71,232

and

XRT (6 failures) = $27,000 × 6 patients = $162,000.

Finally, total costs for the entire ML patient group would be

C (total) = ML + HL + XRT or $1.5 million.

Abbreviations: ML, microlaryngoscopy; HL, hemilaryngectomy; XRT, radiotherapy; C, cost.
(Courtesy of Myers EN, Wagner RL, Johnson JT: *Ann Otol Rhinol Laryngol* 103:28–30, 1994.)

---

and $27,000 per patient with radiotherapy (Table 1). When these costs were extrapolated to a theoretic group of 100 patients, ML plus excision only cost $1.5 million (Table 2), providing savings of up to $2.4 million when compared with hemilaryngectomy ($3.6 million) or irradiation ($3.9 million).

Conclusion.—In T1 glottic carcinoma, ML plus excision provides cure rates similar to open conservation laryngeal surgery or radiotherapy, but with potential for savings. In selected patients, ML with excision is an effective, cost-conscious management option for early vocal cord cancer.

▶ There are 2 important notions to take from this study. The first is that for small T1 glottic lesions, microlaryngoscopic excision appears to be efficacious. The second has to do with recognizing that cost-effectiveness should be considered, to some degree, in therapy decision-making, primarily for the survival of health care and *not* for rationing of care.—G.R. Holt, M.D., F.A.C.S.

Diagnosis, Treatment, and Outcome of Follicular Thyroid Carcinoma
(Emerick GT, Duh Q-Y, Siperstein AE, Burrow GN, Clark OH) (Univ of Calif, San Diego; VA Med Ctr, San Francisco; Yale Univ, New Haven, Conn)
Cancer 72:3287–3295, 1993   130-95-12–3

Background.—Many studies have been published on the diagnosis, treatment, and prognosis of patients with papillary thyroid carcinoma. Relatively few researchers, however, have studied patients with follicular carcinoma.

Patients and Findings.—Sixty-five patients who underwent 96 thyroid operations for pure follicular thyroid carcinoma from 1956 to 1990 were included in the review. There were 43 women and 22 men with a mean age of 45 years. The mean postoperative follow-up was 10.4 years. Initially, 80% had a solitary thyroid nodule. Thirty-seven percent reported symptoms at the initial evaluation. Tumor size was a median of 2.2 cm. Of 20 patients who were undergoing fine-needle aspiration biopsy, 18 had a follicular neoplasm. In the other 2 patients, the specimen was inadequate. Nineteen patients were given thyroid-stimulating hormone (TSH)-suppressive thyroid hormone treatment for an average of 4.5 months before surgery. Tumor size remained the same in 53% of the patients, increased in 26%, and decreased in 11%. Initial surgery in 49% of the patients was lobectomy, total thyroidectomy in 23%, lobectomy plus contralateral partial or subtotal lobectomy in 17%, and lesser procedures in 11%. Twenty-nine patients had a completion total thyroidectomy; therefore, a total of 68% had total thyroidectomy. Only 8% of the 39 patients undergoing intraoperative frozen section were given a correct diagnosis of cancer. Three of the 96 operations resulted in permanent complications. Five percent of the patients died of thyroid cancer since thyroidectomy, and 2 are alive with distant metastatic disease.

Conclusions.—At first examination, patients with follicular thyroid cancer usually have solitary thyroid nodules that are follicular neoplasms by aspiration cytology. These nodules do not regress in response to TSH-suppressive treatment. The treatment of choice for follicular neoplasms is lobectomy followed by completion total thyroidectomy for histologically proven carcinomas greater than 1 cm. Total thyroidectomy permits the use of thyroglobulin and radioiodine scanning in the detection and treatment of metastatic cancer.

▶ I think the philosophy presented in this article for the management of follicular thyroid neoplasms is sound, scientifically supportable, and easily understood. My own experience is that it is sometimes difficult for the cytopathologist to identify a follicular neoplasm solely on fine-needle aspiration.—G.R. Holt, M.D., F.A.C.S.

Serum Thyroglobulin and Iodine-131 Whole-Body Scan in the Diagnosis and Assessment of Treatment for Metastatic Differentiated Thyroid Carcinoma

Lubin E, Mechlis-Frish S, Zatz S, Shimoni A, Segal K, Avraham A, Levy R, Feinmesser R (Beilinson Med Ctr, Petah Tiqva, Israel; Tel Aviv Univ, Israel)
J Nucl Med 35:257–262, 1994   130-95-12–4

Background.—For decades, patients who had undergone thyroidectomy for differentiated thyroid carcinoma (DTC) underwent periodic iodine-131 whole-body scanning. This approach has numerous disadvantages, including the need to suspend therapy for 6 weeks, questionable sensitivity, and low yield in detecting metastases. An experience with serum thyroglobulin (TG) levels in 261 consecutive patients with DTC who had undergone total thyroidectomy and ablation was described.

Methods.—The patients were 178 females and 83 males with histologically confirmed DTC. The mean follow-up was 8 years. Treatment was with near-total thyroidectomy and ablation with ^{131}I, based on the postoperative evaluation. The investigators periodically measured serum TG by using a noncompetitive immunoradiometric assay, with no reduction in replacement therapy. Whole-body ^{131}I scans were obtained after replacement therapy had been suspended for 6 weeks, or when thyroid-stimulating hormone (TSH) levels increased to higher than 50 μU/mL. When radiologic procedures were performed with iodinated contrast media, patients waited no less than 10 weeks before undergoing ^{131}I whole-body scanning.

Results.—Of the 208 patients with serum TG consistently less than 10 ng/mL, 201 had no signs of metastases and were considered true-negatives. Fifty-eight patients with proven metastases were followed-up for a mean of 7 years. Eighty-eight percent of them had high serum TG assays while they were receiving full replacement therapy. Whole-body ^{131}I scan localization was clear in 55% of these patients. In no instance did a patient with a positive whole-body scan have a negative serum TG determination.

Conclusions.—Serum TG had a sensitivity of 88%, specificity of 99%, and accuracy of 97% in the recognition of metastases among these DTC-ablated patients. The recommended protocol for evaluation of DTC patients after surgery and ablation is clinical examination every 6 months for the first 3 years and yearly thereafter; serum TSH and TG measurements at each visit; ultrasound of the neck yearly for the first 3 years and every 2 years thereafter; and chest radiography every 2 years. When any of these raises the suspicion of active disease, ^{131}I whole-body scanning is indicated.

▶ This paper makes a good case for using the serum TG as a screening tool to detect metastatic DTC. A specificity of 99% is excellent. It makes sense both clinically and economically.—G.R. Holt, M.D., F.A.C.S.

New Clinical Severity Staging System for Cancer of the Larynx: Five-Year Survival Rates

Piccirillo JF, Sasaki CT, Wells CK, Feinstein AR (Yale Univ, New Haven, Conn)
Ann Otol Rhinol Laryngol 103:83–92, 1994   130-95-12–5

Background.—Despite its many shortcomings, the tumor, node, metastasis (TNM) morphological staging system remains the classification system for many cancers. Recent studies indicate that the precision of morphological staging in patients with cancer of the larynx can be improved by inclusion of symptom type, symptom severity, and comorbid-

Quantitative Evaluation of Staging Systems

| | *Staging Systems* | | |
Category of Evaluation	*TNM Anatomic (1988)*	*Functional Severity*	*Clinical Severity*
Monotonicity of survival gradient	Yes	Yes	Yes
Range of overall survival gradient	43%	68%	60%
Proportionate reduction in predictive errors	11%	29%	29%
Proportionate reduction in variance	0.094	0.240	0.219
χ^2 For linear trend	15.55	47.30	30.47

(Courtesy of Piccirillo JF, Sasaki CT, Wells CK, et al: *Ann Otol Rhinol Laryngol* 103:83–92, 1994.)

ity. The prognostic importance of staging symptoms and comorbidity in patients with laryngeal cancer was studied and an attempt was made to create a new composite staging system that combines clinical and morphological data to improve the precision of TNM staging.

Methods.—Between 1973 and 1985, 193 patients were treated for cancer of the larynx. The anatomical extent of the tumor was defined by using the TNM morphological staging system. Symptoms were classified into 4 symptomatic stages: local, perilocal, extralocal, and distant symptoms. Associated diseases, termed comorbidities, were noted.

Results.—Total 5-year survival was 66%. By TNM stage, 5-year survival was 78% for stage I, 67% for stage II, 60% for stage III, and 35% for stage IV. Within each TNM stage, a new functional severity (FS) staging system that combined symptom severity and comorbidity produced a consistent prognostic gradient and predicted 5-year survival more effectively than did TNM anatomical staging alone. With the FS staging system, the 5-year survival rates were 83% for the alpha group, 58% for the beta group, and 15% for the gamma group. When the FS stages were combined with TNM stages, a powerful 4-category composite clinical severity (CS) staging system was created: CS stage A, formed by the union of TNM stage I and FS stage alpha; CS stage B, formed by TNM stage II Hand FS stage alpha; CS stage C, by TNM stage III and FS stage beta; and CS stage D, by TNM stage IV and FS stage gamma. The corresponding 5-year survival rates for the new CS staging were 88%, 80%, 63%, and 28%, respectively. Quantitative evaluation of the TNM, FS, and CS staging systems indicated that all 3 had a monotonic survival gradient, but, for every other feature, FS and CS systems were qualitatively superior to the TNM systems (table).

Conclusion.—Clinical variables in a formal staging system can strikingly improve prognostic accuracy in patients with cancer of the larynx. The CS staging system, combining the FS and TNM anatomical stages, is more prognostically precise than TNM anatomical staging alone.

▶ It has always seemed to me that the TNM system needed "fine-tuning," particularly with respect to the individual patient. The symptoms a patient has when he or she is first seen are very significant, and this new composite clinical severity staging system seems quite promising. Let's support its evaluation.—G.R. Holt, M.D., F.A.C.S.

Mucosal Melanoma of the Head and Neck: The Impact of Local Control on Survival

Lee SP, Shimizu KT, Tran LM, Juillard G, Calcaterra TC (Univ of Calif, Los Angeles)

Laryngoscope 104:121–126, 1994   130-95-12–6

Objective.—As yet, there is no consensus on the optimal treatment for mucosal melanoma of the head and neck. To gain more insight into the management of this uncommon disease, patient medical histories were assessed retrospectively.

Patients.—Between 1955 and 1991, 35 patients were treated for primary mucosal melanoma. The tumor was located at the nasal fossa, paranasal sinuses, and nasopharynx in 80% of patients and involved the oral cavity or oropharynx in 20%. All but 1 patient had localized disease; 1 had cervical lymph node involvement, and none had distant metastases. The median follow-up was 45 months (range, 32 to 225 months).

Treatment.—Primary treatment consisted of radical surgery in 15 patients and local resection in 11; 11 of these 26 surgical patients received either adjuvant radiation therapy or systemic treatment (chemotherapy or immunotherapy). Six patients received primary radiation therapy, and another 2 received primary systemic therapy.

Outcome.—After the initial treatments, only 7 of the 34 (21%) patients achieved local control, with a median actuarial local control of 23.7 months and 5-year relapse-free rate of 17%. The rate of local recurrence was high (27 of 34), but only 5 had distant disease develop before local recurrence. Actuarial probability of survival in patients with their disease controlled locally was significantly longer than among patients with persistent local disease. Only 5 of 21 (24%) patients who had local relapse were salvaged successfully. The median disease-free survival rate was 57 months, and the 5-year survival rate was 45%.

Conclusion.—These findings highlight the importance of achieving local control to significantly improve survival in the management of mucosal melanoma of the head and neck. Aggressive local treatments should be initiated when the disease is first diagnosed in patients. Contrary to previous opinions, mucosal melanoma of the head and neck is not necessarily incurable if local control can be achieved. Surgery remains the mainstay of treatment, and the search for effective systemic treatment should be continued.

▶ The message of this study is clear: Control local disease. Difficulty occurs when the otolaryngologist is faced with a tumor that is located in the nasopharynx, where exposure is difficult and functional morbidity abounds.—G.R. Holt, M.D., F.A.C.S.

Management of Ectopic Thyroid Nodules

Kozol RA, Geelhoed GW, Flynn SD, Kinder B (Veterans Affairs Med Ctr, Allen Park, Mich; Wayne State Univ, Detroit; George Washington Univ, Washington, DC; et al)
Surgery 114:1103–1107, 1993   130-95-12–7

Purpose.—Confusion about the malignant nature of low-grade papillary carcinoma of the thyroid gland led to the long-standing surgical dictum that so-called lateral aberrant thyroid actually represents a metastatic papillary carcinoma. It has been further suggested that ipsilateral thyroid lobectomy plus isthmusectomy should be performed when lateral aberrant thyroid tissue is discovered. Sixteen cases of ectopic thyroid tissue in which there was no evidence of carcinoma were reported.

Findings.—The cases were identified from a review of occurrences of benign lateral aberrant thyroid. Most of the nodules were found between the thyroid lobe and carotid sheath; none were lateral to the carotid sheath. In 7 patients, the ectopic tissue was discovered during the evaluation and treatment of hyperparathyroidism, whereas the other 9 cases were identified during the evaluation and treatment of thyroid disorders or cervical nodules. The histologic findings of the nodules were benign in 15 cases. In the remaining case, the ectopic thyroid nodule has remained unchanged after 4 years of follow-up scanning. Thyroid resection was performed to look for occult carcinomas in 8 patients; in all of these patients, histologic examination revealed only normal thyroid or benign nodules.

Conclusions.—Lateral aberrant thyroid tissue is not necessarily malignant. Therapy for these nodules should be guided by their histologic condition along with intraoperative examination of the ipsilateral lobe of the thyroid. Medical teaching should exclude the inaccurate surgical dictum that lateral aberrant thyroid tissue represents metastatic cancer.

▶ I always appreciate the thoughts of free-thinkers. These authors make an excellent case through their examination of "lateral aberrant thyroid nodules" to question a long-held notion. We should reconsider.—G.R. Holt, M.D., F.A.C.S.

Symptom-Directed Selective Endoscopy and Cost Containment for Evaluation of Head and Neck Cancer
Benninger MS, Enrique RR, Nichols RD (Henry Ford Hosp, Detroit)
Head Neck 15:532–536, 1993   130-95-12–8

Background.—Patients with squamous cell carcinoma of the head and neck commonly have synchronous and metachronous neoplasms of the upper aerodigestive tract. Routine screening for these lesions is commonly performed by panendoscopy; however, the diagnostic yield and cost-effectiveness of this procedure have been questioned. The tumor identification rates and cost-effectiveness of panendoscopy vs. symptom-directed selective endoscopy were assessed prospectively.

Methods.—The study included 100 consecutive patients with newly diagnosed, untreated squamous cell carcinoma. Before any further evaluations were performed, all patients' symptoms were assessed to determine which specific studies might be selected to aid in identifying second primary neoplasms. Subsequently, all patients underwent chest radiography, barium esophagography, direct pharyngolaryngoscopy, esophagoscopy, and bronchoscopy with bronchial washings. The 2 approaches were compared for their rate of identification of primary neoplasms and their cost-effectiveness.

Results.—Six patients were found to have a total of 7 synchronous primary neoplasms; 1 of the patients had 3 separate tumors. Synchronous pharyngeal neoplasms were identified in 5 cases, 2 of which were asymptomatic, and oral cavity neoplasms were found in 2 cases. In 3 patients, all with symptoms of dysphagia and odynophagia, 2 primary cervical esophageal tumors and 1 synchronous esophageal tumor were found. Chest radiography detected 2 pulmonary metastases in patients whose bronchoscopies and bronchial washings had been negative. The use of selective, symptom-directed evaluations would have reduced the total cost by one third and minimized excessive diagnostic procedures and potential morbidity.

Conclusions.—Direct pharyngolaryngoscopy and chest radiographs appear to be indicated for all patients with squamous cell carcinoma of the neck to diagnose synchronous primary neoplasms. However, esophagoscopy, esophagography, and bronchoscopy may be better reserved for patients with corresponding symptoms. Bronchial washings do not appear to be helpful in searching for additional primary tumors. With further study, indirect video pharyngolaryngoscopy may prove to be a useful alternative to direct operative pharyngolaryngoscopy.

▶ Can we all agree that a chest radiograph is a baseline need for evaluating the patient who has head and neck cancer? After that, it is up to the clinician who cares for the patient to decide what further evaluation is appropriate (managed care not withstanding). These authors offer some symptom-directed, common sense guidelines for our consideration.—G.R. Holt, M.D., F.A.C.S.

Assessment of Quality of Life in Head and Neck Cancer Patients
Hassan SJ, Weymuller EA Jr (Univ of Washington, Seattle)
Head Neck 15:485–496, 1993   130-95-12–9

Background.—Concern about quality of life (QOL), as well as survival among patients with cancer, has been increasing during the past decade. The ideal QOL questionnaire should be short and easy to understand. The University of Washington (UW) QOL Head and Neck questionnaire, the Sickness Impact Profile (SIP), and the Karnofsky scales were recently investigated.

Methods.—Seventy-five patients with head and neck cancer were selected to assess the UW QOL. The SIP and Karnofsky scales, already established evaluation tools, were used for comparison. Each assessment tool was administered several days before surgery, immediately after surgery, and 3 months after surgery.

Findings.—Ninety-seven percent of the patients found the UW QOL scale to be more acceptable than the SIP because it was more concise and easier to complete. Using the SIP as a gold standard, the UW QOL scale had a mean criterion validity of .849. The Karnofsky average criterion validity was .826. The reliability coefficients for the UW QOL, Karnofsky scales, and SIP scale were more than .9, .8, and .87, respectively. In addition, the UW QOL was more effective at detecting change than the Karnofsky and the SIP.

Conclusions.—The validity and reliability of the UW QOL scale are comparable to those of the Karnofsky and SIP scales. The UW QOL was more acceptable to patients and provided the best indicator of change in their QOL.

▶ Whatever the final form a QOL questionnaire takes for patients with head and neck cancer, it can be a valuable tool. Above all, in my opinion, it focuses the clinical management team on the issue of QOL, and allows many possibly overlooked issues regarding the patient's well-being to be addressed.—G.R. Holt, M.D., F.A.C.S.

Results of Primary and Adjuvant CT-Based 3-Dimensional Radiotherapy for Malignant Tumors of the Paranasal Sinuses
Roa WHY, Hazuka MB, Sandler HM, Martel MK, Thornton AF, Turrisi AT, Urba S, Wolf GT, Lichter AS (Univ of Michigan Med Ctr, Ann Arbor)
Int J Radiat Oncol Biol Phys 28:857–865, 1994   130-95-12–10

Background.—Radiotherapy may be used to treat primary malignant neoplasms of the paranasal sinuses when surgery is not an option. Computed-tomography–based three-dimensional (3-D) radiotherapy provides comprehensive visualization of the tumor-bearing region and surrounding normal anatomy, thus permitting accurate targeting of the tumor and its extensions in relation to normal tissues. Clinical experience with CT-based 3-D treatment planning was reported.

Patients and Methods.—Thirty-nine patients with advanced-stage malignant tumors of the paranasal sinuses underwent CT-based 3-D radiotherapy between 1986 and 1992. Fifteen patients whose tumors were unresectable received primary radiotherapy at a median prescribed total dose of 68.4 Gy. The remaining 24 patients received postoperative adjuvant treatment for close margins of less than 5 mm, microscopic, or gross residual disease at median prescribed total doses of 55.8 Gy, 59.4 Gy, and 67.8 Gy, respectively. In 37 patients, globe-sparing fields were used in the primary treatment plans. The most frequently used treatment technique involved a 4-field arrangement comprising anterior, right, and left lateral photon fields, and an interorbital electron field. Patients were treated primarily with 6-MV x-rays from a linear accelerator using isocentric methods. The interorbital electron boost was given using 6- or 9-MeV electrons, and all fields were treated daily. Isodose displays in axial planes were regularly generated for isodose prescriptions. Isodose plans in the sagittal and/or coronal planes were also generated in 24 patients. The median follow-up was 4.5 years, within a range of 19 to 86 months.

Results.—At 3 years, the local control rate was 32% for the 15 patients with unresectable tumors. Local recurrences were noted in 3 of 14 patients with microscopic residual disease at 26, 63, and 74 months from initial irradiation, and in 4 of 5 patients with gross residual disease at a median of 2 years. None of the 5 patients irradiated for close surgical margins experienced local recurrences. The adjuvant group had local control rates of 75% at 3 years and 65% at 5 years. The overall actuarial survival rate was 65% at 3 years and 60% at 5 years. None of the first sites of local disease progression were thought to have occurred outside the high-dose region. Late complications included mild osteoradionecrosis in 1 patient, limited optic neuropathy in 1 patient, and a possible radiation-induced cataract in 1 patient. No irradiation-related blindness was noted.

Conclusions.—Although additional therapeutic modalities are needed to improve local control and survival rates in patients with advanced paranasal sinus carcinomas, CT-based 3-D radiotherapy can preserve critical structures unaffected by tumor invasions and achieve the expected local control rates when used as all or part of initial treatment.

▶ We must make modern biotechnology work for us in the care of patients. This article shows how it can be done.—G.R. Holt, M.D., F.A.C.S.

Is a Surgical Resection Leaving Positive Margins of Benefit to the Patient With Locally Advanced Squamous Cell Carcinoma of the Head and Neck: A Comparative Study Using the Intergroup Study 0034 and the Radiation Therapy Oncology Group Head and Neck Database

Laramore GE, Scott CB, Schuller DE, Haselow RE, Ervin TJ, Wheeler R, Al-Sarraf M, Gahbauer RA, Jacobs JR, Schwade JG, Campbell BH (Univ of Washington Med Ctr, Seattle; American College of Radiology, Philadelphia; Ohio State Univ, Columbus; et al)

Int J Radiat Oncol Biol Phys 27:1011–1016, 1993   130-95-12–11

Background.—An untested tenet of management of patients with advanced tumors of the head and neck has been that surgery has no role unless there is a high probability of achieving clear margins. Patients with squamous cell carcinomas of the head and neck who had surgical resection that left positive margins followed by postoperative adjuvant therapy were compared with patients who received radiotherapy alone.

Methods.—In a multigroup, cooperative clinical trial testing the efficacy of adjuvant chemotherapy for patients with resectable squamous cell carcinoma of the head and neck, 109 patients were excluded because they had positive surgical margins. They were followed prospectively for local or regional control and survival. Eight of these patients received no further treatment, 6 received postoperative chemotherapy alone, 71 received radiotherapy alone, and 24 received both radiotherapy and chemotherapy. The median dose of radiation was 60 Gy. This group was matched with a control group of patients with cancer of the head and neck through a computer database. These patients received radiotherapy only, with a median dose of 66 GY. The groups were matched for tumor site, tumor stage, nodal status, Karnofsky performance status, and closest age.

Results.—The group with a positive margin had a significantly higher rate of local/regional control (44% vs. 24%) at 4 years. The overall survival rate at 4 years was not significantly different (29% in the patients with a positive margin vs. 25% in the patients receiving only radiotherapy).

Conclusions.—Although survival does not seem to be improved after incomplete excision and adjuvant therapy compared with radiation therapy alone, significant improvements were found in local/regional control of the tumor. This finding may be applicable for palliative treatment.

Until appropriate clinical trials are done, caution should be used when considering changing resectability criteria.

▶ The standard of care requires that we obtain frozen section margins and resect tissue until the margins are reported to be negative.—G.R. Holt, M.D., F.A.C.S.

Does the Method of Management of Papillary Thyroid Carcinoma Make a Difference in Outcome?
DeGroot LJ, Kaplan EL, Straus FH, Shukla MS (Univ of Chicago)
World J Surg 18:123–130, 1994   130-95-12–12

Background.—A previous study examined the data on a group of 269 patients with papillary thyroid carcinoma over a period of 12 years, showing that the major predictors of adverse outcome were increasing extent of spread of disease at time of first diagnosis, increasing age at diagnosis, and increasing size of the primary lesion. Using the same data, an attempt was made to determine whether a prognostic classification scheme can be used to predict an appropriate surgical approach, what the effect of treatment is on prognosis, and if patients with an "excellent" prognosis benefit from more extensive surgery and radioactive iodide (^{131}I) ablation.

Method.—Data were used from the previous study of 269 patients with papillary thyroid carcinoma treated at the University of Chicago since the early 1970s.

Results.—Prognostic classification schemes developed by the American Joint Commission, Cady et al., Hay et al., the European Thyroid Association, and the study's own clinical class scheme each divided patients into risk category groups. However, all systems failed to segregate some apparently low-risk patients who eventually die of thyroid carcinoma. Considering the excellent, but not perfect precision of the prognostic schemes, the need for detailed pathologic analysis, and ideally postoperative thyroid scanning, the prognostic classification schemes do not permit the decision regarding extent of surgery. Significantly fewer deaths and recurrences were seen in patients who were operated on by 3 experienced surgeons at the University of Chicago than in patients operated on by other surgeons and not routinely ablated. However, when groups were restricted to those consisting only of patients who underwent more extensive surgery, postoperative ^{131}I ablation, or both, little difference was seen between the 2 groups. The difference in prognosis, comparing patients treated at the University of Chicago and those treated elsewhere, was principally caused by the routine use of more extensive surgery and postoperative radioactive iodide ablation. An excellent prognosis was seen in patients younger than age 45 with intrathyroidal disease or positive neck nodes and tumors less than 2.5 cm in diameter. The use of ^{131}I ablation and extensive surgery were related to a significant reduction in recurrences.

Conclusion.—These data support the use of lobectomy plus contralateral subtotal lobectomy or near-total thyroidectomy in treating thyroid cancers larger than 1 cm in size and in patients older than age 45. They also suggest that the use of ^{131}I ablation postoperatively provides the best prognosis in terms of reduction in deaths and recurrences.

▶ Even though the outcome of thyroid cancer treatment is generally good, we need to remember that patients can still die of papillary carcinoma. In general, I tend to favor the aggressive approach surgically (total thyroidectomy), with ^{131}I ablation for residual uptake on the postoperative scan.—G.R. Holt, M.D., F.A.C.S.

A Critical Review of Radiotherapy in the Management of T1 Glottic Carcinoma

Morris MR, Canonico D, Blank C (Madigan Army Med Ctr, Tacoma, Wash)
Am J Otolaryngol 15:276–280, 1994   130-95-12–13

Background.—It is commonly thought that T1 glottic carcinoma can be treated with either cordectomy or radiation therapy (RT) with similar expectations relative to tumor control. Therefore, in many institutions, RT has become a popular treatment choice for this condition. The efficacy of RT in the management of patients with T1 glottic cancer was assessed.

Method.—A retrospective evaluation of 43 patients with T1 glottic carcinoma between 1974 and 1989 was done, providing a minimum of 4 years' follow-up for each patient. Two patients were treated with surgery, and 1 died of an unrelated cause. Forty patients were treated initially with RT; however, 2 were lost to follow-up. The parameters examined included incidence of tumor control, need for and type of subsequent salvage surgical procedures, quality of voice, and survival rate.

Results.—Thirty-eight patients completed RT and were available for follow-up. Of these, 10 (26%) had a primary site recurrence in the larynx, and 2 (5.6%) had a regional recurrence in the cervical lymphatics. The average time between treatment and recurrence was 34 months. Salvage surgery for treatment failures included 1 cordectomy, 3 vertical partial laryngectomies, and 6 total laryngectomies (15.6%). Death from T1 glottic cancer occurred in 1 (2.6%) patient. Speech results were judged to be good in 24% of the patients but impaired in 66%; harshness, low pitch, and inefficient breath support were the principal causes of impairment. No patient was considered to have a poor voice.

Conclusion.—Radiation therapy does not appear to be as effective as cordectomy in managing T1 carcinoma. First, initial tumor control is likely to be superior after surgery. Second, a literature review indicates that more than twice as many patients will die of local failure, and more than twice as many will require total laryngectomy for tumor control if RT is used instead of cordectomy. This means that 1 of 12 patients treated with radiation will have some adverse effect if CRT replaces surgery.

▶ Cordectomy with frozen section control and thyroplasty reconstruction appears to be a quite viable alternative to RT for T1 lesions. What would you want if it were your larynx?—G.R. Holt, M.D., F.A.C.S.

Surgical Reporting Instrument Designed to Improve Outcome Data in Head and Neck Cancer Trials
Weymuller EA Jr, Ahmad K, Casiano RR, Schuller D, Scott CB, Laramore G, Al-Sarraf M, Jacobs JR (Univ of Washington, Seattle; Radiation Therapy Oncology Group Statistical Unit, Philadelphia)
Ann Otol Rhinol Laryngol 103:499–509, 1994   130-95-12-14

Background.—Variability in the reporting of surgical data is a major source of uncertainty in the interpretation of multi-institutional studies of combined therapy for head and neck cancer, and it contributes to the consistent failure of multi-institutional protocols to find a separation between control and study arms. A computer-based, anatomically-oriented reporting instrument that improves the quality of surgical data available to multi-institutional protocols was reviewed.

Results.—According to the recommendations in the literature, a standardized format is required to categorize preoperative staging and surgical reporting objectively. All information would be presented in anatomical terms through a common computer-based form to report information related to preoperative imaging, final preoperative staging, and surgical extirpation. In this way, 3 successive aspects of patient evaluation and treatment could be categorized and computer-coded for subsequent analysis. The benefits of this method would include more consistent staging, which would ensure comparison of like tumors; discordance between radiologic stage and clinical stage, which could permit investigation into their relative benefits; comparison of operative resection data with preoperative staging data to ensure that similar tumors received similar surgery at the different institutions. In addition, surgical staging and operative data could be stratified along with other clinical, pathologic, and immunologic data.

Conclusion.—This system would permit analysis of a more uniform subset of patients and provide a more confident analysis of the therapeutic intervention under analysis. It is possible that in the long run, this format could become the foundation of a centralized national registry that would allow access to many more cases and institutions, providing they utilize the accepted form of patient evaluation and treatment.

▶ This multicenter report advances the appeal of a uniform system of record-keeping and central collection of data. I think it is a super idea.—G.R. Holt, M.D., F.A.C.S.

Devascularization of Craniofacial Tumors by Percutaneous Tumor Puncture
Casasco A, Herbreteau D, Houdart E, George B, Tran Ba Huy P, Deffresne D, Merland JJ (Hôpital Lariboisière, Paris)
AJNR 15:1233–1239, 1994   130-95-12–15

Purpose.—Preoperative embolization of hypervascular tumors reduces the tumor blood supply and decreases intraoperative bleeding. Until 1992, only very experienced interventional neuroradiologists were able to embolize hypervascular tumors arising in or extending to the base of the skull. The clinical experience with a new devascularization technique for hypervascular head and neck tumors is reported.

Patients.—Since 1992, 17 hypervascular tumors, including 10 nasopharyngeal angiofibromas, 3 calvarial metastases, 2 hemangiopericytomas, and 2 glomus tumors have been devascularized by direct percutaneous tumor puncture or via natural orifices. Alcohol was used for embolization of metastases that were not managed surgically. A mixture of NBCA, lipiodol, and tungsten powder was used for preoperative embolization. Tumor resection was performed 24–48 hours after embolization.

Results.—Total tumor devascularization was achieved in 14 tumors, and devascularization greater than 90% was attained in 3 tumors. Reflux of blood after direct puncture of the tumor was obtained in all cases. All tumors were completely resected. The black staining caused by the tungsten powder facilitated complete excision. None of the patients required blood transfusions.

Conclusions.—Percutaneous embolization is technically easier than conventional devascularization procedures. The technique facilitates complete tumor excision and consequently decreases the risk of recurrence.

▶ What if the alcohol enters the sphenoid or ethmoid artery systems, which are branches of the internal carotid artery? Base-of-skull and periorbital tumors would seem to be at risk for this complication.—G.R. Holt, M.D., F.A.C.S.

Locally Invasive Papillary Thyroid Carcinoma: 1940–1990
McCaffrey TV, Bergstralh EJ, Hay ID (Mayo Clinic and Found, Rochester,

Minn)
Head Neck 16:165–172, 1994   130-95-12–16

Purpose.—Invasion of the upper aerodigestive tract by well-differenti-ated thyroid carcinoma is an infrequent but significant cause of morbid-ity. Symptoms of airway insufficiency, dysphagia, and hemoptysis can re-sult from invasion of the recurrent laryngeal nerves, larynx, pharynx, and esophagus. The impact of invasion by papillary thyroid carcinoma on survival was evaluated retrospectively.

Findings.—The review included 262 patients treated for invasive papil-lary thyroid carcinoma during a 50-year period. The invaded sites were muscle in 53% of the patients, the laryngeal nerve in 47%, the trachea in 37%, the esophagus in 21%, the larynx in 12%, and other sites in 30%. Fifty-six percent of the patients underwent complete removal of the en-tire tumor. Survival was 79% at 5 years, 63% at 10 years, and 54% at 15 years; 20% of the patients died of papillary carcinoma. On Cox propor-tional-hazard analysis, invasion of the trachea and the esophagus was the factor with a significant effect on survival. Completeness of resection ap-proached significance, but muscle, laryngeal, and recurrent laryngeal nerve invasion had no significant independent effect.

Conclusions.—In patients with papillary thyroid carcinoma that in-vades adjacent structures, survival appears to depend on the site invaded. Complete surgical excision of the tumor may improve survival, but func-tional aerodigestive tract structures should not be sacrificed unless con-servative resection would leave behind gross tumor or intraluminal ex-tension is present. Aerodigestive tract invasion is an indication for aggressive adjuvant therapy.

▶ This review covered 50 years of experience! Although imaging and nerve conduction studies have become more sophisticated in that time, the basic surgical principles and techniques have remained relatively constant, so this study still has relevance for us today.—G.R. Holt, M.D., F.A.C.S.

Intraoperative Monitoring of the Facial Nerve: An Aid in the Manage-ment of Parotid Gland Recurrent Pleomorphic Adenomas

Olsen KD, Daube JR (Mayo Clinic and Found, Rochester, Minn)
Laryngoscope 104:229–232, 1994   130-95-12–17

Background.—The goals of surgery for recurrent pleomorphic ade-noma (RPA) of the parotid gland are to remove the tumor completely while preserving facial nerve function. Continuous intraoperative facial nerve monitoring is a useful adjunct technique for patients undergoing skull-base surgery. This technique has been applied to patients undergo-ing RPA surgery.

Methods.—Of 7 patients evaluated for a probable RPA, 4 underwent total parotidectomy with preservation of the facial nerve. All patients underwent intraoperative monitoring of electromyographic (EMG) activity from 4 muscles innervated by the facial nerve: the orbicularis oris, oculi, frontalis, and mentalis. The same wires used to record neurotonic discharges were also used to record compound muscle action potentials (CMAP) in response to nerve stimulation.

Results.—Preoperative nerve conduction and EMG studies were entirely normal in 4 of the 7 patients; the remaining 3 had signs of old facial neuropathies. All patients had neurotonic discharges of varying intensity and duration. In most cases, the discharges were moderate to intense and short and long; they generally occurred in association with surgical manipulation. There were no recurrent tumors during 10–15 months of follow-up. Postoperative facial nerve function was normal in 5 patients and essentially normal in another. One patient with preoperative grade 5 function and a massive RPA was left with grade 6 function.

Conclusion.—Intraoperative facial nerve monitoring is a beneficial adjunct to surgery for RPAs. The goals of monitoring are to enhance nerve identification and preservation with minimal nerve trauma. Although it is not a replacement for surgical experience, intraoperative facial nerve monitoring is a useful adjunct for patients who need reoperation in the parotid area and in whom preservation of facial nerve function is a realistic goal.

▶ I think that the application of the facial nerve monitor in the difficult situation of parotid gland reoperation was a great idea. It is often difficult to find the facial nerve in the scar tissue that is inevitably present, and anything that can help the surgeon find its location is appreciated.—G.R. Holt, M.D., F.A.C.S.

Surgical Management of the Temporomandibular Joint in Resection of Regional Tumors

Kreutziger KL (Ochsner Clinic, New Orleans, La)
South Med J 87:215–224, 1994   130-95-12–18

Background.—Ablative surgery for tumors is the most common cause of loss of temporomandibular joint (TMJ) integrity and function. Patients with primary tumors of bone, regional tumors of the oral cavity or mandibular erosion, or soft tissue tumors around the joint require different types of resections. The surgeon must understand the anatomical structure of the TMJ to use joint structures as resectional margins, to preserve uninvolved structures for maximal postoperative function, and to achieve reconstruction of ablated structures. The surgical management and rehabilitation of the TMJ is illustrated in a review of 14 patients requiring ablative resection.

Findings.—Five categories of surgical defects were identified among the 14 cases. The first category involves mandibular resection without entry into the TMJ structures. This type of defect involves a loss of mandibular arch integrity with varying amounts of adjacent soft tissue and muscle resection. The surgical goals are to maintain or re-establish occlusion and interarch relationships. Scar contracture and condylar drift in a medial-superior direction may be difficult problems to overcome. It is important to maintain the anatomical position of the condyle for immediate or delayed reconstruction.

In the second category, the mandibular condyle is resected with preservation of the meniscus. The inferior joint space is violated, but the intact meniscus preserves the superior joint space and maintains a vertical relationship of the reconstructed mandible to the cranial base.

The third category involves condylar and meniscal resection, with variable involvement of the superior joint space. An interpositional implant is used to separate the autogenously reconstructed condyle from the glenoid fossa; this prevents ankylosis and helps to maintain the vertical dimension of the TMJ.

In the fourth category, the degree of lateral resection determines TMJ involvement. If TMJ capsule resection is used for the deep margin, the superior joint space will be exposed. In this situation, a dermal or temporalis fascia graft can be used to protect the joint and reconstruct the superior joint space. In patients with malignant parotid tumors involving the TMJ, extended lateral resection and subtotal TMJ may be needed. In this situation, en bloc resection of the mandibular condyle, inferior and superior joint spaces, and the parotid gland is required, sometimes with neck dissection. Joint reconstruction followed principles similar to those in category 3. Finally, various TMJ resections may be needed in patients undergoing temporal bone resection. The complex reconstructive problems encountered in this situation are discussed elsewhere. Whenever extensive soft tissue resection is performed, local or regional flaps are needed to provide adequate soft tissue coverage and to prevent scar bands and scar contracture.

Discussion.—In patients with tumors in the region of the TMJ, various types of resection may be required for tumor ablation, including total resection of the TMJ, with or without reconstruction; subtotal resection with preservation of the glenoid fossa and meniscus; capsule resection with dermal graft reconstruction; or subcondylar resection with mandibular reconstruction. In all of these situations, the goal of surgery is reconstruction of all mandibular/TMJ/craniofacial complexes; immediate reconstruction is generally preferred. The surgeon must combine sound surgical principles with expertise in the anatomical features and physiologic function of the TMJ.

▶ For many years, this author has helped teach us about the clinical interface of dental and otorhinolaryngology/head and neck surgery practices. In this article he demonstrates options in managing the TMJ in large tumor resections.—G.R. Holt, M.D., F.A.C.S.

Analysis of Recurrence, Complications, and Functional Results With Free Jejunal Flaps
Bradford CR, Esclamado RM, Carroll WR, Sullivan MJ (Univ of Michigan, Ann Arbor; Ohio State Univ, Columbus)
Head Neck 16:149–154, 1994   130-95-12–19

Background.—Squamous cell carcinoma of the hypopharynx remains an aggressive malignancy with a poor prognosis regardless of treatment. Jejunal interposition provides a means of single-stage reconstruction when total laryngopharyngectomy leaves a complete oro/hypopharyngeal defect. Swallowing function is rapidly restored and the rate of complications is acceptable. The best margin to leave when removing a hypopharyngeal lesion remains uncertain.

Patients.—Recurrences were analyzed in a series of 20 patients who underwent free jejunal flap reconstruction after ablation of advanced laryngeal or hypopharyngeal squamous cell carcinoma in 1986–1991. Thirteen patients had a primary lesion in the hypopharynx, 6 in the larynx, and 1 in the cervical esophagus. Eleven patients had surgery for recurrent tumor and 2 for a second primary tumor. All patients but 1 had received radiotherapy, chemotherapy, or both previously. The average follow-up was 15 months.

Results.—One of 15 patients with new or recurrent cancer resected had persistent disease at the superior margin. Three patients had locoregional recurrences, distant metastasis developed in 1, and 2 had both locoregional and distant disease develop at the same time. Two patients had local recurrences at the distal esophageal margin. Five of the 20 patients (25%) had major complications and 2 of them died. There were 3 failures, 2 of which occurred intraoperatively and 1 of which was delayed. Swallowing function returned in about 1 month on average.

Recommendation.—Jejunal flap reconstruction is indicated only when it is feasible to achieve a distal margin of at least 2 cm above the cervical esophagus and when the distal esophagus is normal.

▶ This procedure is difficult and fraught with complications, some of which can be catastrophic. The authors tell us that we must be as certain as possible to have a disease-free 2-cm superior margin and no disease of the distal esophagus.—G.R. Holt, M.D., F.A.C.S.

Oral Tongue Cancer in Young Adults Less Than 40 Years of Age: Rationale for Aggressive Therapy
Sarkaria JN, Harari PM (Univ of Wisconsin, Madison)
Head Neck 16:107–111, 1994   130-95-12–20

Introduction.—Squamous cell carcinoma (SCC) of the tongue is rare in young adults, little information is available on the cause and management of a disease that carries a poor prognosis in the young. The literature on cases of SCC of the tongue in adults younger than age 40 years was reviewed.

Methods.—At the University of Wisconsin Hospital and Clinics, 6 patients, aged 17 to 39, had SCC of the tongue develop between 1971 and 1991. Three patients had stage I disease, 1 had stage II disease, and 2 had stage III disease.

Results.—Between 1968 and 1993, 152 cases of SCC of the oral tongue were reported in the literature. The disease stage identified for 132 patients was 37% at stage I, 27% at stage II, 20% at stage III, and 16% at stage IV. Although 64% of patients had early stage disease, 71 patients experienced progression of their disease, and 47% died of the disease. In the 6 University of Wisconsin patients, 4 used chewing tobacco or smoked cigarettes. Five of the 6 had primary surgery and were treated with chemotherapy and/or radiotherapy. Five patients had recurrences. Two patients with stage I and 2 with stage III disease died of their disease.

Conclusion.—Younger people with SCC of the tongue had higher recurrence rates and higher mortality rates than older people. Although the reason for the increased mortality among younger patients is unknown, it is possible that their cancers may be more aggressive, genetic predisposition may be a factor, or treatment may be less aggressive than in older patients. More information needs to be developed on the etiology of the disease in younger patients. The treatment approach in this group of patients should be more aggressive.

▶ Some of my most disappointing and heart-rending patients have been young adults with oral cancer. Particularly for nonsmoking women, the cure and survival rates are very depressing. Although it is very hard to do sometimes, surgical aggressiveness seems to be best for the patient.—G.R. Holt, M.D., F.A.C.S.

Early Glottic Carcinoma Treated With Open Laryngeal Procedures
Thomas JV, Olsen KD, Neel HB III, DeSanto LW, Suman VJ (Mayo Clinic and Found, Rochester, Minn; Mayo Clinic, Scottsdale, Ariz)
Arch Otolaryngol Head Neck Surg 120:264–268, 1994   130-95-12–21

Introduction.—Between 1976 and 1986, 159 patients with early glottic carcinoma without impaired vocal cord mobility underwent primary curative resection via an open laryngeal procedure. The surgical procedures included 82 frontolateral partial laryngectomies, 61 laryngofissures with cordectomy, 12 hemilaryngectomies, and 4 anterior commissure procedures. The recurrence rate and long-term survival of these patients were analyzed using the Kaplan-Meier product-limit method. The median follow-up was 6.6 years (range, 2.5 months to 14.6 years).

Results.—The probability of surviving 3 and 5 years beyond the day of surgery was estimated to be 91% and 84%, respectively. Eleven (7%) patients had a local recurrence and 4 (2.5%) had regional or distant metastasis. Of those with local recurrence, 1 had a recurrence at 41 months and another at 74 months, and 2 had cancer on the opposite cord. All those cancers probably represented a second laryngeal primary tumor; hence, it is likely that only 7 (4.4%) patients experienced a true local recurrence. Among those with recurrent laryngeal cancer, 10 (6%) underwent a laryngectomy and 1 had an anterior commissure procedure. Three patients were ultimately salvaged after retreatment. The probability of remaining free of local recurrence 3 and 5 years after surgery was 94% and 93%, respectively.

Conclusion.—Open laryngeal procedures continue to be an excellent treatment for selected cases of early glottic carcinoma. These procedures are versatile and effective for managing the wide spectrum of larger T1 glottic carcinomas, particularly those with involvement of the anterior commissure.

▶ In years past, open laryngeal surgery for vocal cord malignancy lost favor—perhaps, in part, because of better x-ray therapy and an increased use of microlaryngeal endoscopy. However, I agree with the authors that we need to revisit open laryngeal surgery and look at its potential benefits for the patient.—G.R. Holt, M.D., F.A.C.S.

The Role of Surgery Following Radiotherapy Failure for Advanced Laryngopharyngeal Cancer: A Prospective Study
Davidson J, Briant D, Gullane P, Keane T, Rawlinson E (St Michaels Hosp, Toronto; Toronto Hosp; Princess Margaret Hosp, Toronto)
Arch Otolaryngol Head Neck Surg 120:269–276, 1994   130-95-12–22

Introduction.—In 1982, 212 patients with histologically proven squamous cell carcinoma of the hypopharynx (any stage) or a stage III or IV squamous cell carcinoma of the larynx participated in a randomized controlled trial comparing conventional radical radiotherapy with split-course radiotherapy and simultaneous chemotherapy. Of these, 88 underwent potentially curative surgical salvage after radiotherapy failure. The results of prospective follow-up of these 88 patients, in terms of complications, recurrences, tumor measures, and survival, were evaluated. The Median follow-up was 4.4 years (range, .5 to 6.9 years).

Results.—Forty-two (48%) of the patients had surgical complications. The most common complication was pharyngocutaneous fistula (27%), mainly among patients who underwent partial or total pharyngectomy. Neither the addition of a neck dissection nor the site of the primary tumor influenced the complication rate. Recurrences developed at the primary site only in 62% of patients, in regional lymph nodes only in 19%, and at both sites in 19%. Overall, surgery for recurrent-persistent disease salvaged 26 (30%) of the 88 patients. The tumor, node, metastasis (TNM) stage of the recurrent tumor and the site of recurrence (local, regional, or both) significantly affected survival, whereas TNM stage of the original tumor, time to recurrence, age, sex, or primary site did not affect survival. Overall, the 5-year postsurgical survival rate was 35%, with 41% of patients retaining functional larynges.

Conclusion.—Primary radiotherapy with surgery for the salvage of recurrent-residual disease is a reasonable treatment policy for patients with advanced laryngopharyngeal squamous cell carcinoma. Although the long-term survival is not impressive, approximately 2 in 5 patients will retain a functional larynx. As yet, there is no evidence that a treatment approach that sacrifices the larynx will improve the survival of these patients. When primary treatment fails, the recurrent tumor should be restaged, because the measures of the recurrent tumor, and not those of the original tumor, correlate best with survival.

▶ This study emphasizes two major philosophic points. First, radiation therapy alone will not cure all advanced tumors. Second, we need to restage a recurrent tumor at its current extent, not where it was initially. Also, in a managed care or capitated setting, we must resist the temptation to pick the best therapy for a patient with head and neck cancer on the basis of economics rather than efficacy.—G.R. Holt, M.D., F.A.C.S.

Lobectomy Versus Total Thyroidectomy for Differentiated Carcinoma of the Thyroid: A Matched-Pair Analysis
Shah JP, Loree TR, Dharker D, Strong EW (Mem Sloan-Kettering Cancer Ctr, New York)
Am J Surg 166:331–335, 1993   130-95-12–23

Purpose.—Patients with carcinoma of the thyroid, compared with patients with other malignancies, are typically low-risk and do well regardless of treatment regimen. Poor prognosis is associated with tumor size and extrathyroid extensions but not multifocal lesions. Surgical excision of 1 lobe or the total gland is controversial, and prospective, randomized trials are needed to resolve such debates. However, the need for long-term follow-up limits the use of a trial. A matched-pair analysis of patient records for a 50-year period yielded subgroups of patients with nearly identical prognostic factors.

Methods.—The sample was developed from records of 931 patients undergoing surgical treatment from 1930 to 1980 at the Sloan-Kettering Cancer Center. As age is the most important prognostic factor, patients younger than 45 years of age were excluded, leaving 429 patients, with 196 having a total thyroid lobectomy and 104 having a total thyroidectomy. The remaining patients had subtotal procedures and were excluded. Patients were then matched according to age, metastatic stage, extrathyroidal extensions, tumor size, and histologic findings. There were 31 patients in the total thyroidectomy group without a match, which was not unexpected as this group had the more aggressive disease. This left 73 pairs of patients matched. Survival rates were analyzed on both the matched pairs and unmatched patients.

Findings.—Patient ages ranged from 45 to 76 years. The matching process yielded pairs of patients with similar distant metastases, extrathyroidal extensions, tumor size, follicular tumors, nodal stage, gender, and focality. Unmatched patients were older, and a greater proportion had distant metastases, extrathyroidal extensions, and follicular lesions. In the matched group, the 20-year survival rate was 82% in the lobectomy group and 73% in the thyroidectomy group. The difference was not significant. In the unmatched group, the survival rate for patients having lobectomy was 79%, statistically similar to the matched group. For those having total thyroidectomy, the survival rate was 38%, significantly below the matched group.

Summary.—In a matched-pair selection of patients with carcinoma of the thyroid, total thyroidectomy offered no survival advantage over lobectomy. The definition of "low risk," the use of radioiodine therapy, and recurrence rates are topics of debate. Selective use of total thyroidectomy is suggested. Lobectomy can be considered if the tumor is 4 cm or less, restricted to the thyroid gland, and without contralateral involvement or distant metastasis.

▶ For the past 25 years of my medical career, I have read and heard the debates regarding lobectomy vs. total thyroidectomy. Unfortunately, the issue is still unresolved, and the best guide continues to be the surgeon's judgment and experience.—G.R. Holt, M.D., F.A.C.S.

Fine Needle Aspiration Cytology of Salivary Gland Lesions Reported Immediately in a Head and Neck Clinic
Roland NJ, Caslin AW, Smith PA, Turnbull LS, Panarese A, Jones AS (Royal Liverpool Univ Hosp, England)
J Laryngol Otol 107:1025–1028, 1993   130-95-12–24

Background.—Finding a mass in the area of the major salivary glands poses several diagnostic problems. Although it is important to know the diagnosis before surgery, authorities disagree about the value and place of fine-needle aspiration cytology (FNAC) as a diagnostic tool. The relationship of the cytologic findings of aspirates performed and reported in a specialist head and neck oncology clinic with clinical and histologic findings was investigated.

Methods.—Fine-needle aspiration cytology was performed on 92 patients with salivary gland lesions. The aspirates were examined immediately by a cytopathologist, and the reports were conveyed to the surgeon. The results of FNAC were compared with the histologic results in those patients who underwent surgery and, also, with the clinical course of the disease at subsequent clinic visits in patients not undergoing surgery.

Findings.—The lesions from which aspirates indicated no positive diagnosis were all subsequently diagnosed as benign, for a sensitivity of 90.9% and a specificity of 100%. The positive and negative predictive values were 100% and 98.1%, respectively. Among benign cases, FNAC gave the correct diagnosis in 51 of 56, or 91.1%. An incorrect cytologic diagnosis was made in 5 cases, 1 of which was a false negative result. Among malignant cases, FNAC yielded no false positive findings. Histologic tumor classification was predicted in all 10 malignant aspirates.

Conclusions.—This rapid report system at FNAC is safe, free of complications, and useful in treatment planning. Close cooperation between the surgeon and pathologist is essential.

▶ It is clear that FNAC has become a standard of care for evaluating masses in the head, face, and neck. With rapid reporting, a treatment plan can be developed very quickly, and therapy may then be initiated in a timely fashion. I hope that open biopsies will not be entertained by primary care providers in a managed care setting when FNAC is as reliable and safer.—G.R. Holt, M.D., F.A.C.S.

13 Comprehensive Otolaryngology

Altered Dental Sensation Following Intranasal Surgery
MacDougall G, Sanderson RJ (Royal Infirmary, Edinburgh)
J Laryngol Otol 107:1011–1013, 1993   130-95-13–1

Objective.—Some patients complain of pain or paresthesia of the upper teeth or gums after intranasal surgery. When a 10-year review of the literature failed to identify the cause, an attempt was made to evaluate and quantify this problem prospectively.

Methods.—Sixty consecutive patients, aged 18 to 60 years, were evaluated 1 to 3 weeks after routine intranasal surgery. The affected area in patients who complained of altered sensation of the teeth or gums was tested by tapping the teeth with a metal spatula or touching the gums with a cotton wool probe.

Results.—Of the 83 intranasal procedures performed, 36% resulted in altered dental sensation after surgery. It was apparent that patients who underwent a particular procedure complained of altered sensation in a specific area. All patients who complained of premaxilla sensation had undergone a submucous resection or septoplasty, whereas all patients who complained of altered teeth sensation had undergone intranasal antrostomy as part of the surgery. All patients with dental pain or paresthesia recovered fully, but this took as long as 8 weeks in some.

Discussion.—Altered dental sensation is common after intranasal surgery, particularly intranasal antrostomy or septal surgery. The nasopala-

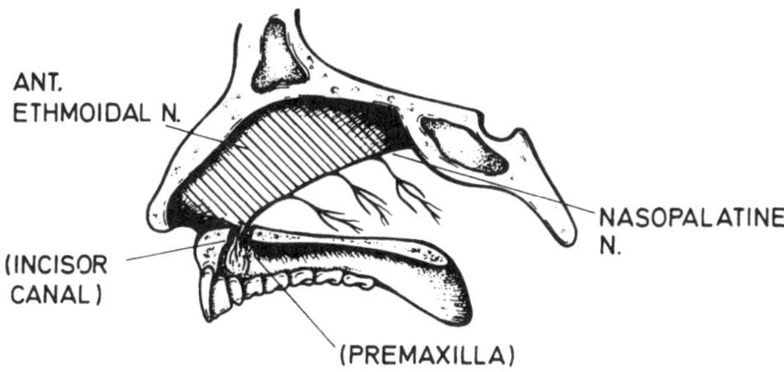

Fig 13–1.—Sensory supply of the nasal septum. (Courtesy of MacDougall G, Sanderson RJ: *J Laryngol Otol* 107:1011–1013, 1993.)

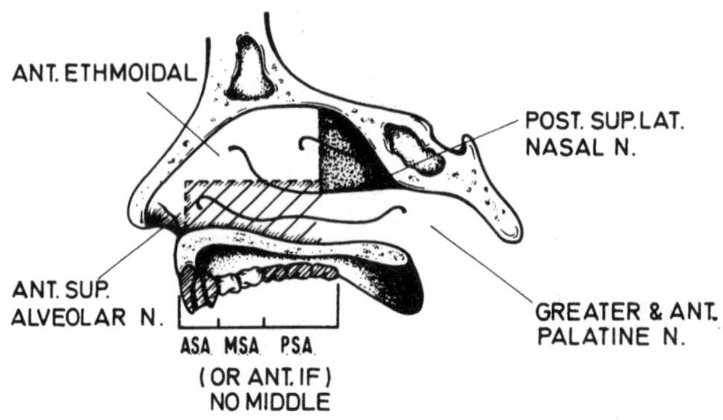

Fig 13–2.—Sensory supply of the lateral wall of the nose. (Courtesy of MacDougall G, Sanderson RJ: *J Laryngol Otol* 107:1011–1013, 1993.)

tine nerve, which supplies the posteroinferior half of the nasal septum, passes through the incisor canal to supply the mucous membrane of the premaxilla (Fig 13-1). Hence, the nerve is divided during a submucous resection (Killian's incision) but may be preserved within the mucoperichondrial flap during a septoplasty (hemitransfixion incision). The anterosuperior alveolar nerve supplies the lateral wall of the nose, a small area of the anterior nasal septum, the floor of the nasal cavity, and the mucous membranes of the anterior antral wall, as well as the canine and incisor teeth (Fig 13-2). The middle or anterior superior alveolar nerves supply the premolar teeth, and the posterosuperior alveolar nerves supply the molar teeth. Because there is a well formed anastomosis among all alveolar nerves, surgery to the lateral nasal walls may damage these nerves, resulting in referred pain in the teeth.

▶ This paper reviews the neuroanatomy and helps us understand why just about any intranasal or antral surgery performed along the inferior half of the nasal cavity can lead to hypesthesia. Fortunately, most problems resolve with time.—G.R. Holt, M.D., F.A.C.S.

Obstructive Sleep Apnea Syndrome: A Surgical Protocol for Dynamic Upper Airway Reconstruction

Riley RW, Powell NB, Guilleminault C (Stanford Univ, Calif)
J Oral Maxillofac Surg 51:742–747, 1993   130-95-13–2

Purpose.—Although uvulopalatopharyngoplasty (UPPP)—the primary treatment for obstructive sleep apnea syndrome (OSAS)—is an excellent method of controlling snoring, recent reviews suggest that it improves OSAS in only half of patients. Multiple upper airway sites appear to play a role in the obstructive process, including the soft palate, the pharyngeal walls, and the base of the tongue. Maxillofacial surgery in conjunction with UPPP has been used to correct the multiple sites of obstruc-

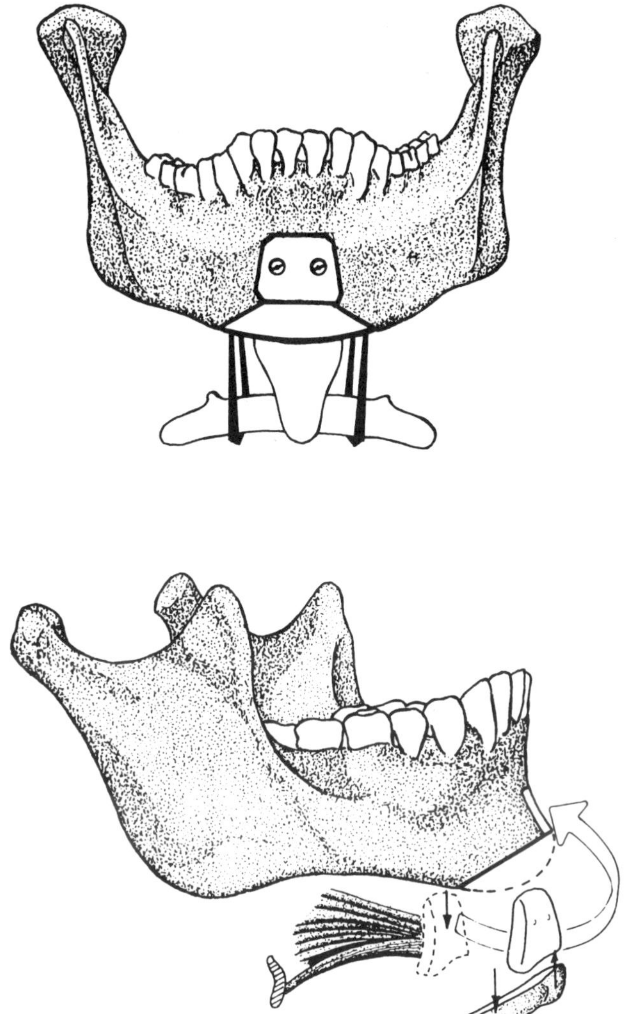

Fig 13–3.—Diagram of mandibular osteotomy/genioglossis advancement with hyoid myotomy/suspension. (Courtesy of Riley RW, Powell NB, Guilleminault C: *J Oral Maxillofac Surg* 51:742–747, 1993.)

tion; the protocol includes a mandibular osteotomy/genioglossus advancement with hyoid myotomy/suspension (GAHM) (Fig 13–3) and, when this fails, maxillary and mandibular advancement osteotomy (MMO) (Fig 13–4). A surgical protocol for dynamic upper airway reconstruction in OSAS was presented.

Methods.—A presurgical evaluation of 239 consecutive patients was done to document the diagnosis and isolate the obstructed areas; included were fiberoptic pharyngoscopy, cephalometric analysis, and poly-

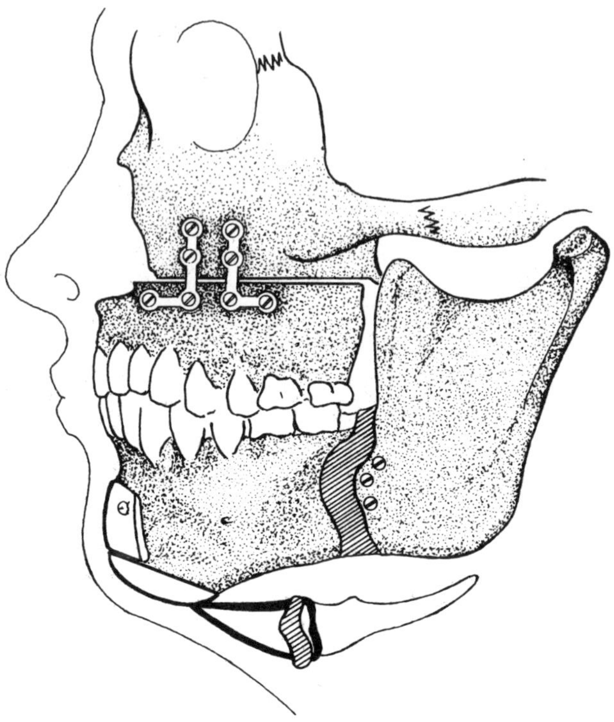

Fig 13–4.—Diagram of maxillary and mandibular osteotomy. (Courtesy of Riley RW, Powell NB, Guilleminault C: *J Oral Maxillofac Surg* 51:742–747, 1993.)

graphic monitoring. Treatment was directed to the obstructive site in a 2-phase surgical protocol, beginning with GAHM. If surgical failure was documented at 6 months by polysomnography, MMO was offered (Fig 13-5). The results of this protocol were compared with those of a series of patients using nasal continuous positive airway pressure (CPAP).

Results.—The success rate with phase 1 therapy was 61%; most of these patients required both GAHM and UPPP. Twenty-four patients went on to phase 2 therapy, for which the success rate was 100%. Surgery was as effective as nasal CPAP, as determined by analysis of changes in sleep architecture and sleep-disordered breathing. The success rates in phase 1 were almost as high as 80% for patients with mild-to-moderate OSAS, compared with about 40% for those with severe OSAS. Postoperative morbidity was low for all surgical procedures.

Conclusions.—The surgical protocol reported for OSAS yields more than a 95% long-term success rate, the highest of any protocol reported. The comprehensive presurgical evaluation, permitting a logical approach to reconstruction of the upper airway, is a vital part of treatment.

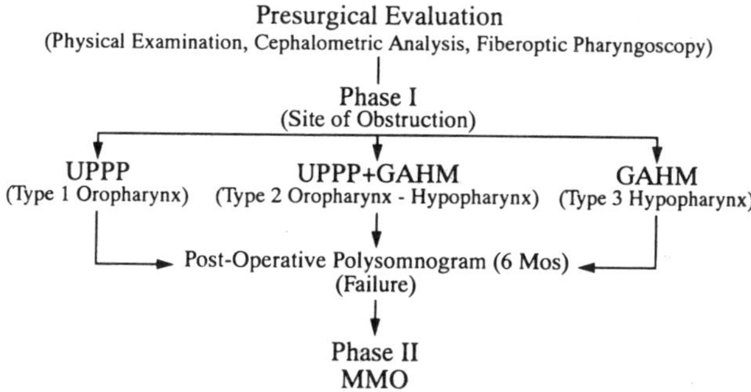

Fig 13–5.—Surgical protocol. (Courtesy of Riley RW, Powell NB, Guilleminault C: *J Oral Maxillofac Surg* 51:742–747, 1993.)

▶ For severe OSAS, particularly for those patients who fail UPPP/septoplasty, this surgical protocol is worth considering. Remember that immediate postoperative airway and oxygenation monitoring is important in patients with severe OSAS, particularly after extensive surgical procedures such as those described here.—G.R. Holt, M.D., F.A.C.S.

Peritubal Adenoidectomy

Drake AF, Fischer ND (Univ of North Carolina, Chapel Hill)
Laryngoscope 103:1291–1292, 1993   130-95-13–3

Background.—Most otolaryngologists use an adenotome or adenoid curette to do an adenoidectomy. A Bovie electrocautery may also be used to cauterize this lymphoid tissue. A method of using a curved uterine curette to complete the adenoidectomy was described.

Technique.—The new technique addresses the concern about incomplete tissue removal, which may cause persistent symptoms, predispose to regrowth, and necessitate another procedure. In this technique, a midline resection of adenoid tissue is initially done using the adenoid curette, which is selected to fit the nasopharynx between the torus tubarius on either side. Therefore, adenoid tissue is left laterally, and direct trauma to the tori is avoided. A 5-mm curved uterine curette is then used bilaterally from the level of the eustachian tube orifice inferiorly to the lower extent of the nasopharynx. A large amount of tissue often is removed along with the central mass. The uterine curette is bent, allowing the tip to reach into the pharyngeal recess, a procedure called peritubal adenoidectomy. Immediate perioperative antibiotics are given, and hemostasis is achieved.

Conclusions.—With this new method, surgeons can remove lymphoid tissue laterally in the nasopharynx and inferior to the fossae of Rosenmüller, which may be left using conventional techniques. The new technique has been used for more than 10 years with no known nasopharyngeal stenosis or increased incidence of eustachian tube dysfunction.

▶ In "experienced" hands, the uterine curette may be helpful in removing adenoid tissue from the peritubal area. However, damage to the torus tubarius can also occur if it is improperly handled. The use of perioperative antibiotics should be optional.—G.R. Holt, M.D., F.A.C.S.

Is the Sleep Apnoea/Hypopnoea Syndrome Inherited?
Douglas NJ, Luke M, Mathur R (City Hosp, Edinburgh, Scotland)
Thorax 48:719–721, 1993   130-95-13–4

Background.—The etiology of the sleep apnea/hypopnea syndrome (SAHS) remains unclear. Because snoring, a prerequisite for SAHS, runs in families, it was hypothesized that SAHS may be inherited. In a pilot study, it was determined whether there is an increased frequency of irregular breathing during sleep in relatives of nonobese patients with SAHS (more than 15 apneas + hypopneas (per hour of sleep).

Methods.—In a prospective study, questionnaires were sent to all first-degree relatives of 20 consecutive new patients with SAHS. Those living within 150 miles of Edinburgh were invited for overnight monitoring of their breathing, sleep, and oxygenation patterns in the sleep laboratory.

Findings.—Of the 76 eligible first-degree relatives, 40 consented to have overnight sleep studies. Of these, 10 had more than 15 apneas + hypopneas per hour of sleep, and 8 had more than five 4% desaturations per hour. These "affected" relatives were older but were not more obese than others, had more frequent arousals from sleep and lower minimal oxygen saturations, more frequently were described as loud snorers, and had more witnessed apneas than the unaffected relatives. Except for a difference in gonion-gnathion-hyoid angle and uvular width, none of the affected relatives had skeletal deformities on cephalometry.

Summary.—First-degree relatives of nonobese patients with SAHS demonstrate increased irregular breathing and desaturation during sleep, and the frequencies are significantly higher than in the British population. The increased uvular width in affected relatives may reflect either increased fat deposition or mucosal or muscular changes, which, like the difference in gonion-gnathion-hyoid angle, may be secondary to abnormal breathing during sleep. The inherited anomaly may be altered soft tissue or fat deposition in the neck, or a defect of the control of upper airway caliber rather than an inherited skeletal defect. These preliminary findings provide sufficient evidence of a familial predisposition to SAHS to warrant further studies.

▶ Physiognomy may play a role in obstructive sleep apnea and SAHS, and family members tend to be built similarly. Other issues, such as a tendency for facial trauma/accidents, views on tonsillectomy, ethyl alcohol intake, and dietary habits may also play a role in the familial explanation.—G.R. Holt, M.D., F.A.C.S.

Bacteriology of Tonsil and Adenoid and Sampling Techniques of Adenoidal Bacteriology

Gaffney RJ, Timon CI, Freeman DF, Walsh MA, Cafferkey MT (Beaumont Hosp, Dublin; St James' Hosp, Dublin; Trinity College, Dublin)
Respir Med 87:303–308, 1993   130-95-13–5

Background.—Despite the ubiquitous nature of recurrent acute tonsillitis and adenotonsillitis, the underlying pathogens are poorly understood. The results of a previous study in which an operative pernasal swab was used to predict tonsil core pathogens were confirmed and extended, and the relationship between the bacteriologic findings of the adenoid and the tonsil was studied. A direct adenoid swab was also compared with the pernasal swab.

Methods.—All patients admitted for elective adenoidectomy or adenotonsillectomy during a 16-month period were studied. After anesthesia was induced, pernasal and direct swabs of the adenoid were taken, as were swabs of the tonsils if tonsillectomy was being done. After removal, adenoid curettings were crushed, and samples were cultured. After removal, tonsils were carefully dissected under sterile conditions, and their inner cores were cultured.

Results.—Elective adenoidectomies were done in 53 patients; 122 patients had adenotonsillectomies. The average age of the 86 males and 89 females was 5.6 years. Pathogenic bacteria were isolated from all but 3 of the adenoid specimens, with *Haemophilus influenzae* (nontypeable) being the most common (76.7% of specimens). Mixed pathogens, most commonly *H. influenzae* and *Staphylococcus aureus*, were isolated in 37.6% of specimens. Direct adenoid swab and curettings cultures were available in 77 patients, and 48 patients (62.3%) had the same results. Comparison of pernasal adenoid swab and curettings cultures, available in 143 patients, showed identical pathogens in 76 patients (52.1%). Tonsil core and adenoid curettings were available in 122 patients; a common pathogen was found in 112 patients (91.8%), whereas an identical pathogen was found in 69.7%. Of 102 patients with both tonsil core cultures and pernasal swab cultures, results were the same in 43 (44.7%).

Conclusions.—*Haemophilus influenzae* is closely associated with hypertrophy of the adenoid and the tonsil. A pernasal swab is preferable to a throat swab as a reliable indicator of both tonsil and adenoid bacteriologic findings in children with hypertrophy of the adenoid and recurrent acute tonsillitis.

▶ For some time, I have believed that we need to recognize and legitimatize the term "adenoiditis." How many times do we need to see a child with purulent nasal drainage, swollen adenoids, and tender neck nodes before we suspect an infection of the adenoids?—G.R. Holt, M.D., F.A.C.S.

Outpatient Tonsillectomy and Adenoidectomy: Complications and Recommendations

Schloss MD, Tan AKW, Schloss B, Tewfik TL (McGill Univ, Montreal; Montreal Children's Hosp)
Int J Pediatr Otorhinolaryngol 30:115–122, 1994   130-95-13–6

Background.—In the face of increasing pressure to control health care costs, the use of outpatient surgery for children requiring tonsillectomy with adenoidectomy is becoming more popular. The complications resulting from such procedures and how they could be avoided were studied, and the parental views and concerns of home care of postoperative children were assessed.

Method.—To assess complications, a retrospective chart analysis of 555 cases on tonsillectomy and adenotonsillectomy was carried out. The patients' age, sex, and detailed history were recorded, along with preoperative assessment, examination, and type of operation, the technique, intraoperative blood loss, length of hospitalization (if required), complications, and management. To evaluate parental concerns, a questionnaire was given to the families of 49 patients to ask their opinions on providing postoperative care.

Results.—Of the 555 patients undergoing tonsillectomy and adenotonsillectomy, 103 (19%) were scheduled for inpatient procedures. The remaining 452 patients (81%) underwent ambulatory surgery. Of these, 91 (20%) had at least 1 complication: 17 required emergency room management only, whereas 74 patients were admitted on the day of surgery or later. A total of 282 scheduled outpatients underwent surgery by the traditional knife dissection techniques, and 170 underwent electrocautery dissection. Those outpatients who underwent knife dissection averaged 68 mL of blood loss. The patients who had electrocautery dissection averaged 26 mL of blood loss. These data were similar to the inpatient group.

The complications encountered in the outpatient group included intraoperative hemorrhage (less than 1%), primary postoperative hemorrhage (3.5% in the outpatients vs. 1.9% in the inpatients), secondary postoperative hemorrhage (5.1% in the outpatients vs. 1.9% in the inpatients), and aerodigestive tract complications (10% of outpatients vs. 12.6% of inpatients). In the study of parental attitudes and concerns, about 15% of the patients had a high degree of nervousness regarding the surgery, with another 68% indicating somewhat lesser anxiety. More than 80% believed that their child would cooperate well with the surgery and convalescence. Most revealing, however, was the parents' anxiety about their child's first postoperative night. Sixty percent of parents reported being somewhat worried, and only 25% were relieved that in-hospital care was provided. Twenty percent of the parents were terrified of having to care for their child postoperatively, with an additional 58% expressing some concern over this possibility. Only 4% of the parents felt relief at being able to care for the child at home.

Conclusion.—This comparative study indicates that the physician providing care for children undergoing tonsillectomy or adenotonsillectomy must understand and address the relative social circumstances as well as the factors influencing postoperative complication rates. A triad, including recent history of upper airway infection, knife dissection techniques, and increased intraoperative blood loss of 100 mL or more, provides selection criteria for the performance of these procedures on an inpatient basis because of increased risk of postoperative hemorrhage. The effect on family lifestyle as the result of a surgical procedure and postoperative care of the child can be seen and hypothesized from the data provided.

▶ Call me old-fashioned (and many do), but I do not send my tonsillectomy and adenotonsillectomy patients home the same day. I have used the dissection and suture technique for nearly 25 years, and it has served me and my patients well. This article did not address the risk of dehydration in outpatients. It has been my experience that it takes about 21–22 hours to get them to take adequate fluids.—G.R. Holt, M.D., F.A.C.S.

The Functional Role of the Tonsils in Speech
Finkelstein Y, Nachmani A, Ophir D (Meir Hosp, Kfar Saba, Israel; Tel Aviv Univ, Israel)
Arch Otolaryngol Head Neck Surg 120:846–851, 1994   130-95-13–7

Background.—Much information is available regarding the role of the tonsils in infectious disease and obstructive sleep apnea, but little consideration is given to their role in speech. Illustrative cases of various interrelations between the tonsils and the activity of the venopharyngeal (VP) valve in speech were presented.

Case 1.—In this patient, markedly hypertrophic tonsils veil a bifid uvula. A careful peroral examination, including prodding of the uvula, is required in candidates for adenotonsillectomy with hypertrophic tonsils.

Cases 2 and 3.—In patients with markedly hypertrophic tonsils, bilateral convexity of the nasal aspect of the velum can be observed as the velum is pushed posteriorly by the tonsils. On videofluoroscopic lateral view, the tonsils take an oval shape and remain between the anterior and posterior tonsillar pillars below the velum, at rest and during closure of the VP valve.

Case 4.—Extension of the hypertrophic tonsils posteriorly to the velum and upward into the VP isthmus may occur in patients with VP insufficiency. In contrast to the normal tonsil that remains stationary below the velum, as the velum elevates in these patients during closure of the VP valve, the tonsils rise with the velum. The superior tonsillar poles protruding in both portal areas of the VP isthmus obstruct superoposterior velar movement. Thus, a central gap forms between the superior poles of the tonsils, the velum, and the posterior pharyngeal wall. The tonsillar poles seal the VP isthmus only during short phonetic efforts, deglutition, or gagging.

Case 5.—Unilateral extension of the superior tonsillar pole was discovered in 1 patient with an unoperated submucous cleft palate. Deep diastasis of velar musculature was seen with a circular VP closure pattern. Sealing of the VP valve was achieved through approximation of its walls and the velum to the tonsillar pole. Subsequent speech evaluation revealed only borderline hypernasality.

Case 6.—The tonsils may be significant for VP closure in patients with palatal defects who have had pharnygeal flap surgery, and who tend to snore and have obstructive sleep apnea. The flap is too narrow and low for the correction of VP insufficiency. Tonsillectomy brings a notable improvement of symptoms.

Conclusion.—The morphological features and closure of the VP valve are closely associated with the tonsils. The tonsils may influence VP valving and, consequently, may affect speech patterns. Combination nasendoscopic and multiview videofluoroscopic studies of the mechanical properties of the tonsils during speech are required in patients with tonsillar hypertrophy who are seen with VP insufficiency, and also in patients with palatal anomalies who are candidates for tonsillectomy.

▶ Nowhere is this point made more clear than when we must decide whether to remove the tonsils of a professional (or aspiring) singer. There is a risk of altering the voice, although in most cases the benefits of reducing infections outweigh this risk.—G.R. Holt, M.D., F.A.C.S.

Teleconsultation of Patients With Otorhinolaryngologic Conditions: A Telendoscopic Pilot Study
Pedersen S, Hartviksen G, Haga D (Univ Hosp of Tromsø, Norway; Norwegian Telecom Research, Tromsø, Norway; Alta Primary Care Centre, Norway)
Arch Otolaryngol Head Neck Surg 120:133–136, 1994   130-95-13–8

Background.—Through audiovisual communication with expert medical centers, telemedicine systems substantially improve the quality of the assistance service provided in remote regions. The design and preliminary results of remote endoscopic examination trials were reported.

Methods and Findings.—This diagnostic test was done in 3 phases. In phase 1, a general practitioner was instructed in otorhinolaryngologic assessment methods; in phase 2, remote endoscopic assessments were simulated and the diagnoses were compared with findings from a standard examination; and in phase 3, the general practitioner performed real telendoscopic examinations. The last 2 phases involved a convenience sample of 24 patients. Although the video image is compressed before it is transmitted over the telecommunications network, the quality of the transmitted images was found to be the same as the quality of images from a standard endoscopic assessment.

Conclusions.—Teleconsultation for otorhinolaryngologic conditions may be used in the clinic with the same degree of reproducibility as in conventional consultation. With this technology, patients in remote areas can be given better service at a lower cost.

▶ Military medicine is currently fascinated with telemedicine for remote outposts and distant conflicts. I suppose if we really thought about it, we could find an application for underserved areas of the United States. However, there is no substitute for doing the examination yourself to obtain the level of confidence needed for proper diagnosis: "I have to see it for myself."—G.R. Holt, M.D., F.A.C.S.

The Aetiology of Lateral Cervical (Branchial) Cysts: Past and Present Theories
Golledge J, Ellis H (Univ of Cambridge, England; Bedford Gen Hosp)
J Laryngol Otol 108:653–659, 1994   130-95-13–9

Objective.—Although cysts of the lateral neck were first described almost 200 years ago, there is no general agreement as to their definition and etiology. Theories of origin include the Branchial Theory, Precervical Sinus Theory, Pharyngeal Pouch Theory, and the Lymph Node Theory. The clinical and histologic aspects of excised lateral neck cysts were examined to determine how they arise and develop.

Methods.—The records of 20 patients (age, 14–49 years) with excised lateral neck cysts were examined.

Results.—Most patients complained of neck swelling. Approximately 40% reported a history of swelling and pain that stopped after treatment with antibiotics. In 85% of patients, the cyst was in front of the upper sternocleidomastoid, lying in the cervical fascia. All cysts had stratified squamous epithelial lining and contained lymphoid tissue. Half showed reactive hyperplasia (Fig 13-6).

Conclusion.—It is suggested that epithelium from the palatine tonsil, which penetrates the lymph node, causes the transformation that later results in a cyst.

▶ Read the arguments and make your decision. Your opinion is as good as that of anyone else.—G.R. Holt, M.D., F.A.C.S.

INCLUSION THEORY

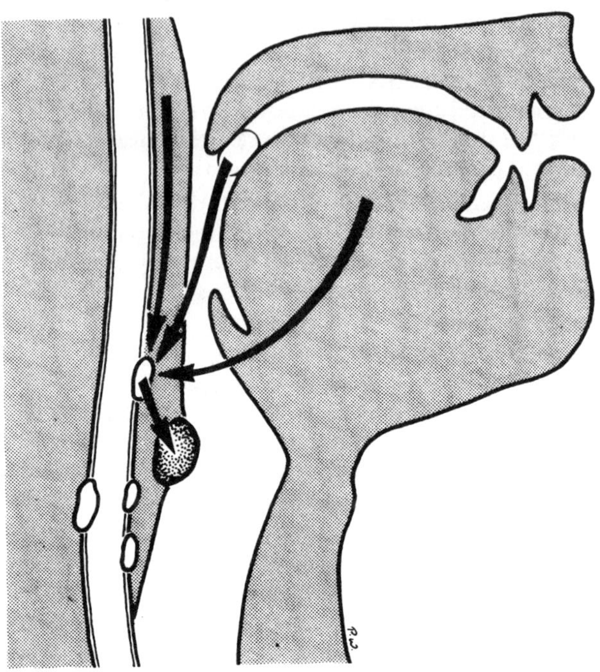

Fig 13–6.—Diagram to illustrate how squamous epithelium from the palatine tonsil could enter a cervical lymph node via the lymphatics and stimulate cystic transformation to a lateral cervical cyst. (Courtesy of Golledge J, Ellis H: *J Laryngol Otol* 108:653–659, 1994.)

Value of Radiography in the Management of Possible Fishbone Ingestion

Sundgren PC, Burnett A, Maly PV (Univ of Lund, Malmoe, Sweden; Malmoe Gen Hosp, Sweden)
Ann Otol Rhinol Laryngol 103:628–631, 1994   130-95-13–10

Purpose.—Patients with complaints of fishbone ingestion are routinely treated by endoscopic examination, preceded by a radiographic examination. Because fishbone can be radiolucent, the results of radiographic examination are often inconclusive. The records of patients with a history of fishbone ingestion were retrospectively reviewed to assess the value of radiographic examination before endoscopy.

Patients.—The study population consisted of 42 patients, ages 2–82, with complaints of fishbone ingestion. All patients underwent an oral examination, a radiographic examination, and endoscopy. The radiographic examination included plain films, barium swallow studies, and water swallows. Endoscopy was performed as soon as possible under general anesthesia.

Results.—Fifteen of the 42 patients (36%) had pathologic findings at endoscopic examination, radiographic examination, or both. Eleven patients (26%) had pathologic findings on endoscopy. Of these 11, 7 had fishbones removed, 2 had fish meat removed, 1 had an almond removed, and 2 had mucosal tears. Of the 7 fishbones removed at endoscopy, 5 (71%) were missed by the primary radiologist. Two expert radiologists who reviewed the radiographs also missed 2 bones (29%).

Conclusions.—Radiographic examination in patients with complaints of fishbone ingestion provides no valuable information and only delays endoscopic examination and fishbone removal. Patients with a short history of symptoms of fishbone ingestion should proceed directly from oral examination to endoscopic examination.

▶ This paper makes sense and fits with our clinical impression of the usefulness of radiography in fishbone ingestion. However, I do not think Sweden has quite the same number of personal injury attorneys that we have in the United States.—G.R. Holt, M.D., F.A.C.S.

IgE-Mediated Allergy From Vegetable Allergens

Ortolani C, Pastorello EA, Farioli L, Ispano M, Pravettoni V, Berti C, Incorvaia C, Zanussi C (Ospedale Niguarda Ca' Granda, Milan, Italy; Univ of Milan, Italy)
Ann Allergy 71:470–476, 1993   130-95-13–11

Introduction.—Oral mucosal contact with some fruits and vegetables causes allergic symptoms in sensitized subjects. The symptoms of fruit and vegetable allergies are commonly associated with allergic rhinitis, especially birch pollen allergy. A critical reassessment of food allergy to fruits and vegetables was presented.

Discussion.—Studies demonstrate that allergy to fresh fruits and vegetables is IgE-mediated. The symptoms generally occur immediately and involve the areas in direct contact with the food. Most of the clinical features are local and include oral pruritus and swelling of the lips and tongue. However, systemic symptoms such as urticaria, asthma, or anaphylactic shock may also occur. Systemic symptoms may be particularly severe in patients allergic to celery. Because cross-reactive antigens of pollens and foods are frequent, clinical associations between food allergy and allergic rhinitis are commonly noted. Age of onset of allergic rhinitis is closely associated with the onset of food allergy. An IgE-mediated allergy is generally diagnosed by skin tests and the detection of specific IgE in serum; however, fruit and vegetable allergens are easily denatured by common procedures of allergenic extraction. Further study is needed to better standardize diagnostic tests using fresh fruits and vegetables. Double-blind placebo-controlled food challenge is the "gold standard" for the diagnosis of food allergies. These tests are difficult to perform with fresh fruits and vegetables, however.

Summary.—Sensitized subjects may experience IgE-mediated allergic symptoms to fresh fruits and vegetables. The main clinical features are local, but systemic symptoms also occur. Allergic rhinitis is the most important risk factor for the development of fruit and vegetable allergies.

▶ The otolaryngologist should now begin to suspect a relationship between nasal allergic patients and certain food allergies. The problem may be more common than we think.—G.R. Holt, M.D., F.A.C.S.

Ambulatory Pediatric Tonsillectomy and the Identification of High-Risk Subgroups

Rothschild MA, Catalano P, Biller HF (Mount Sinai School of Medicine, New York)
Otolaryngol Head Neck Surg 110:203–210, 1994   130-95-13–12

Background.—Tonsillectomy is one of the procedures that has been targeted for cost reduction in recent years, but the cost-effectiveness and safety of ambulatory tonsillectomy remain under discussion. A number of insurance carriers currently do not reimburse for inpatient tonsillectomy, but in some cases, the hospital will absorb this cost in the interest of patient safety and comfort.

Objective.—The records of 153 consecutive patients, younger than 19 years, who underwent tonsillectomy in 1989 and 1990 were reviewed in an attempt to identify those at relatively high risk. Tonsillectomy was performed either by blunt and sharp dissection or by electrocautery.

Patients.—Nearly one fourth of the patients were 3 years of age or younger; the mean age was 8.3 years. Half the patients underwent surgery for recurrent tonsillitis, but 81% of patients aged 3 and younger and half of those 4 to 8 years of age had surgery because of obstructive sleep apnea syndrome. An attending otolaryngologist performed 41% of the operations, and residents did the remaining procedures under close supervision.

Results.—Patients younger than 4 years of age resumed oral intake after a mean of 26.5 hours, compared with 16.5 hours for older patients, a significant difference. Mean times to discharge were 59 and 31.5 hours, respectively. Five patients operated on for sleep apnea (7%) had evidence of airway compromise in the immediate postoperative period. No patient had bleeding before being discharged.

Recommendation.—Children aged 3 and younger are more likely not to tolerate oral feedings for a longer time after tonsillectomy. Those with obstructive sleep apnea may have airway problems after the procedure. Under these circumstances, the benefits of admission to the hospital justify the higher cost.

▶ I am sorry, but I still keep my tonsillectomy patients in the hospital for 23 hours after surgery, because it has been my experience that they start taking adequate oral fluids only about 21–22 hours after surgery. We need to identify the high-risk groups pointed out in the article.—G.R. Holt, M.D., F.A.C.S.

The Human Adenoid: A Morphologic Study

Winther B, Innes DJ (Univ of Virginia Health Sciences Ctr, Charlottesville)
Arch Otolaryngol Head Neck Surg 120:144–149, 1994   130-95-13–13

Introduction.—Although adenoid tissue is present in adults, the epithelium is difficult to distinguish from the neighboring mucosa. In studies of volunteers infected with the human rhinovirus, the virus was detected on the surface of the adenoid more frequently, for a longer period of time, and within 24 hours of infection compared with 4 other nasal cavity sites. The mechanism by which antigens interact with adenoid mucosa in adults was examined.

Methods.—Samples from 13 adenoids were taken from children younger than 12 years of age. Epithelial cells were examined by 3 types of microscopy—light, transmission electron, and scanning electron—and by cryofractography.

Results.—Clefts between the ridges on the anterior surface of the adenoid were filled with mucus. Lymphoid follicles beneath the epithelium were filled with lymphocytes. Cells on the ridges of the surface were 62% ciliated, 34% nonciliated flat, and 4% goblet, the cells in the clefts were 73% nonciliated flat cells, 26% ciliated, and 1% goblet. Lymphocyte presence was highest in the areas where nonciliated flat cells predominated. Basement membrane was easily recognized under the ciliated epithelium. No inflammation was observed. Multiple microfold surface cells (M cells) were visible in the lymphoepithelium under the electron microscope. The M cells were covered with fuzzy microvilli and joined by connections that may permit cells to move between the epidermis and the lamina propria. Lymphocytes were present beneath the M cells, and the space between lymphocytes was filled with proteinaceous material.

Conclusion.—The epithelium of the adenoid mucosa is made up of ciliated and nonciliated flat cells, and it contains M cells and channels for lymphocyte passage between the epidermis and the lamina propria.

▶ It is interesting to envision the adult adenoid tissue as a functioning transport and antigen recognition system that has continued immune "service" to our upper aerodigestive tracts.—G.R. Holt, M.D., F.A.C.S.

Mycobacterial Cervical Adenitis in Children: Medical and Surgical Management

Hawkins DB, Shindo ML, Kahlstrom EJ, MacLaughlin EF (Univ of Southern California, Los Angeles)
ENT J 72:733–742, 1993   130-95-13–14

Series.—Eighty-five children and adolescents were seen over 20 years for chronic cervicofacial adenitis suggesting a mycobacterial origin and a positive tuberculin skin test, isolation of mycobacteria from aspirated or surgical material, or histopathologic findings of mycobacterial infection. There were 39 males and 46 females (mean age, 5.5 years) in the series.

Clinical and Bacteriologic Findings.—Three fourths of the patients had had adenopathy for more than 3 weeks. Most often, a firm or hard mass was present; however, a number of patients had indurated or fluctuant masses. Most patients had a mass high in the anterior region of the neck. Tuberculin purified protein derivative skin testing was positive in 95% of 79 evaluable patients. One fifth of 80 patients had chest x-ray adnormalities, and 2 had findings consistent with miliary tuberculosis. Mycobacterial organisms were detected in 62% of cases.

Management.—Twenty-three patients received antituberculosis drug treatment only. Thirteen others had diagnostic biopsy or drainage of an abscess initially, followed by antituberculosis drug therapy. Forty-nine patients received drug treatment initially, with or without needle aspiration, and later underwent surgery.

Outcome.—All but 5% of the patients who received only antituberculosis drug treatment were cured, as were half the patients who had initial surgical treatment followed by drug therapy. All patients who underwent secondary surgical treatment were cured. The overall cure rate was 93%. Postoperative hematomas were not a problem because wounds were routinely drained for 24 hours after surgery.

Conclusions.—A significant number of children and adolescents in this series had cervical adenitis caused by *Mycobacterium tuberculosis.* Even patients with atypical infection do not always require operative treatment; 4 of 18 patients who were cured by chemotherapy alone had such organisms.

▶ With a national increase in the incidence of tuberculosis, we must be vigilant in observing its presentation in the neck. It is also worrisome that some strains appear to be resistant to our antituberculosis drugs.—G.R. Holt, M.D., F.A.C.S.

Eye Protection in Ear, Nose and Throat Surgery
Prior AJ, Montgomery PQ, Srinivasan V (Whipps Cross Hosp, Leytonstone, London)
J Laryngol Otol 107:618–619, 1993   130-95-13–15

Background.—Contamination of the surgeon with infectious agents can result from a needle stick or through contamination of mucous membrane or traumatized skin. There is a case report of conjunctival contamination, and The Royal College of Surgeons of England considers the cornea as a potential entry portal for HIV. A 10% to 70% incidence of contamination has been reported for general and orthopedic surgeons and during necropsies.

Methods.—Risk of contamination through the conjunctiva was quantified by examining blood splashes that landed on the protective glasses of otolaryngologic surgeons. The safety glasses of 3 surgeons were examined after a total of 260 procedures. Glasses were examined for number, size, and location of splashes.

Results.—The overall contamination rate was 15%. Ninety-two percent of the splashes from contaminated cases occurred on the outside of the glasses, and the remaining splashes were internal. The average number of splashes was 3.1 per contaminated operation. These splashes were small, with two thirds being less than .5 mm in diameter. Surgeons were aware of splashes only 31% of the time. Side shields decreased the risk by a factor of 10.

Conclusions.—The use of safety glasses during otolaryngologic surgical procedures resulted in a 15% risk of contamination, which was reduced when side shields were also used. The results demonstrate that eye protection, initially regarded as inconvenient, should be used to offer conjunctival protection to surgeons during ear, nose, and throat procedures. For absolute protection when operating on high-risk groups, goggles are preferred over safety glasses.

▶ We practice in a very risky environment in both the office and the hospital. We can no longer ignore the risks of HIV transmission and must do everything possible to protect ourselves, our staff, and our families from a tragedy. Somehow, there does not seem to be the same risk to the personal injury attorneys, does there?—G.R. Holt, M.D., F.A.C.S.

14 Environmental Health and Epidemiology

Risk of Multiple Primary Tumors Following Oral Squamous-Cell Carcinoma

Jovanovic A, Van Der Tol IGH, Schulten EAJM, Kostense PJ, De Vries N, Snow GB, Van Der Waal I (Free Univ Hosp/Academic Centre for Dentistry, Amsterdam, The Netherlands)

Int J Cancer 56:320–323, 1994   130-95-14–1

Introduction.—Various studies reporting the incidence of multiple primary tumors (MPT) in patients who have squamous cell carcinoma (SCC) of the lip and oral cavity have estimated the percentage to be 10% to 27%. The incidence of MPTs in patients with SCC and in the general population was compared to determine the relative risk of MPTs after SCC of the lip and oral cavity.

Methods.—The records of 727 patients with no previous history of malignancy, who had been treated for SCC of the lip or oral cavity, were reviewed. Data were collected regarding MPT location, synchronicity or metachronicity of the MPTs, and patient demographics. This information was compared with data from the general population-based cancer registry taken from the appropriate person-year of follow-up. Risk was determined by calculating the ratio of the numbers of observed tumors in the SCC population to the numbers of expected tumors in the general population.

Results.—During the 2,860.2 person-years of follow-up, 96 of the 727 patients with SCC had 114 MPTs develop. Of these MPTs, 80% appeared in the respiratory and upper digestive tract (RUDT), and 13% were synchronous. In women, most of the MPTs occurred in the oral cavity; in men, the MPTs occurred all over the RUDT. Patients with SCC of the lip and oral cavity have a significantly increased risk of another primary cancer developing in the oral cavity or pharynx (74.7 for men, 190.4 for women) and in the upper esophagus (24.6 for men, 45.3 for women). The risk of lung or larynx cancer developing is less elevated, and the risk of non-RUDT cancers developing is not increased.

Discussion.—Because patients with SCC of the lip and oral cavity have a much greater risk of subsequent primary lesions developing, management strategies should include identification of risk factors, early detection, and chemoprevention. These patients should be advised to avoid known risk factors, such as smoking and drinking alcohol, and to increase their consumption of fruit and vegetables. Further study is required to identify risk factors, optimal screening methods, and the most effective chemopreventive agent.

▶ This study supports what clinicians have determined through experience: Oral carcinoma is associated with an increased risk for cancer farther down the throat. Although we must encourage behavior modification, this effort would be more productive in those who are just starting to smoke and drink.—G.R. Holt, M.D., F.A.C.S.

Gender Differences in Sleep Disordered Breathing in a Community-Based Sample
Redline S, Kump K, Tishler PV, Browner I, Ferrette V (Case Western Reserve Univ, Cleveland, Ohio; Cleveland Veterans Affairs Med Ctr, Ohio; Harvard Med School, Brockton, Mass)
Am J Respir Crit Care Med 149:722–766, 1994   130-95-14–2

Introduction.—Studies of patients referred for clinical evaluation and polysomnography have suggested that most patients with sleep-related breathing disorders are men. However, some recent epidemiologic evidence suggests that this reported male preponderance may be greatly overestimated. This issue was assessed as part of a community-based study of the genetic epidemiology of sleep apnea.

Methods.—The study included 2 groups of subjects: a laboratory sample of 36 index probands with laboratory-confirmed obstructive sleep apnea syndrome, and a community sample including 196 of their family members and 157 of their neighbors. In addition to physical examination and symptom questionnaires, each participant completed overnight in-home monitoring of airflow, oximetry, heart rate, and chest wall impedance. Individuals with a respiratory disturbance index (RDI) of 15 or greater were considered to have sleep-disordered breathing (SDB). The findings were analyzed for associations between sex, SDB, and symptoms of SDB.

Results.—By the study definition, SDB was present in 38% of the male and 15% of the female participants. Whereas women outnumbered men in the laboratory sample by a ratio of 8:1, the corresponding ratio in the community sample was only 2:1—26% men vs. 13% women. Women in the laboratory sample tended to be younger and heavier than men. In contrast, women with SDB from the community sample tended to be older than the men, 63 vs. 47 years, and 75% were postmenopausal. In the community sample, men and women with SDB were not different in body mass. Women were 2 to 3 times less likely to report symptoms of snoring, snorting, gasping, and apnea than men, after adjustment for RDI.

Conclusions.—This community-based study confirms the suggestion that the male preponderance in SDB is not as great as previously reported. Older women are commonly affected by SDB, often in the absence of morbid obesity. Underreporting of SDB symptoms may be the reason why it is clinically recognized less frequently in women. However, apnea is more severe in men than in women, as identified from a community sample.

▶ Men, now you have some scientific information to take home! Seriously, it seems that more women are being seen with sleep disorders, and the earlier "apparent" male predominance may be changing.—G.R. Holt, M.D., F.A.C.S.

Determinants of Papillary Cancer of the Thyroid
Wingren G, Hatschek T, Axelson O (Univ Hosp, Linköping, Sweden)
Am J Epidemiol 138:482–491, 1993   130-95-14–3

Background.—Reported differences in the incidence, geographic distribution, trends, clinical course, and causes of the various types of thyroid cancer suggest that they should be considered separate biological entities. The various exposures, occupations, and medical aspects of papillary cancer were studied in a case-control study.

Methods.—One hundred four patients in whom papillary thyroid cancer was diagnosed between 1977 and 1987 and 387 randomly selected control patients were included. Information was obtained by questionnaire.

Findings.—Women with papillary cancer had worked as dentists or dental assistants, telephone operators, teachers, and day nursery personnel more often than did women without cancer. The former group also reported a greater occupational exposure to chemicals and video display terminals. The 11 men with papillary cancer more often worked as mechanics and metal workers and had more occupational contact with solvents. Among women, additional factors associated with increased risk were the presence of private well water at the birth address: leisure time exposure to combustion smoke; low intake of cruciferous vegetables and seafood; and a family history of goiter, heart disease, biliary disorder, or female genital cancer. Also associated with an increased risk were repeated dental examinations and diagnostic radiographic assessments, especially to the head, neck, or upper back-chest area. Among women younger than 50 years at diagnosis, an increased risk was associated with pregnancy soon after puberty. There were also tendencies toward a decreasing risk with increasing age of first pregnancy and an increasing risk with a greater number of pregnancies. Multiparity appeared to potentiate the effect from previous radiographic assessment.

Conclusions.—These findings confirm some of the known or suspected risk factors for thyroid cancer. Some new factors were also found to be associated with an increased risk, including solvents, various chemicals, some occupational exposures, well water, diagnostic radiographic assessment, some diseases other than goiter in the family, and pregnancy soon after puberty.

▶ Each practitioner can be a clinical researcher in his/her own office. Simply develop environmental and occupational questionnaires and review the data to look for correlations, trends, or suspicions. We are all potential epidemiologists.—G.R. Holt, M.D., F.A.C.S.

How Effective is Nicotine Replacement Therapy in Helping People to Stop Smoking?

Tang JL, Law M, Wald N (Wolfson Inst of Preventive Medicine, London; St Bartholomew's Hosp Med College, London)
BMJ 308:21–26, 1994　　　　　　　　　　　　　　　　　　　130-95-14–4

Introduction.—Various forms of nicotine replacement therapy have been used in smoking cessation trials. The results from 40 randomized controlled trials were analyzed to determine and compare the efficacy of the different forms.

Methods.—The trials analyzed included 28 using nicotine 2-mg chewing gum, 6 using nicotine 4-mg chewing gum, 6 using a nicotine transdermal patch, and 1 each using nicotine nasal spray and nicotine inhaler. The study subjects were either self-referred volunteers or invited. Treatment efficacy was determined by computing the difference between the percentages of treated and control patients who had stopped smoking at 1 year.

Results.—Nicotine 2-mg chewing gum had a treatment efficacy of 6% overall. Efficacy was greater among self-referred (11%) than among invited (3%) patients. In 6 of the trials, the level of nicotine dependence was assessed and efficacy was significantly higher in high-dependence (16%) than in low-dependence (2%) smokers. Nicotine 4-mg chewing gum was superior to 2-mg gum among high-dependence smokers, enabling about 33% to give up smoking. There was no difference in efficacy between 2-mg and 4-mg gum among low-dependence smokers. Overall efficacy for the nicotine transdermal patch was 9%, with greater efficacy among self-referred (12%) than among invited (6%) patients, and greater efficacy using a 21-mg patch than with a 14-mg patch. Efficacy was only slightly related to nicotine dependence. The nasal spray had 15% efficacy and the inhaler had 12% efficacy with self-referred volunteers, but these forms caused habituation.

Discussion.—Nicotine replacement therapy was more effective among self-referred patients who may be assumed to be more highly motivated. Both nicotine chewing gum and the transdermal patch are effective in smoking cessation treatment. Among the most highly nicotine-dependent smokers (those who crave a cigarette upon waking), the most effective form of nicotine replacement therapy currently is nicotine 4-mg chewing gum.

▶ This interesting study showed a 9% success rate with the use of nicotine transdermal patches. That sounds lousy to me. I am not sure that I have ever gotten anyone to stop smoking over the long haul by using any of the nicotine preparations—old or new. Maybe I am not convincing enough.—G.R. Holt, M.D., F.A.C.S.

Global Monitoring of Positive Surgical Outcome: A Feasibility Study at the Royal National Throat Nose and Ear Hospital

Ryan RM, East CA, White C (Royal Natl Throat Nose and Ear Hosp, London)
Ann R Coll Surg Engl 76:234–237, 1994   130-95-14–5

Background.—Assessment of clinical outcome is increasingly being considered crucial to monitoring quality in health care. The usefulness and feasibility of documenting positive outcome in every surgical patient were assessed.

Method.—During a 6-month period, every patient awaiting surgery at the Royal National Throat, Nose, and Ear Hospital in London was asked to define in simple terms his/her subjective goals of the operation. These goals were documented in the patient notes, along with the surgeon's diagnosis and objective goal, which may or may not be the same as the subjective goal of the patient. After surgery, both surgeons and patients answered the question, "Has this operation achieved the stated goal?"

Results.—A total of 1,490 patients defined their goals of surgery. Of these, 530 had their operation and came to early postoperative follow-up during the same 6-month period. Because this is a feasibility study, the results are the following conclusions drawn to date: First, some gauge of positive outcome was found to be documented after every operation. Second, the data could be broken down when a certain number of cases were followed by both subjective and objective success, and a proportion were failures both subjectively and objectively. Third, the system required simplicity and had to restrict itself to primary goals that were defined as precisely as possible and were well understood by the patient. Finally, it was obvious that some operations do not lend themselves to short-term assessment and require subsequent postal communication with the patient to obtain details of subjective outcome.

Conclusion.—The early conclusions drawn from this study indicate that it is feasible to collect useful data about positive outcome after every surgical procedure. The logistics of such a system are relatively simple, and the information provided is helpful when used as pointers to more detailed study, rather than as end points in themselves. This system is particularly suitable for otolaryngology, in which many procedures are carried out with relatively clear objectives. However, the system of individual outcome monitoring could equally be applied to any surgical specialty.

▶ I like the notion of simplifying outcomes studies to answer a single question: "Was the therapeutic goal for this patient achieved?" Will the hospitals' quality assurance communities buy it? Maybe they would if we obtained sufficient information to give us the appropriate feedback.—G.R. Holt, M.D., F.A.C.S.

Disappearance of Epiglottitis During Large-Scale Vaccination With *Haemophilus influenzae* Type B Conjugate Vaccine Among Children in Finland
Takala AK, Peltola H, Eskola J (Natl Public Health Inst, Helsinki; Children's Hosp, Finland; Helsinki Univ, Stenbäckinkatu, Finland)
Laryngoscope 104:731–735, 1994   130-95-14–6

Background.—Haemophilus influenzae type B is the major pathogen causing epiglottitis in children (80% of all cases) and adults (53% of all cases). Because of the localization of the infection and inflammation, epiglottitis may proceed rapidly to airway obstruction, with mortality as high as 6% in children. The effect of vaccination of Finnish children with *H. influenzae* type B–conjugate vaccine on the incidence of epiglottitis from 1985 to 1992 was reported.

Methods.—As part of clinical trials for this conjugate vaccine, intensified surveillance of invasive disease was established in 1985 in Finland. Each laboratory in the country had a liaison who prospectively sent to the national laboratory all bacterial isolates recovered from blood, CSF, or otherwise sterile body fluids recovered from children, as well as *H. influenzae* isolates from Finns 16 years of age and older. Clinical data from the hospitals were sent with these isolates. All hospital records for children with invasive bacterial disease during the 1985–1989 period were retrospectively reviewed. The conjugate vaccine trials began in 1986, and vaccination coverage of 94% to 98% of infants was achieved. By 1992, 85% of all children in Finland younger than 5 years of age were protected against *H. influenzae* type B.

Results.—In the prevaccination period, the annual incidence of epiglottitis among all children was 5.3/100,000; among children younger than 5 years, it was 13.2/100,000. The annual incidence among adults was .08/100,000 during the prevaccination period. During the vaccination period, as the proportion of children younger than 5 years vaccinated with the conjugate increased, the number of cases of epiglottitis decreased in a significant, linear trend. No decreasing trend was seen among children 7–15 years of age or among those older than 16 years of age. All but 1 patient who contracted epiglottitis during the vaccination period was unvaccinated. The 1 vaccinated child was 18 months old, had received vaccine doses at 4 and 6 months of age, and was due for a booster when he became ill.

Conclusions.—Most cases of epiglottitis among children can now be prevented safely and efficiently with the *H. influenzae*-conjugate vaccine.

▶ In addition to having all of our children obtain vaccinations against polio, mumps, measles, and tetanus, we need to consider a mandatory *H. influenzae*-conjugate vaccine.—G.R. Holt, M.D., F.A.C.S.

Second Cancers Following Oral and Pharyngeal Cancers: Role of Tobacco and Alcohol

Day GL, Blot WJ, Shore RE, McLaughlin JK, Austin DF, Greenberg RS, Liff JM, Preston-Martin S, Sarkar S, Schoenberg JB, Fraumeni JF Jr (Natl Cancer Inst, Bethesda, Md; New York Univ Med Ctr, NY)
J Natl Cancer Inst 86:131–137, 1994   130-95-14–7

Background.—An unusually high risk of second primary cancers is seen in patients with oral and pharyngeal cancers. Extensive cytologic changes and subsequent multifocal cancers seem to occur after carcinogenic exposure of the epithelial lining of the aerodigestive tract (i.e., oral cavity, pharynx, esophagus, and larynx) and lungs. The major carcinogens implicated have been alcohol and tobacco smoke. The relationship between alcohol intake and smoking and the development of second primary cancers in patients with oral and pharyngeal carcinomas were evaluated.

Methods.—A nested case-control study design was used within a multicenter cohort analysis of 1,090 patients with oral cancers. Patients who had second cancers 6 months or more after their initial diagnosis were included. The analysis included 80 patients and 189 matched controls taken from the cohort sample. Among the cases and controls, 70% were men and 30% were women. Patients were interviewed through a structured questionnaire at enrollment in the initial 1984–1985 cohort study regarding tobacco, alcohol, and other suspected risk factors for oral cancer. To ascertain changes in drinking and smoking habits and other factors, a follow-up telephone interview was conducted an average of 5 years later as part of the nested case-control study. Patients were followed through June 30, 1989 for second cancers. Conditional logistic regression was used to estimate odds ratios (ORs) and 95% confidence intervals (CIs).

Findings.—A history of tobacco smoking was reported in 93% of cases and 88% of controls. The risk of a second aerodigestive tract cancer rose with the intensity and duration of smoking. A threefold increase in risk was seen for smoking 40 or more cigarettes a day, and a fourfold risk was seen for 40 or more years of smoking. An OR of 4.7 was seen in smokers with 40 or more cigarettes per day for 20 or more years. In patients who quit smoking 1 or more years before initial diagnosis, the risk of a second cancer was similar to lifelong nonsmokers. Risks, although elevated for drinkers, were not statistically significant. However, there was a statistically significant trend in risk with increasing beer consumption. Smoking combined with alcohol intake suggests a multiplicative effect on risk.

Conclusions.—A dose-response relationship between risk of a second aerodigestive tract cancer and smoking was demonstrated. It seems wise to advocate avoidance of tobacco smoking and alcohol intake to prevent oral and other aerodigestive tract cancers.

▶ If we could do away with smoking, excessive drinking, and bad judgment, just think how much better life would be for all of us.—G.R. Holt, M.D., F.A.C.S.

Costs of Hay Fever in the United States in 1990
McMenamin P (Battelle Med Technology Assessment and Policy Research Ctr, Washington, DC)
Ann Allergy 73:35–39, 1994   130-95-14–8

Background.—The total cost of hay fever was estimated, focusing on the use of terfenadine in treatment.

Methods.—Using existing data, the direct and indirect costs of hay fever were estimated. Direct cost included physician visits, diagnostic tests, and medications, whereas indirect cost included measurement of lost productivity. Information was collected from the National Health Interview Survey (NHIS) to estimate the number of individuals with hay fever. The National Ambulatory Medical Care Survey (NAMCS) was used to estimate the treatments prescribed. The value of productivity lost because of hay fever was estimated from a 1989 national survey of allergy sufferers conducted for Marion Merrell Dow, Inc. Health Care Financing Administration (HCFA) data on total national health expenditures and the cost of drugs provided information needed to estimate the total cost of medication provided, purchased, and used by this group.

Findings.—The 1988 NHIS data revealed that 22.4 million patients, or 9.3% of the population, are affected by hay fever. All data were adjusted to represent 1990 estimates. In 1985, 9.8 million physician visits occurred for hay fever. Adjusted to 1990 dollars, this translates into an annual cost of $881 million in physician visits. Prescriptions were ordered during 92% of those visits. Only 29% of those with hay fever did not see a physician. Combined physician and medication costs were estimated to be $1.16 billion. Productivity lost because of allergic rhinitis totaled 3.4 million days, or $639 million per year, which included work days lost and reduced productivity at work and home. The total cost of illness of 1990 was calculated to be $1.8 billion.

Conclusion.—The total cost of hay fever represents a significant cost. Nearly 75% of this amount results from physician visits and lost productivity. The increased availability of effective over-the-counter (OTC) medications to reduce physician cost and the use of nonsedating medication to maintain productivity levels are encouraged. Patient education may also be warranted to encourage proper use of OTC drugs and symptom management.

▶ The cost of treating food, grass, pollen, and cedar allergies, etc., make an indentation on the gross national product. How will managed care change this?—G.R. Holt, M.D., F.A.C.S.

The Retreat of *Hemophilus influenzae* Type B Invasive Disease: Analysis of an Immunization Program and Implications for OTO-HNS
Beck RA, Kambiss S, Bass JW (Dwight D Eisenhower Army Med Ctr, Ft Gordon, Ga; Tripler Army Med Ctr, Honolulu, Hawaii)
Otolaryngol Head Neck Surg 109:712–721, 1993   130-95-14–9

Objective.—The most common cause of bacterial meningitis during the first 5 years of life is *Hemophilus influenzae* type b (Hib). Other invasive Hib diseases include epiglottitis, cellulitis, sepsis, pneumonia, and osteomyelitis (Fig 14–1). First marketed in 1985 and improved since then, Hib vaccines are being given to children at increasingly younger ages. Because there have been no studies to analyze the effects of widespread Hib immunization in a population representative of the United States at large, a sample of children treated for Hib meningitis or epiglottitis at United States Army medical facilities was studied.

Methods and Results.—A total of 373 children 5 years of age or younger was treated from 1986 to 1991—290 for Hib meningitis and 83 for Hib epiglottitis. The combined incidence of these diseases in children 4 years of age or younger decreased 86%, from 59/100,000 in 1986 to 8/100,000 in 1991. The greatest incidence of disease was in children less than 1 year of age; they also showed the largest decrease after vaccines were licensed for use in this age group. The number of cases of bacterial meningitis caused by other organisms was unchanged. Only about 3% of the study group represented recognized vaccine failures. Economic modeling suggested that vaccination was cost effective.

Conclusions.—The Hib vaccination is significantly reducing the incidence of invasive Hib disease. This trend will have an important impact on health care systems and otolaryngology head and neck surgery. Training programs will be affected because the expertise of otolaryngologists

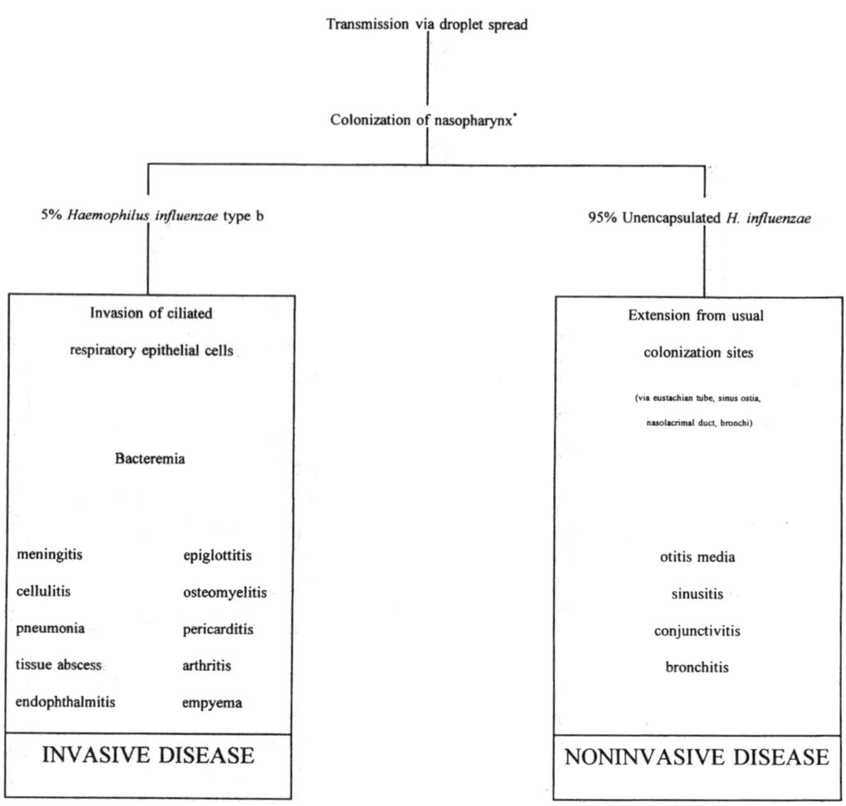

Fig 14–1.—Pathogenesis of *Hemophilus influenzae* disease. *By 2 to 5 years of age, virtually all children have been colonized with 1 or more strains of *H. influenzae*. (Courtesy of Beck RA, Kambiss S, Bass JW: *Otolaryngol Head Neck Surg* 109:712–721, 1993.)

is needed to manage the neurologic sequelae and the emergent airway associated with invasive Hib disease.

▶ It is very encouraging to see this report on a decrease in Hib infections. Unfortunately, the vaccine is not yet in widespread distribution, so we will likely be called on to manage the airway in affected children for some time.—G.R. Holt, M.D., F.A.C.S.

A Protective Association Between the HLA-A2 Antigen and Nasopharyngeal Carcinoma in US Caucasians

Burt RD, Vaughan TL, Nisperos B, Swanson M, Berwick M (Fred Hutchinson Cancer Research Ctr, Seattle; Michigan State Univ, East Lansing; et al)
Int J Cancer 56:465–467, 1994   130-95-14–10

Objective.—There is wide variation worldwide in the incidence of nasopharyngeal carcinoma (NPC), with some Chinese populations being at 50 times higher risk than white Americans. It is possible that histocompatibility leukocyte antigen (HLA) molecules, which present foreign antigens to the immune system, might influence NPC risk through their role in mediating response to the Epstein-Barr virus. Recent research has suggested that NPC risk might be modified in individuals with the HLA-A2 antigen. Data from a collaborative population-based case-control study of NPC and from other sources were used to examine the association between this antigen and NPC in white Americans.

Methods.—The case-control study included 42 American adult whites with diagnosed NPC and 2 external matched control groups. Histocompatibility leukocyte antigen typing studies were performed in all subjects; linkage disequilibrium among subjects with only an A2 at the HLA-A locus was assumed to identify presumptive homozygotes for A2.

Findings.—Risk of NPC was considerably lower in individuals with the A2 antigen than in those with other antigens at the A locus (odds ratio, .46). Presumptive homozygotes for A2 demonstrated a greater strength of this protective association. Comparison of the case patients with American whites studied as part of the Collaborative Transplant Study or the Ninth International Histocompatibility Workshop yielded similar results. Similar findings were also reached on statistical summary of odds ratios for A2 from a number of previous studies in non-Chinese subjects (odds ratio, .69). Among patients with squamous cell carcinomas, the odds ratio was .56; among 7 patients with undifferentiated tumors, the odds ratio decreased to .14.

Conclusion.—The presence of the HLA-A2 antigen has a protective effect against NPC. The rationale for this effect may relate to the ability of the HLA-A2 antigen to efficiently present the Epstein-Barr virus gene product LMP-2, which is present in NPC tumor cells. The HLA-specific immune response to Epstein-Barr virus may thus be a productive area for future NPC research.

▶ Although NPC is not frequently seen in most parts of the country, the information that HLA-A2 antigen can be "protective" against this cancer opens up the possibilities of using at-risk testing and genetic therapy for susceptible populations.—G.R. Holt, M.D., F.A.C.S.

Ingestion of Caustic Cosmetic Products

Stenson K, Gruber B (Univ of Illinois, Chicago)
Otolaryngol Head Neck Surg 109:821–825, 1993   130-95-14–11

Objective.—Young children often will ingest any substance or liquid that is available, including cosmetics and hair care products that may contain caustic chemicals used as scenting agents. Twelve children, all of

Common Caustic Hair Conditioning Products

Product name	Caustic agent	Warning	Child-proof container
Rave home permanent	NH_4OH	−	−
Ogilvie home permanent	NH_4OH	−	−
Revlon Realistic	NaOH	+	−
Luster S-Curl	NaOH	+	−
Excelle	$Ca(OH)_2$	−	−
Gentle Treatment	$Ca(OH)_2$	+	−
Duke Texturizing Cream	NaOH	+	−
Soft and Beautiful	$Ca(OH)_2$	+ *	−

* Warning does not specify "Keep Out of Reach of Children."
(Courtesy of Stenson K, Gruber B: *Otolaryngol Head Neck Surg* 109:821–825, 1993.)

whom were seen in a 6-year period and who underwent endoscopic examination of the aerodigestive tract after having ingested alkali-containing cosmetic products were studied.

Clinical Aspects.—The children, age 2 years–25 months, were black. Most of them ingested a hair care product that contained sodium hydroxide or calcium hydroxide (table). These products are marketed to black persons as hair "activators" or "relaxers." The children had swollen lips, facial erythema, and occasional facial burns when seen in the emergency room. Oral blisters and a swollen tongue were observed. Burns were limited to the face, mouth, and oropharynx, except in a child who ingested a solution used in fingernail decorating and was seen with laryngeal and esophageal burns requiring intubation. All the children swallowed normally after 6–8 weeks, and none had an esophageal stricture.

Discussion.—Only a few patients suspected of ingesting a caustic agent have significant esophageal damage. Child-proof containers may be used; nevertheless, many caustic products still are available to curious children. The indications for using child-proof containers should be expanded, and product control should be tightened.

▶ These authors point out the caustic and potentially dangerous chemistry of so-called hair "activators" and "relaxers." Otolaryngologists should try to inform the community about the risks to small children who might have access to these products.—G.R. Holt, M.D., F.A.C.S.

Non-Melanoma Skin Cancer in Renal Transplant Recipients: The Extent of the Problem and a Strategy for Management
Glover MT, Niranjan N, Kwan JTC, Leigh IM (Royal London Hosp)
Br J Plast Surg 47:86–89, 1994   130-95-14–12

Introduction.—There is a high incidence of warts and skin cancer on the hands of renal transplant patients. The incidence of disease increases with the length of time since transplantation. Exposure to sunlight appears to increase the incidence of nonmelanoma skin cancer (NMSC). Ways of improving the management of renal transplant patients by educating them to avoid overexposure to sunlight and by emphasizing early detection and aggressive treatment of their malignant lesions were examined.

Methods.—Patients who had undergone renal transplant were assigned a risk status according to their skin type, and each patient had a physical examination.

Results.—Of the 291 patients, 30 to 67 years of age, who received transplants, 59% had warts. Patients having had a transplant for more than 5 years and those with fair skin and more sun exposure had more warts. One or more NMSC was detected in 64 patients—13 with both squamous cell carcinoma (SCC) and basal cell carcinoma (BCC), 29 with SCC, and 21 with BCC. In patients with transplants for more than 10 years, the incidence of NMSC was 40%. Forty-two patients had multiple SCC lesions, and 34 patients had multiple BCC lesions. An additional 20 patients had epithelial dysplasia. No patient had had a diagnosis of skin cancer before receiving a renal transplant. Severe, extensive dysplasia was treated by excision and grafting in 4 patients. In 6 other patients, systemic retinoid therapy was given.

Conclusion.—Educating renal transplant patients to avoid ultraviolet radiation is the most important component in preventing skin cancer. Annual dermatologic examinations, surgical excision of cancerous lesions, and long-term therapy with systemic retinoids are important to control recurrence of aggressive SCC.

▶ The theoretical likely causes of rapidly progressive ectodermal dysplasia in some renal transplant recipients are many (e.g., immunosuppression, free radicals, and tumor-promoting drugs). Clinically, these patients are problematic (having multiple excisions, poor control of lesions, anesthetic risks, and reduced clearance of some medications), and they require close follow-up as well as vigorous education regarding negative effects of ultraviolet light exposure.—G.R. Holt, M.D., F.A.C.S.

Thyroid Cancer Among Persons Given X-Ray Treatment in Infancy for an Enlarged Thymus Gland

Shore RE, Hildreth N, Dvoretsky P, Andresen E, Moseson M, Pasternack B
(New York Univ Med Ctr, NY; Univ of Rochester, Rochester, NY)
Am J Epidemiol 137:1068–1080, 1993   130-95-14–13

Background.—There has long been an interest in the association between ionizing radiation and thyroid cancer. However, there remain unresolved issues, such as the dose-response curve, risks at low dosages, effects of dose fragmentation, time factors, and risk modification. The use of x-ray treatment for thymus gland enlargement was first described in 1907 under premises later determined to be unfounded. Therefore, numerous infants with normal thymus glands were irradiated. The purpose was to follow patients who received such radiation to see whether there was a relationship between their treatment and thyroid cancer.

Methods.—A total of 2,657 infants who received radiation for an enlarged thymus gland and 4,833 siblings were studied. The minimum follow-up was 5 years. A questionnaire about cancer, benign tumors, and other factors was mailed, and 86% of both irradiated and control subjects completed the questionnaire. Medical conditions were verified by a pathologist and the New York State Cancer Registry. Cancer rates were compared with published rates of the state of New York and divided according to 6-year intervals beginning at 5 years of age, with the final age group being 47 years or older.

Results.—Thyroid doses were estimated for 91% of irradiated individuals. Dosages ranged from .03 to more than 10 Gy with a mean of 1.36 Gy and a median of .3 Gy. There were 37 diagnosed cases of thyroid cancer in the irradiated group vs. 5 in the sibling control group, with a standardized incidence ratio of 24.3 for the irradiated group compared with 1.8 for the sibling controls. The dose-response relationship was basically linear, with the relative risk of thyroid cancer adjusted for sex and age. The risk ratio decreased with time but was still increased 45 years after radiation. The most significant risk factor was older age at first childbirth. Interaction between possible risk factors and radiation suggested that Jewish individuals, and women with older ages at menarche or at first childbirth were at greater risk for thyroid cancer.

Conclusion.—There was basically a linear dose-response relation for thyroid cancer, even at radiation doses less than .3 Gy. This risk persists for at least 4 or 5 decades.

▶ This article has personal significance, as I and both of my siblings received irradiation for "enlarged thymus glands" when we were children. Fortunately, 2 of us have passed the 45-year postirradiation mark, but for all those who have not, we must continue to be highly vigilant.—G.R. Holt, M.D., F.A.C.S.

Subject Index*

A

Aboulker stent
  for laryngotracheal stenosis in children,
    93: 213
Abscess
  brain
    mortality and morbidity in, 93: 115
    otogenic, 93: 114
  peritonsillar, needle aspiration of, in
    children, 94: 275
Abuse
  child, otolaryngologic manifestations of,
    94: 288
  physical, of children, otolaryngology
    perspective, 93: 291
Acoustic
  neuroma (*see* Neuroma, acoustic)
  trauma, 93: 18
    drilling causing, 93: 37
    from trumpets in symphony orchestra,
     93: 20
  tumor
    facial nerve neuroma presenting as,
     95: 86
    surgery, hearing conservation,
     endoscopy of internal auditory
     canal during, 94: 94
Acquired immunodeficiency syndrome (*see*
  AIDS)
Acyclovir
  in herpes zoster oticus, 93: 55
Adductor
  spasmodic dysphonia, unilateral vs.
    bilateral injections of botulinum
    toxin in, 95: 219
Adenitis
  mycobacterial cervical, in children,
    management, 95: 272
Adenocarcinoma
  middle ear, 95: 76
  neck, metastatic, 93: 227
  of sinonasal cavities, wood dust
    exposure increasing risk of, 94: 159
Adenoid
  bacteriology of, 95: 263
  carcinoma, cystic, stage means more
    than grade, 94: 264
  morphology of, 95: 271
Adenoidectomy
  outpatient, complications and
    recommendations, 95: 264
  pain reduction with bupivacaine in
    children, 94: 282
  peritubal, 95: 261
Adenoids

cystic carcinoma, flow cytometry of,
  93: 240
hypertrophy assessment, 93: 321
immunoglobulin-secreting cells in,
  93: 317
radiological assessment methods with
  endoscopy, 93: 300
Adenoma
  middle ear, 95: 76
    case report, 94: 87
  parotid, recurrent pleomorphic, facial
    nerve intraoperative monitoring in,
    95: 247
Adenotonsillectomy
  laryngospasm after, 93: 197
  in otitis media, secretory, 95: 104
  outpatient, for children, 93: 292
  in sleep apnea, obstructive, respiratory
    compromise after, in children,
    93: 313
  for upper airway obstruction and
    prematurity history, 93: 299
Adhesive
  cyanoacrylate and fibrin tissue, current
    status of, 94: 198
Adolescence
  streptococcal pharyngitis during,
    cefixime and penicillin V for,
    94: 282
  thyroid carcinoma during, differentiated,
    93: 263
Adrenaline
  for nasal surgery, catecholamine levels
    after, 93: 319
Adriamycin
  in head and neck cancer, advanced,
    93: 279
Aerobics
  high impact, inducing vestibulopathy,
    95: 10
Aerodigestive tract
  tumors, upper, neck staging procedure
    for, 93: 248
  upper, chemical industry pollution of,
    93: 155
Aesthetic
  procedures, blood contact risk through
    surgical gloves in, 95: 203
Age
  in bone conduction threshold change by
    total footplate stapedectomy,
    94: 72
  immunoglobulin-secreting cells in
    adenoids and, 93: 317
  influence on stapedectomy results,
    93: 49

---

* *All entries refer to the year and page number(s) for data appearing in this and the
previous edition of the* YEAR BOOK.

in joint noises prevalence, 94: 289
at repair and speech outcome in cleft
    palate, 93: 171
Aged
    acoustic neuroma of, disappearing
        recurrent, in woman, 94: 92
    dysphonia in, physiology vs. disease,
        93: 205
    temporomandibular joint noises in,
        94: 290
    vocal quality in, 93: 206
Agenesis
    kidney, in Potter's syndrome in infant,
        94: 58
AIDS
    carcinoma in, squamous cell, 94: 235
    cochlear ultrastructural findings in,
        95: 35
    head and neck tumors in, 94: 235
    Kaposi's sarcoma in, 94: 235
    lymphoma in, malignant, 94: 235
    salivary lymphoepithelial lesions and,
        93: 233
    (See also HIV)
Air
    bone gap
        bone conduction implant and, 93: 68
        stapedectomy improving, 93: 49
    caloric test with continuous thermal
        change, 95: 6
    conduction hearing aid, 93: 26
    intrusion to scala vestibuli of cochlea,
        causing inner ear injury, 95: 59
Airway, 93: 195, 94: 211, 95: 217
    collapse
        site in obstructive sleep apnea, airway
            pressure monitoring in, 95: 217
        and tracheobronchomalacia in
            children, 93: 215
    complication in thyroid surgery, 94: 224
    CPAP, reducing gastroesophageal reflux
        in obstructive sleep apnea, 93: 294
    endoscopy in bacterial tracheitis in
        children, 95: 229
    gaining, in subglottic stenosis, 93: 201
    lower, responsiveness, and intranasal
        corticosteroids for allergic rhinitis
        in mild asthma, 94: 155
    management in laryngeal paralysis,
        endoscopic laser medial
        arytenoidectomy for, 94: 214
    manifestations of gastroesophageal
        reflux, in children, 93: 218
    perichondrium in, free and vascularized,
        chondrogenic potential of, 95: 157
    resection in thyroid cancer, 93: 256
    resistance

nasal, and middle ear pressure in
    upper respiratory tract infection,
    94: 153
in tracheostomy tubes, 95: 221
in sleep apnea, obstructive, 93: 199
thyroid carcinoma invading, resection,
    93: 255
upper
    in children with velopharyngeal
        inadequacy, pharyngeal flap in,
        95: 184
    dimensions, posture and sleep
        apnea/hypopnea syndrome,
        93: 197
    narrowing in obstructive sleep apnea,
        flexible fiberoptic
        nasopharyngoscopy of, 94: 284
    obstruction, adenotonsillectomy for,
        and prematurity history, 93: 299
    obstruction, and tonsillar
        hypertrophy, 93: 289
    reconstruction, in obstructive sleep
        apnea syndrome, 95: 258
    transplant, 93: 203
Alar
    spreader grafts for pinched nasal tip
        correction, 94: 199
Alcohol
    polyvinyl, for embolization in
        arteriovenous malformation of face,
        93: 260
    in second cancers after oral and
        pharyngeal cancers, 95: 281
Allergen
    nasal challenge with, unilateral,
        terfenadine in, 95: 171
    vegetable, IgE mediated allergy from,
        95: 269
Allergic
    reactions, immunologic aspects and
        inflammatory mechanisms of,
        94: 301
    rhinitis (see Rhinitis, allergic)
Allergy
    histamine and cold air challenges in,
        nasal response to, and rhinovirus 39
        infection, 95: 178
    IgE mediated, from vegetable allergens,
        95: 269
    interface of allergy in sinus disease,
        93: 145
    respiratory, upper, in chronic or
        recurrent sinusitis, 93: 146
Allograft
    in tracheal replacement (in dog),
        94: 145
Alloplastic
    implant

in facial plastic and reconstructive
surgery, 94: 208
qualities of, 93: 87
Amniotic fluid
middle ear contamination by, model of,
94: 101
Amoxicillin
continuous vs. intermittent, in otitis
media prevention, 93: 78
Anaerobic bacteria
therapy against in chronic suppurative
otitis media, 95: 118
Anastomosis
hypoglossal-facial nerve, for facial nerve
palsy after cerebellopontine angle
tumor surgery, 94: 83
Anesthesia
general, for laryngeal microsurgery, with
small-bore endotracheal tubes,
blood gas analysis in, 95: 226
inducing in subglottic stenosis, 93: 201
local vs. general, for functional
endoscopic sinus surgery, 94: 165
spinal
auditory function after, 94: 25
low-frequency hearing loss after, as
perilymphatic hypotonia, 93: 21
Anesthetic
Carden tube for surgery around a
tracheostome, 95: 224
effects of intranasal cocaine vs.
xylometazoline/lidocaine solution,
94: 164
practices in ambulatory aesthetic
surgery, 95: 213
Angiofibroma
nasopharyngeal, juvenile, treatment,
93: 249
Angiogenic
growth factors, in soft tissue wound
healing, 93: 131
Angiography
magnetic resonance, of tinnitus,
pulsatile, 95: 49
Anomalies
malformed ear, congenital, cochlear
implant in, 94: 45
vascular malformations of head and
neck, MRI of, 94: 246
Anthropometry
before and after lip and palate repair,
94: 197
Anthroposcopy
before and after lip and palate repair,
94: 197
Antibiotics
IV, for otitis media, chronic suppurative,
without cholesteatoma, 94: 124

oral, in sinusitis, intranasal flunisolide
spray as adjunct to, 95: 172
for otitis media, acute, in children,
outcome, 94: 105
parenteral, serious infections in children
requiring, infectious disease team
approach for, 94: 124
prophylactic eardrops, and ventilation
tubes, 93: 79
with steroids for ear drops to reduce
postoperative otorrhea and
ventilation tube blockage, 94: 111
Antibodies
autoantibodies against neutrophil
constituents in subglottic stenosis
diagnosis, 94: 219
neutralizing, to transforming growth
factor β for scarring control in
adult wounds, 93: 130
Antidepressant
for tinnitus, 93: 31
Antigens
HLA-A2, protective association with
nasopharyngeal carcinoma, 95: 284
mediated histamine release from blood
in allergic rhinitis, astemizole in,
94: 156
Antihypertensives
in sleep pattern and sleep apnea,
93: 198
Antrostomy
inferior, vs. natural ostiotomy in sinusitis
(in rabbit model), 95: 136
Antrum
bacteriology of, in chronic maxillary
sinusitis, 95: 179
AO plate
with myocutaneous flap, instead of
revascularized tissue transfer, for
mandibular reconstruction, 95: 185
Aphthous stomatitis
features of, and steroids in, 93: 312
triamcinolone in, 93: 312
Apnea, sleep (*see* Sleep apnea)
Arm
free flap, lateral, in head and neck
reconstruction, 94: 176
Arteries
carotid, emergency coverage, superiorly
based trapezius flap for, 94: 239
facial, flap, 93: 180
maxillary and ethmoidal arterial
occlusion in epistaxis, 93: 155
stapedial, persistent, in middle ear,
95: 79
supply
of anterior ear, 93: 68
of endolymphatic duct and sac, 94: 5

thyroid, anatomical variations, 93: 218
Arteriography
  magnetic resonance, to distinguish soft
     tissue hemangioma from vascular
     malformation, 93: 187
Arteriovenous
  malformation of face, embolization in,
     93: 259
Artifacts
  CT imaging, from craniomaxillofacial
     internal fixation devices, 95: 132
Arytenoid
  adduction, and Silastic medialization,
     94: 231
Arytenoidectomy
  medial, endoscopic laser, for airway
     management in laryngeal paralysis,
     94: 214
Ascorbic acid
  in allergic rhinitis, 93: 147
Aspiration
  biopsy, fine needle, in head and neck
     masses, cytopathology in, 94: 244
  cytology, fine needle, of salivary gland
     lesions, 95: 254
  fine needle, vascular proliferation of
     thyroid complicating, 94: 248
  needle, of peritonsillar abscess in
     children, 94: 275
Aspirin
  intolerance, easy bruisability and
     DDAVP response, 94: 276
Astemizole
  in antigen-mediated histamine release
     from blood in allergic rhinitis,
     94: 156
  interactions with, possible, 95: 169
Asthma
  mild, allergic rhinitis in, intranasal
     corticosteroids for, 94: 155
  nose response to exercise in, 95: 163
Atelectasis
  of ear, surgery of, 93: 91
  surgery, with ventilation tube, 93: 92
Atherosclerosis
  carotid, irradiation as risk factor for,
     93: 231
Atresia
  of auditory canal, external acquired,
     surgery results, 94: 119
  aural, congenital
    grading system for, 93: 59
    long-term surgery results, 95: 96
    surface contour three-dimensional
      imaging in, 94: 100
  esophageal, with tracheomalacia
     absence, 93: 204
Audiant XA-II implant

experiences with, 95: 124
Audiological
  department, children under 4 referred
     to, 93: 13
Audiometry
  consequences of ear blast injury, 95: 44
Auditory
  brain stem responses, intraoperative, to
     guide prosthesis positioning, 93: 90
  canal
    external, atresia of, acquired, surgery
      results, 94: 119
    internal, endoscopy of, during hearing
      conservation acoustic tumor
      surgery, 94: 94
    internal, facial neuroma of, 94: 84
  function after spinal anesthesia, 94: 25
  temporary threshold shift in rock
     musicians after heavy metal concert,
     94: 37
  threshold and round window fistula (in
     guinea pig), 93: 40
Aural atresia (*see* Atresia, aural)
Auricular
  cartilage grafts in laryngotracheal
     reconstruction, 94: 222
Autoantibodies
  against neutrophil constituents in
     subglottic stenosis diagnosis,
     94: 219
Autograft
  jejunal, revascularized, for tracheal
     replacement (in dog), 94: 143
  vs. xenograft for tympanoplasty,
     95: 117
Automobile
  company, hearing loss at, follow-up,
     94: 36
Avulsion
  facial nerve at stapedectomy, 93: 51

B

Baclofen
  in trigeminal neuralgia, 93: 303
Bacteria
  anaerobic, therapy effective against in
     chronic suppurative otitis media,
     95: 118
  round window membrane and, 93: 33
  tympanogenic labyrinthitis, meningitis
     and sensorineural damage, 93: 33
Bacterial
  tracheitis, in children, airway endoscopy
     in, 95: 229
Bacteriology
  of adenoid, 95: 263

sampling techniques, 95: 263
of antrum in chronic maxillary sinusitis,
  95: 179
of tonsil, 95: 263
Balance
  pathology resource registry, 94: 23
  rehabilitation therapy, 94: 20
Ballooning
  surgery of endolymphatic sac for
    Ménière's disease, 95: 22
Barometric
  pressure changes damaging cochlea,
    93: 35
Barotrauma
  of inner ear, 93: 35
    in scuba divers, long-term follow-up
      with continued diving, 94: 55
Basal cell
  carcinoma in young adults, 93: 185
Base
  super-base bone anchored hearing aid,
    93: 25
Baton
  graft for short nose, 94: 206
Behind-the-ear device
  experiences with, 95: 124
Bell's palsy, 93: 56
  infection in, 93: 57
  paranasal sinus disease in, inflammatory,
    MRI of, 94: 80
Benzoylecgonine
  screening, intranasal cocaine in, 93: 144
Biochemistry
  of neutralization, 95: 168
Bioengineering
  molecular, of biomaterials, 93: 128
Biofeedback
  for tinnitus, chronic, 94: 39
Biologic
  grafts in facial plastic and reconstructive
    surgery, 94: 208
Biology
  molecular, and polymers, 93: 128
Biomaterials
  molecular bioengineering of, 93: 128
Biopsy
  brush, in mucociliary transport
    disorders, 93: 152
  cervical node, open, indications for, in
    HIV, 94: 288
  fine needle aspiration, of head and neck
    masses, cytopathology in, 94: 244
  frozen section, in oral cavity carcinoma,
    93: 230
  of nasal mucosa, brush, for electron
    microscopy, 93: 152
  vs. modern technology, 95: 3
Biostatistics

in otolaryngology journals, 93: 123
Blast
  injury of ear, vestibular and audiometric
    consequences of, 95: 44
Bleomycin
  in cystic lymphangioma, 93: 262
Blepharoplasty
  eyelid, lower, transconjunctival
    approach, experience, indications
    and technique, 95: 199
Blindness
  after maxillofacial blunt trauma, optic
    nerve decompression surgery in,
    95: 190
Blood
  contact risk through surgical gloves in
    aesthetic procedures, 95: 203
  gas analysis in laryngeal microsurgery
    with small-bore endotracheal tubes,
    95: 226
  histamine release from,
    antigen-mediated, in allergic
    rhinitis, astemizole in, 94: 156
  patch, epidural, facial nerve paralysis
    after, 94: 80
  pressure, high, and tinnitus, 93: 8
Blue
  ear drum in children, initial evaluation,
    93: 76
Bone
  air gap (see Air bone gap)
  anchored
    hearing aid, super-base, 93: 25
    reconstruction of irradiated head and
      neck cancer, 94: 186
  bone-inducing factor, recombinant,
    mandibular reconstruction with,
    93: 122
  bovine, demineralized, for composite
    graft for growing cricoid
    reconstruction (in rabbit), 94: 147
  calvarial (see Calvarial bone)
  conduction
    hearing aid, traditional, modification
      of, 94: 42
    hearing device, implant, in
      sensorineural hearing loss, 93: 24
    implant, transcutaneous vs.
      percutaneous, 93: 66
    threshold change by total footplate
      stapedectomy, and age, 94: 72
  craniofacial, growth, pressure in
    regulation of, 95: 139
  flap, vascularized, in oromandibular
    reconstruction, 95: 132
  graft (see Graft, bone)
  matrix, incomplete coverage by lining
    cells (in mammals), 94: 24

olecranon bone graft for nasal
augmentation, 93: 190
petrous, fracture, in children,
management, 95: 50
scanning in postradiotherapy jaw
osteonecrosis, 93: 172
temporal (*see* Temporal bone)
Botox
storage causing degradation in potency,
94: 221
Botulinum toxin
in facial dyskinesia, 93: 192
point-touch technique of injection for
spasmodic dysphonia, 94: 220
type A, crystalline preparation of,
storage causing degradation in
potency, 94: 221
unilateral vs. bilateral injections in
adductor spasmodic dysphonia,
95: 219
Brain
abscess
mortality and morbidity in, 93: 115
otogenic, 93: 114
herniation into middle ear
cleft, 93: 112
spontaneous, histopathology of,
93: 113
stem, intraoperative auditory brain stem
responses in prosthesis positioning
guiding, 93: 90
Branchial
cysts, etiology theories, 95: 267
Branemark implant
in cleft palate, 93: 160
Breathing
sleep disordered, gender differences in,
95: 276
work of, in tracheostomy tubes, 95: 221
Bronchi
tracheobronchial (*see* Tracheobronchial)
tracheobronchomalacia
airway collapse in children and,
93: 215
classification system for, 93: 216
Bronchopulmonary
suction, 93: 195
Bronchoscopy
laryngobronchoscopy, rigid,
complications in children, 94: 227
Bruisability
easy, aspirin intolerance and DDAVP
response, 94: 276
Bupivacaine
for tonsillectomy and adenoidectomy
pain reduction, in children, 94: 282

C

Caloric
function return of ear after vestibular
nerve section, 93: 10
Calvarial
bone
elevated IGF-II and TGF-beta
concentrations in, 95: 138
graft harvest, techniques,
considerations and morbidity,
94: 172
defects, reconstruction with
hydroxyapatite cement, 93: 135
graft, split, for nasal reconstruction,
94: 190
Cancer
cervical nodes, neoplastic spread in,
MRI vs. CT in, 93: 254
glottic, partial laryngectomy after
radiotherapy, 93: 196
head and neck (*see* Head and neck
cancer)
laryngopharyngeal, radiotherapy failure,
surgery after, 95: 252
larynx (*see* Larynx, cancer)
nose (*see* Nose cancer)
oral cavity (*see* Oral cavity cancer)
oral (*see* Oral cancer)
paranasal sinus
CT-based 3-dimensional radiotherapy
of, 95: 241
in metal industry, 93: 147
and occupational exposures, 94: 157
pharyngeal
second cancer after, tobacco and
alcohol in, 95: 281
vitamin supplement to reduce risk of,
93: 302
precancer of larynx vs. oral leukoplakia,
93: 201
salivary gland, elective treatment of neck
in, 93: 248
sinonasal, occupational risk factors for,
93: 148
sinus, and formaldehyde occupational
exposure, 94: 158
skin
non-melanoma, after kidney
transplant, 95: 287
skin carcinoma risk after, 94: 253
staging with panendoscopy, 93: 278
thyroid (*see* Thyroid cancer)
tongue, oral, under 40 years, aggressive
therapy, 95: 251
Cannulation

long-term, in subglottic stenosis,
94: 212
Canthus
medial, basal cell carcinoma, limits of
microscopically controlled excision
of, 94: 195
Capillary
vascular malformations, tunable
pulsed-dye laser for, 95: 202
Capsule
gene sequences in pharyngeal isolates of
nontypeable
Hemophilusinfluenzae, 95: 150
Carbamazepine
in trigeminal neuralgia, 93: 303
Carbon dioxide
laser, microspot microslad for, 93: 284
Carcinogenesis
oral, and vitamin E, 93: 303
Carcinoma
adenoid cystic
flow cytometry of, 93: 240
stage means more than grade,
94: 264
basal cell, aggressive-growth in young
adults, 93: 185
canthus, medial, basal cell, limits of
microscopically controlled excision
of, 94: 195
glottic
early, open laryngeal procedures for,
95: 251
T1, radiotherapy of, 95: 244
T1 and T2, surgery and radiotherapy
of, 93: 229
head and neck (*see* Head and neck
carcinoma)
hypopharynx, hypothyroidism after
treatment, 93: 234
larynx (*see* Larynx, carcinoma)
nasopharyngeal (*see* Nasopharyngeal
carcinoma)
oral, squamous cell, multiple tumor risk
after, 95: 275
oral cavity
neck dissection and frozen section
biopsy in, 93: 230
squamous cell, supraomohyoid neck
dissection in, 93: 247
pharyngolaryngeal, with palpable nodes,
93: 239
skin, risk after skin cancer, 94: 253
squamous cell
in AIDS, 94: 235
cell line growth and hyperbaric
oxygen therapy, 94: 143
temporal bone, squamous cell, surgery
efficacy in, 95: 41

thyroid (*see* Thyroid carcinoma)
tongue, advanced, total glossectomy
without total laryngectomy in,
94: 269
Carden
anesthetic tube for surgery around
tracheostome, 95: 224
Cardiovascular
effects of pseudoephedrine in
hypertension, 93: 312
risk factors in snoring, 94: 292
Care
home, after tracheostomy in children,
93: 207
"Carhart's notch," 94: 73
Carotid
artery coverage, emergency, superiorly
based trapezius flap for, 94: 239
atherosclerosis, irradiation as risk factor
for, 93: 231
canal dehiscence, prevalence in middle
ear, temporal bone in, 95: 98
system, external, occipital branch
supplying endolymphatic duct and
sacs, 94: 6
Cartilage
auricular, for graft in laryngotracheal
reconstruction, 94: 222
cricoid
four-quadrant division in
laryngotracheal reconstruction,
94: 217
intrinsic response to vertical division,
95: 142
graft, irradiated, in nose, 94: 196
new cartilage formation, chondrocytes
seeding synthetic polymers for,
93: 127
tragal and conchal palisade, in
tympanomastoid reconstruction,
93: 93
Cassette
players, personal, causing noise-induced
hearing loss, 93: 18
Catecholamine
levels after adrenaline for nasal surgery,
93: 319
Caustic
cosmetic products, ingestion of,
95: 285
Cecum
foramen, core-out toward, in
thyroglossal duct cyst operation,
93: 296
Cefixime
for streptococcal pharyngitis during
childhood and adolescence,
94: 282

Ceftazidime
  in otitis media with cholesteatoma,
      93: 109
Cell(s)
  differentiation after respiratory epithelia
      free graft, 93: 132
  growth on collagen, 93: 132
  hair (*see* Hair cell)
  line growth, squamous cell carcinoma,
      and hyperbaric oxygen therapy,
      94: 143
  lining, incomplete coverage of bone
      matrix by (in mammals), 94: 24
Cement, hydroxyapatite (*see*
      Hydroxyapatite cement)
CEOEs
  in children, 93: 14
Cephalexin
  in streptococcal throat infections, group
      A beta-hemolytic, 94: 302
Cerebellopontine angle
  facial neuroma of, 94: 84
  tumor surgery, facial nerve palsy after,
      hypoglossal-facial nerve
      anastomosis for, 94: 83
Cerebral
  palsy, drooling in, treatment, 93: 287
  symptoms after whiplash injury of neck,
      94: 277
Cerebrospinal fluid
  findings in facial palsy, acute idiopathic
      peripheral, 94: 81
  otorhinorrhea, technique to avoid, with
      translabyrinthine removal of
      acoustic neuroma, 95: 88
  pressure, in hearing loss after
      neurosurgery, 95: 34
Cerumen, 93: 62
Cerumenolytic
  nonprescription, 93: 62
Cervical
  cysts, lateral, etiology theories, 95: 267
  exploration for primary
      hyperparathyroidism, 94: 245
  lymphadenitis, mycobacterial, curettage
      of, 93: 308
  lymphadenopathy, in AIDS, 93: 285
  mycobacterial adenitis, in children,
      management, 95: 272
  node
    biopsy, open, indications for, in HIV,
        94: 288
    dissection in melanoma, 93: 253
    enlargement in Kawasaki disease,
        93: 310
    evaluation in head and neck cancer,
        93: 230

metastases, CT and palpation in,
    93: 245
necrosis and neoplastic spread in,
    MRI vs. CT, 93: 254
recontouring, submentoplasty to
    enhance, in face lift, 94: 203
tuberculosis, contemporary
    management, 93: 292
Chemoradiation
  in head and neck cancer, 93: 265
Child abuse
  otolaryngologic manifestations of,
      94: 288
Children
  under 16, tympanostomy tube proposed
      for, 95: 105
  adenitis, mycobacterial cervical,
      management, 95: 272
  adenoidectomy, pain reduction with
      bupivacaine, 94: 282
  adenotonsillectomy in obstructive sleep
      apnea, respiratory compromise
      after, 93: 313
  blue ear drum in, initial evaluation,
      93: 76
  CEOEs in, 93: 14
  cholesteatoma, open vs. closed
      techniques with, 93: 101
  cochlear loss in, 93: 18
  consumer product aspiration and
      ingestion by, 93: 216
  DPOEs in, 93: 14
  ear abnormalities, osseointegrated
      implants in, 94: 43
  endonasal sinus surgery, 93: 149
  eustachian tube
    goblet cell and gland distributions,
        and otitis media, 93: 74
    lumen lining of roof, 93: 74
  under four referred to audiological
      department, 93: 13
  gastroesophageal reflux, airway
      manifestations, 93: 218
  gastropharyngeal reflux, pharyngeal pH
      monitoring in, 94: 284
  Goode's tympanostomy tubes for,
      long-term results, 94: 113
  hearing impaired, otoacoustic emissions
      in, 93: 14
  hearing loss, noise-induced, 93: 18
  Hemophilus influenzae type B
      large-scale vaccination, epiglottitis
      disappearance during, 95: 280
  histiocytosis X of head and neck in,
      93: 276
  Hunter's syndrome with
      tracheobronchomalacia, endoscopy
      in, 94: 226

infections, serious, requiring parenteral
    antibiotics, infectious disease team
    approach for, 94: 124
Kawasaki disease, five-year experience,
    93: 309
laryngobronchoscopy, rigid,
    complications of, 94: 227
laryngocele, 93: 208
laryngotracheal
    reconstruction, rib cartilage graft in,
        93: 201
    reconstruction, with four-quadrant
        cricoid cartilage division, 94: 217
    stenting stenosis, stenting for,
        93: 213
lymphangioma, cystic, bleomycin in,
    93: 263
mandibular fracture patterns in, 94: 180
measles epidemic,
    laryngotracheobronchitis
    complicating, 94: 218
middle ear
    disease with sensorineural hearing
        loss, 94: 65
    effusion, vestibular disturbances and,
        93: 44
motion sickness, experimental, 95: 8
mucopolysaccharidoses, head and neck
    complications in, 93: 307
nasal cavity fiberoptic exam, 93: 320
nasopharyngeal
    angiofibroma treatment, juvenile,
        93: 249
    fiberoptic exam, 93: 320
ossicular replacement prosthesis, total
    and partial, 95: 123
ostiomeatal unit development,
    radiography of, 94: 156
otitis media
    acute, antibiotics for, outcome after,
        94: 105
    acute, recurrent, language
        development in, follow-up for
        seven years, 94: 108
    acute, risk factors for, temporal aspect
        control in, 94: 103
    with cholesteatoma, outpatient
        management, 93: 108
    chronic, conservative surgical
        approach to, 94: 128
    chronic, noncholesteatomatous,
        surgery results, 94: 128
    chronic suppurative, incidence and
        risk factors, 93: 110
    chronic suppurative, without
        cholesteatoma, medical treatment,
        94: 123

with effusion, pars tensa
    micropathologic changes in,
    95: 112
otitis-prone, treatment failure with
    tympanostomy tube and
    Hemophilus influenzae, 93: 81
otorrhea, postoperative,
    antibiotic/steroid ear drops to
    reduce, 94: 111
otoscopy, clinical and histologic
    correlation, 93: 71
palate impalement injuries, case review,
    94: 189
peritonsillar abscess, needle aspiration
    of, 94: 275
petrous bone fracture, management,
    95: 50
physical abuse, otolaryngology
    perspective, 93: 291
respiratory tract symptoms and illness,
    lower, and nasal disorders, 94: 159
rhabdomyosarcoma of head and neck,
    93: 231, 250
rheumatic fever in developing countries,
    94: 286
rhinopharyngitis, nasopharyngeal pH
    monitoring in, 93: 286
rhinoplasty with external approach,
    93: 187
saccular cyst, 93: 208
sinonasal disease, endonasal sinus
    surgery for, 93: 150
sinusitis, chronic, nasal mucociliary
    transport of, 94: 162
sleep apnea
    obstructive, polysomnographic and
        clinical findings in, 93: 304
    syndrome, obstructive, habitual
        snoring and, early tonsil surgery in,
        94: 299
streptococcal
    pharyngitis, cefixime and penicillin V
        for, 94: 282
    throat infections, group A
        beta-hemolytic, cephalexin for,
        94: 303
stridor, CT and MRI in, 93: 209
subglottic stenosis, auricular cartilage
    graft for laryngotracheal
    reconstruction in, 94: 223
T tubes for, insertion retrospective
    review; 94: 114
temporal bone fracture, 93: 44
    oblique, 93: 45
thyroid carcinoma, differentiated,
    93: 263
thyroid disorder evaluation with
    iodine-123 scintigraphy, 93: 311

tonsillectomy
  ambulatory, and high-risk subgroup
    identification, 95: 270
  outpatient, 93: 292
  pain reduction with bupivacaine,
    94: 282
  vomiting after, metoclopramide
    reducing, 93: 316
tonsillitis, chronic, immunoglobulin E
  in, 93: 318
tracheitis, bacterial, airway endoscopy
  in, 95: 229
tracheobronchial
  disruption, mortality in, 93: 203
  injuries, 93: 203
tracheobronchomalacia and airway
  collapse, 93: 215
tracheostomy, and home care, 93: 207
tracheotomy of, long-term, granuloma
  excision in, 94: 228
tympanoplasty, type 1, 95: 116
velopharyngeal inadequacy, pharyngeal
  flap for upper airway in, 95: 184
ventilation
  tube blockage, antibiotic/steroid ear
    drops for, 94: 111
  tube removal in, tympanic membrane
    perforation after, 94: 115
Cholesteatoma
  in children, open vs. closed techniques
    with, 93: 101
  congenital, 93: 100
    differentiating from acquired
      cholesteatoma, 95: 100
    identification and diagnosis, 93: 101
    twelve case review, 95: 78
  ear canal, 93: 62
    debridement, 93: 64
    differentiated from hyperkeratosis
      obturans, 93: 64
  fibroblast alterations, induction of
    neoplastic-like phenotype, 94: 132
  in intact canal wall tympanoplasty, for
    recurrence prevention, 95: 121
  mesotympanic, posterior, management,
    93: 102
  model (in animal), 94: 130
  morphologic development (in gerbil),
    94: 131
  with otitis media
    ceftazidime in, 93: 109
    in children, outpatient management,
      93: 108
  petrous apex, diagnostic and treatment
    dilemmas, 94: 133
  recurrent and residual, surgery of,
    93: 106

  residual, endoscopy guiding otosurgery
    to prevent, 94: 134
  single-stage management, 93: 107
  tympanoplasty in, transcanal, 93: 105
Chondrocytes
  seeding synthetic polymers provide
    template for new cartilage
    formation, 93: 127
Chondrogenic
  potential of free and vascularized
    perichondrium in airway, 95: 157
Chorda
  tympani damage, unilateral, effect on
    taste, 95: 90
Cigarette smoking (*see* Smoking)
Cilazapril
  in sleep apnea, 93: 199
Cilia
  activity in eustachian tube and influenza
    A virus (in chinchilla), 94: 105
  nasal, ultrastructural changes due to
    common cold, 94: 154
Ciliated
  epithelium, recovery of, and
    ultrastructural changes in nasal cilia
    due to common cold, 94: 154
Ciprofloxacin
  as topical otic preparation, 93: 66
  vs. gentamicin in chronic otitis media,
    93: 65
Cisplatin
  in head and neck cancer, advanced,
    93: 278
Cleft
  lip
    bilateral, columellar elongation in,
      93: 186
    fetal, endoscopic creation and repair
      of, 94: 150
    repair, major vermilion deficiency
      after, bipedicled axial cross-lip flap
      to correct, 95: 206
  lip and palate repair, anthropometry and
    anthroposcopy before and after,
    94: 197
  middle ear, brain herniation into,
    93: 112
  palate
    Branemark implant in, 93: 160
    palatoplasty for, long-term speech
      results, 94: 179
    repair, age at repair and speech
      outcome in, 93: 171
    Wardill-Kilner technique, experience
      with, 95: 194
Clonazepam
  in tinnitus, 93: 30
  in trigeminal neuralgia, 93: 303

CO$_2$ laser
  microspot microslad for, 93: 284
Cocaine
  intranasal
    in benzoylecgonine screening,
      93: 144
    vasoconstrictive and anesthetic effects
      of, vs. xylometazoline/lidocaine
      solution, 94: 164
    for nasal surgery, ventricular fibrillation
      after, 93: 315
    vs. lidocaine with oxymetazoline for
      nasal procedures, 95: 165
Cochlea
  damage
    due to barometric pressure changes,
      93: 35
    otitis media induced, cochlear
      polyamines marking, 95: 62
  duct, stapedotomy and, 93: 50
  dysfunction in perilymph fistula (in
    guinea pig), 93: 39
  electrophysiology, effect of vasodilating
    agent topical application, 94: 66
  hair cell (see Hair cell)
  implant, 93: 3
    22-electrode, 93: 28
    binaural, 94: 48
    coating by hand, 93: 26
    device, inexpensive, 93: 26
    in ear malformations, congenital,
      94: 45
    with labyrinthectomy, 94: 47
    multichannel, otopathology with,
      95: 28
    multichannel, performance of
      prelingually or postlingually
      deafened adults with, 95: 30
    in postlingual deafness, 93: 27
    single-channel vs. multichannel,
      94: 45
    surgical pitfalls, 94: 48
    for tinnitus suppression, 95: 63
  loss in children, 93: 18
  nerve microvascular decompression,
    restoration of useful hearing after,
    94: 28
  pathology in presbycusis, 94: 35
  polyamines, marking otitis media
    induced cochlear damage, 95: 62
  scala vestibuli of, air intrusion to,
    causing inner ear injury, 95: 59
  spinal anesthesia and, 93: 21
  ultrastructural findings in AIDS, 95: 35
Cold
  air challenge in allergy, nasal response
    to, and rhinovirus 39 infection,
    95: 178

common, ultrastructural changes in
  nasal cilia due to, 94: 154
Collagen
  cell growth on, 93: 132
  injectable
    in glottic insufficiency, 93: 206
    in larynx, 93: 207
    in vocal fold problems, 93: 207
  sponge containing fibroblasts,
    keratinocytes proliferated and
    differentiated on, as new skin
    equivalent, 95: 152
  for vocal cord augmentation, 93: 212
Columellar
  elongation in bilateral cleft lip, results,
    93: 186
Communicative development
  after tracheostomy in infant, 93: 205
Composite graft
  survival, pharmacologic and surgical
    enhancement (in rabbit), 94: 141
Computed tomography
  of acoustic neuroma, and histology,
    94: 92
  artifacts, imaging, from
    craniomaxillofacial internal fixation
    devices, 95: 132
  based 3-dimensional radiotherapy of
    paranasal sinus cancer, 95: 241
  of cervical nodes, necrosis and
    neoplastic spread in, 93: 254
  for DentaScan imaging of mandible and
    maxilla, 94: 270
  development of, radiation exposure and
    cost containment, 93: 142
  of endolymphatic sac tumors, 94: 19
  guided stereolithography, new in
    craniofacial surgery, 95: 148
  in head and neck carcinoma, squamous
    cell, vs. MRI, 93: 254
  of sinuses, screening, technique
    optimization, 93: 141
  in stridor in children, 93: 209
  three-dimensional, in aural atresia,
    congenital, 94: 100
Computer
  reconstruction in facial canal
    dehiscence, 94: 75
Conchal
  palisade cartilage in tympanomastoid
    reconstruction, 93: 93
Consumer product
  aspiration and ingestion by children,
    93: 216
Continuous positive airway pressure
  reducing gastroesophageal reflux in
    obstructive sleep apnea, 93: 294
  in sleep apnea, obstructive, 93: 199

Cor pulmonale
  in obstructive sleep apnea in children,
    93: 305
Corticosporin, 93: 66
Corticosteroids
  in facial palsy, acute idiopathic
    peripheral, 94: 81
  intranasal, for allergic rhinitis in mild
    asthma, 94: 155
  perioperatively, for enhancement of
    composite graft survival (in rabbit),
    94: 141
  topical, in nose, long-term effects,
    94: 166
Cosmetic
  products, caustic, ingestion of, 95: 285
Cost
  considerations in mandibular fracture,
    94: 185
  containment
    and CT development, 93: 142
    in head and neck cancer evaluation,
      95: 239
  effective option, microlaryngoscopic
    surgery for T1 glottic lesions as,
    95: 232
  effectiveness, of parotidectomy,
    outpatient, 93: 283
  of hay fever in U.S. in 1990, 95: 282
  of health care, 93: 4
  inexpensive cochlear implant device,
    93: 26
  of mandibular reconstruction, 94: 175
  of programmable hearing aid, 93: 28
Cotton tipped swab
  effect on earwax occlusion, 95: 96
CPAP (see Continuous positive airway
    pressure)
Cranial
  base surgery, facial nerve management
    in, 94: 267
  base tumors, maxillary removal and
    reinsertion in, 93: 169
  nerve monitoring during otologic and
    neurotologic surgery, 95: 91
Craniofacial
  bone graft, onlay, revascularization and
    resorption in endurance of (in
    rabbit), 95: 157
  bone growth, pressure in regulation of,
    95: 139
  defects, gradual distraction for, 93: 165
  resection, complications and early
    outcome, 93: 277
  surgery, CT guided stereolithography
    new in, 95: 148
  tumors, devascularization by puncture,
    95: 246

Craniomaxillofacial
  internal fixation devices, CT imaging
    artifacts from, 95: 132
Cranioplasty
  hydroxyapatite cement (in cat), 93: 134
Cricoarytenoid
  muscle, posterior, function in
    phonation, laryngeal model in,
    95: 218
Cricoid
  cartilage
    division, four-quadrant, in
      laryngotracheal reconstruction,
      94: 217
    intrinsic response to vertical division,
      95: 142
    growing, reconstruction with bovine
      bone graft and perichondrium (in
      rabbit), 94: 147
Cricopharyngeus
  myotomy in postlaryngectomy
    pharyngeal contraction pressures,
    94: 252
"Crown-cork" technique
  for tympanic membrane reconstruction,
    93: 92
Crystalline
  preparation of botulinum toxin type A,
    storage causing degradation in
    potency, 94: 221
Cuff
  silicone, for peripheral nerve repair (in
    rat), 94: 77
Curettage
  in lymphadenitis, mycobacterial cervical,
    93: 308
Cutaneous (see Skin)
Cyanoacrylate
  adhesive, current status of, 94: 198
Cyst
  branchial, etiology theories, 95: 267
  cervical, lateral, etiology theories,
    95: 267
  saccular, in children, 93: 208
  thyroglossal duct cyst operation,
    core-out toward foramen cecum in,
    93: 296
Cystic
  acoustic neuroma, neuroimaging and
    histology of, 94: 90
  adenoid carcinoma
    flow cytometry of, 93: 240
    stage means more than grade,
      94: 264
  lymphangioma, bleomycin in, 93: 262
  parotid lesion in HIV, 93: 284
Cytokeratin

patterns of middle ear epithelium,
95: 110
Cytokine
attenuating ozone-induced DNA
synthesis in nasal epithelium (in
rat), 93: 156
Cytology
fine needle aspiration
of salivary gland lesions, 95: 254
of thyroid nodules, 93: 271
Cytomegalic
inclusion disease, temporal bone
histopathology 14 years after,
94: 25
Cytometry
flow, of adenoid cystic carcinoma,
93: 240
Cytopathology
in fine needle aspiration biopsy of head
and neck masses, 94: 244

D

Dacron
mesh tube, implantable, for tracheal
replacement, with jejunal autograft
(in dog), 94: 143
Dacryocystorhinostomy
endoscopic laser, 95: 186
Day care
in otitis media risk factors, acute, in
children, 94: 103
DDAVP
response, aspirin intolerance and easy
bruisability, 94: 276
Deafness
postlingual, cochlear implant in, 93: 27
postlinguistic with cochlear implant,
postoperative sentence scores in,
93: 27
prelingually or postlingually,
performance in adults with
multichannel cochlear implant,
95: 30
sensorineural, tinnitus suppression by
electrical promontory stimulation
in, 94: 40
sudden, with vertigo, outcome, 95: 12
Decompression
microvascular
of cochlear nerve, restoration of
useful hearing after, 94: 28
in hemifacial spasm, 93: 56
orbital, for vision preservation in Graves'
ophthalmopathy, 94: 183
sickness, of inner ear, 93: 35

vascular, for surgery of severe tinnitus,
selection criteria and results, 94: 41
Demineralized
bovine bone for composite graft in
growing cricoid reconstruction (in
rabbit), 94: 147
Dental
arch morphology after tonsillar
obstruction and tonsillectomy,
93: 289
sensation alteration after intranasal
surgery, 95: 257
DentaScan
imaging of mandible and maxilla,
94: 270
Dermatophagoides pteryonyssinus
allergic rhinitis due to, immunotherapy
of, subcutaneous, oral and nasal,
humoral response to, 95: 167
Desmopressin acetate
DDAVP response, aspirin intolerance
and easy bruisability, 94: 276
Devascularization
of craniofacial tumors by puncture,
95: 246
Dexamethasone
to prevent laryngeal edema after tracheal
extubation, 93: 212
Dextran
for sudden hearing loss, 93: 23
Diabetes mellitus
hearing loss in, 94: 34
Diet
effect on Ménière's disease, committee
evaluation, 95: 20
Disinfection
of laryngoscope in office practice,
94: 233
Distraction
osteogenesis, 93: 165
in irradiated mandible (in dog),
95: 131
Diuretic
effect on Ménière's disease, committee
evaluation, 95: 20
Diver
scuba, inner ear barotrauma, long-term
follow-up with continued diving,
94: 55
Diving
related inner ear injuries, 93: 35
Dizziness
after vestibular rehabilitation, 93: 9
vestibular autorotation and
electronystagmography testing in,
95: 7
DNA
ploidy

in head and neck cancer, 93: 236
in parotid tumors, adenoid cystic,
93: 240
synthesis, ozone-induced, in nasal
epithelium, endotoxin or cytokines
attenuating (in rat), 93: 156
Docusate
sodium, 93: 62
DPOEs
in children, 93: 14
Dressings
head, in middle ear surgery, 94: 129
Drill
generated noise levels during ear
surgery, 93: 36
Drilling
acoustic trauma due to, 93: 37
Drooling
in cerebral palsy, treatment, 93: 287
parotid duct ligation and submandibular
duct diversion in, 93: 287
team assessment and management,
93: 294
Drops
ear, antibiotic/steroid, to reduce
postoperative otorrhea and
ventilation tube blockage, 94: 111
Drugs
effects on human keloid implants (in
athymic mice), 93: 121
interactions with terfenadine and
astemizole, 95: 169
ototopical, and ototoxicity,
otolaryngologists survey, 94: 109
Dust
level reduction for foundry workers and
textile workers, 93: 148
wood, exposure increasing risk of
adenocarcinoma of sinonasal
cavities, 94: 159
Dye
transport function in eustachian tube,
and influenza A virus (in chinchilla),
94: 105
Dyskinesia
facial
botulinum toxin in, 93: 192
Oculinum in, 93: 192
Dysphonia
in aged, physiology vs. disease, 93: 205
spasmodic
adductor, unilateral vs. bilateral
injections of botulinum toxin in,
95: 219
botulinum toxin point-touch
technique for injection in, 94: 220
electromyography of, 93: 223
Dysplasia

Mondini, bilateral, with normal hearing,
94: 30

E

Ear
abnormalities
in newborn, 94: 101
osseointegrated implant in, in
children, 94: 43
anterior, arterial supply of, 93: 68
behind-the-ear device, experiences with,
95: 124
blast injury, vestibular and audiometric
consequences of, 95: 44
caloric function return after vestibular
nerve section, 93: 10
canal cholesteatoma, 93: 62
debridement, 93: 64
differentiated from hyperkeratosis
obturans, 93: 64
drops, antibiotic/steroid, to reduce
postoperative otorrhea and
ventilation tube blockage, 94: 111
drum, blue, in children, initial
evaluation, 93: 76
external, 93: 59, 94: 99, 95: 95
foreign body removal, case review,
94: 99
infections, chronic, with tympanic
membrane perforation, temporal
bone histopathology in, 94: 125
inner
barotrauma, 93: 35
barotrauma, in scuba divers,
long-term follow-up with continued
diving, 94: 55
decompression sickness, 93: 35
disorders, steroids for, 93: 21
hair cell regeneration in,
ultrastructural evidence (in
mammals), 94: 32
immune disease, laboratory diagnosis,
95: 26
injury, diving-related, 93: 35
injury, due to air intrusion to scala
vestibuli of cochlea, 95: 59
interaction with middle ear, 93: 33,
94: 53, 95: 41
membranous labyrinth injury after
cytomegalic inclusion disease,
94: 28
vertigo, vestibular neurectomy for,
93: 11
irradiated, in nasopharyngeal carcinoma,
tympanomastoidectomy for chronic
suppurative otitis media of, 95: 120

malformations
  congenital, cochlear implant in,
    94: 45
  in Treacher Collins syndrome, *94:* 30
microsurgery, high-definition television
  for, *93:* 60
middle, *93:* 59, *94:* 99, *95:* 95
  abnormalities, in perilymphatic fistula,
    congenital, *94:* 62
  adenocarcinoma, *95:* 76
  adenoma, *95:* 76
  adenoma, case report, *94:* 87
  brain herniation into (*see* Brain
    herniation into middle ear)
  carotid canal dehiscence prevalence
    in, temporal bone in, *95:* 98
  cleft, tegmental dehiscence and brain
    herniation into, *93:* 112
  conductive hearing loss and, *93:* 43
  contamination by amniotic fluid,
    model of, *94:* 101
  disease, with sensorineural hearing
    loss in children, *94:* 65
  effusion, chronic, and spontaneous
    hemotympanum, *93:* 76
  effusion, histamine and prostaglandin
    E_2 in, *93:* 77
  effusion, minimal, indicating
    ventilation tubes in vomiting infant,
    94: 111
  effusion, otitis media with effusion
    due to (in chinchilla), *93:* 77
  effusion, persistent, in otitis media in
    children, *94:* 105
  effusion, vestibular disturbances and,
    in children, *93:* 44
  effusion, vestibular labyrinth and,
    93: 43
  endoscopy of, transtympanic, *93:* 73
  epithelium, cytokeratin patterns of,
    95: 110
  facial canal dehiscence prevalence in,
    95: 79
  fluid of, *93:* 75
  implant device for, contactless
    electromagnetic, for sensorineural
    hearing loss, *95:* 52
  interaction with inner ear, *93:* 33,
    94: 53, *95:* 41
  meningioma, intracranial extension,
    94: 86
  mucosa, lymphocyte migration to,
    95: 111
  persistent stapedial artery in, *95:* 79
  pressure, and nasal airway resistance
    in upper respiratory tract infection,
    94: 153

reconstruction, alloplastic, problems
  with, *93:* 87
status in otitis media, *94:* 104
surgery, head dressings for, *94:* 129
susceptibility to *Pseudomonas*
  infection during acute otitis media,
  94: 106
symptoms while flying, severe
  outcome prevention, *95:* 103
surgery
  drill-generated noise levels during,
    93: 36
  outpatient, postoperative nausea with,
    transdermal scopolamine for,
    95: 11
Eardrops
  antibiotic prophylactic, and ventilation
    tubes, *93:* 79
Earphone
  vs. sound field methods for estimating
    noise attenuation of foam earplugs,
    94: 36
Earplug
  foam, noise attenuation of, earphone vs.
    sound field methods for estimating,
    94: 36
Earwax
  occlusion, effect of cotton tipped swab
    on, *95:* 96
Economic considerations (*see* Cost)
Ectopic
  thyroid nodules, management, *95:* 238
Edema
  larynx, after tracheal extubation,
    dexamethasone to prevent, *93:* 212
Elderly (*see* Aged)
Electrical
  promontory stimulation for tinnitus
    suppression in sensorineural
    deafness, *94:* 40
Electrocochleography
  for Ménière's disease diagnosis,
    vestibular, *94:* 16
  tympanic, in endolymphatic hydrops,
    93: 6
Electromagnetic
  implant middle ear device, contactless,
    for sensorineural hearing loss,
    95: 52
  ossicular replacement device, implant,
    95: 54
Electromyography
  for botulinum toxin injection, *94:* 221
  in dysphonia, spasmodic, *93:* 223
Electron
  microscopy, brush biopsies of nasal
    mucosa for, *93:* 152
Electroneurography

in facial nerve degeneration, and
    histology (in cat), 94: 76
Electronic
  National Electronic Injury Surveillance
    System, emergency room reports
    to, 93: 216
Electronystagmography
  standardization of, 93: 7
  testing in dizziness, 95: 7
  in vestibular disorders, peripheral, 93: 7
Electrophysiology
  cochlear, effect of vasodilating agent
    topical application on, 94: 66
  monitoring of facial nerve,
    intraoperative, is it standard of
    practice, 95: 92
  in perilymphatic fistula, spontaneous,
    94: 61
Embolization
  in arteriovenous malformation of face,
    93: 259
Emergency
  carotid artery coverage, superiorly based
    trapezius flap for, 94: 239
  room reports to National Electronic
    Injury Surveillance System, 93: 216
Endocrine
  multiple endocrine neoplasia type IIb,
    natural course of, 93: 260
Endolymphatic
  duct, arterial supply of, 94: 5
  hydrops (*see* Hydrops, endolymphpatic)
  sac
    absorption activity and barrier
     properties in, ultrastructure and
     morphometry, 95: 15
    arterial supply of, 94: 5
    ballooning surgery in Ménière's
     disease, 95: 22
    immune reaction, vestibular immune
     injury after, 95: 19
    procedure, 93: 11
    surgery, in vertigo in Meniere's
     disease, efficacy, 94: 14
    surgical anatomy, 95: 13
    tumors, radiographic appearance,
     94: 19
Endonasal
  sinus surgery in children, 93: 149
  with sinonasal disease, 93: 150
Endoscopic
  dacryocystorhinostomy, laser, 95: 186
  gastrostomy
    in head and neck cancer, 93: 241
    in head and neck carcinoma, 93: 279
    percutaneous, in head injury, 95: 228
  telendoscopic study, 95: 266
Endoscopy

of adenoids, assessment methods,
    93: 300
airway, in bacterial tracheitis in children,
    95: 229
of auditory canal, internal, during
    hearing conservation acoustic
    tumor surgery, 94: 94
for creation and repair of fetal cleft lip,
    94: 150
guiding otosurgery to prevent residual
    cholesteatoma, 94: 134
head and neck, open tube vs. flexible
    esophagoscopy in, 93: 290
in Hunter's syndrome with
    tracheobronchomalacia, in child,
    94: 226
for laser medial arytenoidectomy in
    airway management of laryngeal
    paralysis, 94: 214
panendoscopy, justifications and
    controversies, 93: 278
in sinus surgery (*see* Sinus surgery,
    endoscopic)
symptom-directed selective, in head and
    neck cancer evaluation, 95: 239
transtympanic, of middle ear, 93: 73
Endotoxin
  attenuating ozone-induced DNA
    synthesis, in nasal epithelium (in
    rat), 93: 156
Endotracheal
  tube, small-bore, for laryngeal
    microsurgery under general
    anesthesia, blood gas analysis in,
    95: 226
Enteral
  feeding in head and neck cancer,
    93: 241
Environmental
  health, 95: 275
Eperisone hydrochloride
  in tinnitus, 93: 30
Epidemiology, 95: 275
Epidermal
  autologous cells, of epithelium, for
    mastoid cavity graft to prevent
    chronic otorrhea, 95: 119
  growth factor for chronic tympanic
    membrane perforation repair,
    95: 115
Epidural
  blood patch, facial nerve paralysis after,
    94: 80
Epiglottitis
  disappearance, during *Hemophilus
    influenzae* type B vaccination in
    children, 95: 280
Epinephrine

for nasal mucosa vasoconstriction,
93: 320
for nasal surgery, ventricular fibrillation
after, 93: 315
Epistaxis
intractable, maxillary and ethmoidal
arterial occlusion in, 93: 155
nasal packing in, 93: 156
Epithelium
cells on fascia lata as living skin
substitute, 93: 137
ciliated, recovery of, and ultrastructural
changes in nasal cilia due to
common cold, 94: 154
from epidermal cells for mastoid cavity
graft to prevent chronic otorrhea,
95: 119
equivalent, for tracheal reconstruction,
95: 141
middle ear, cytokeratin patterns of,
95: 110
migration, and living skin substitute,
93: 137
nasal transitional, endotoxin or
cytokines attenuating
ozone-induced DNA synthesis in (in
rat), 93: 156
respiratory, free grafting of, cellular
differentiation after, 93: 132
tracheal, damage from suction, 93: 195
Erythrocyte
scintigraphy to distinguish soft tissue
hemangioma from vascular
malformations, 93: 186
Esophagoscopy
open tube vs. flexible, in head and neck
endoscopy, 93: 290
Esophagus
atresia, with tracheomalacia absence,
93: 204
cervical, total reconstruction, 94: 237
foreign bodies in, causative factors,
93: 288
spasm and foreign bodies, 93: 288
Ethanol
production workers, mortality study,
93: 152
Ethmoidal
and maxillary arterial occlusion in
epistaxis, 93: 155
Eustachian tube
ciliary activity and dye transport in, and
influenza A virus (in chinchilla),
94: 105
distribution of goblet cells and glands in
otitis media in children, 93: 74
function

localization of, hypothesis concerning,
95: 101
tests, diagnostic potential of, 94: 107
lumen, lining of roof in children, 93: 74
Exercise
conditioning, in peripheral vestibular
disorders, 93: 9
nose response to, in rhinitis and asthma,
95: 163
Expanded skin
long-term histopathologic evaluation,
94: 182
Explant
skin wound, in tissue culture, 93: 137
Extracellular
matrix, tissue engineering with scaffolds
of, 93: 132
Eye
protection, in otolaryngologic surgery,
95: 272
Eyelid
lower, blepharoplasty, transconjunctival
approach, experience, indications
and technique, 95: 199

F

Face
arteriovenous malformation,
embolization in, 93: 259
canal dehiscence
computer reconstruction and
histology, 94: 75
prevalence in middle ear, 95: 79
craniofacial (*see* Craniofacial)
craniomaxillofacial internal fixation
devices, CT imaging artifacts from,
95: 132
dyskinesia
botulinum toxin in, 93: 192
Oculinum in, 93: 192
fracture
association with skull base fracture,
94: 185
microplates for repair, 93: 171
reconstruction, fate of plates and
screws after, 94: 170
growth after tonsillar obstruction and
tonsillectomy, 93: 289
hemangioma, laser for, 94: 258
lift
incision, modified for parotidectomy,
95: 208
infection after requiring hospital
readmission, incidence, treatment
and sequelae, 95: 212

musculoaponeurotic system
suspension in, 94: 203
submentoplasty to enhance cervical
recontouring in, 94: 203
maxillofacial reconstruction, temporalis
myofascial flap for, 93: 161
maxillofacial skeleton, rigidly fixated,
impact tolerances of, 94: 148
midfacial trauma, postoperative
infection rates in, and intermaxillary
fixation, wire fixation and rigid
internal fixation implant, 94: 169
nerve (*see* Nerve, facial)
neuroma of cerebellopontine angle and
internal auditory canal, 94: 84
plastic surgery (*see* Plastic surgery, facial)
reconstruction, biologic grafts and
alloplastic implants in, 94: 208
silicone implant, safety of, 95: 214
trauma management, extended
access/internal approaches for,
94: 177
tumors, 93: 55, 94: 75, 95: 73
Facial
artery flap, 93: 180
Failure to thrive
in sleep apnea, obstructive, in children,
93: 305
Fallopian
canal and stapedectomy, 93: 51
Family
violence and physical abuse of children,
93: 291
Fascia
flap, temporoparietal, in head and neck
reconstruction, 94: 187
lata, epithelial cells on, as living skin
substitute, 93: 137
temporalis, grafts in open secondary
rhinoplasty, 95: 204
vascularized, as transferable bed for
laryngeal reconstruction (in rabbit),
95: 160
Fat
autogenous, for vocal cord
augmentation, 93: 210
Feeding
enteral, in head and neck cancer,
93: 241
Femur
condyle flap in mandibular
reconstruction, 93: 162
Fenestra
microdrill stapedotomy, small, footplate
complication reduction in, 94: 71
stapes surgery, large and small, for
otosclerosis, hearing recovery after,
94: 70

Fetus
cleft lip, endoscopic creation and repair
of, 94: 150
wound healing in, 93: 124
Fever
rheumatic, prevention in Costa Rica,
94: 286
Fiberoptic
exam of nasal cavity and nasopharynx in
children, 93: 320
nasopharyngoscopy, flexible, of upper
airway narrowing in obstructive
sleep apnea, 94: 284
Fibrillation
ventricular, after cocaine and
epinephrine for nasal surgery,
93: 315
Fibrin
tissue adhesive, current status of,
94: 198
Fibroblast
alterations in cholesteatoma, induction
of neoplastic-like phenotype,
94: 132
collagen sponge containing fibroblasts,
keratinocytes proliferated and
differentiated on, as new skin
equivalent, 95: 152
growth factor in healing of traumatic
tympanic membrane perforation,
94: 115
Fibronectin
like substance secretion from head and
neck carcinoma, 95: 145
Fibrosarcoma
lethal, complicating radiotherapy of
benign glomus jugulare tumor,
94: 89
Fibrosis
meatal, medial, experience with,
94: 122
Fine needle aspiration (*see* Aspiration, fine
needle)
Fire
safety of patient in operating room,
95: 196
Fishbone
ingestion, possible, radiography in,
95: 268
Fistula, perilymph
chronic (in guinea pig), 93: 37
cochlear dysfunction in (in guinea pig),
93: 39
congenital, with middle ear
abnormalities, 94: 62
diagnostic tests value, 95: 57
MRI of (in cat), 94: 59

pathogenic mechanisms (in guinea pig),
    93: 40
perilymphatic hydrops and, 93: 38
spontaneous, electrophysiologic
    findings, 94: 61
Flap
  arm free, lateral, in head and neck
    reconstruction, 94: 176
  bone, vascularized, in oromandibular
    reconstruction, 95: 132
  cross-lip, bipedicled axial, to correct
    major vermilion deficiency after
    cleft lip repair, 95: 206
  facial artery, 93: 180
  femoral condyle, in mandibular
    reconstruction, 93: 162
  forehead
    expanded unilateral, for coverage of
      opposite forehead defect, 95: 188
    in nasal reconstruction, anatomic vasis
      for design, 93: 167
  free, in head and neck cancer defect
    repair, 95: 195
  infrahyoid musculocutaneous, in head
    and neck reconstruction, 93: 159
  intraoral
    facial artery flap, 93: 180
    free muscle, skin in, 94: 173
  jejunal, free, recurrence, complications
    and functions results with, 95: 250
  Kerr, in myringoplasty for anterior
    perforation, 93: 84
  myocutaneous
    with AO plate, instead of
      revascularized tissue transfer, for
      mandibular reconstruction, 95: 185
    platysma, indications and caveats,
      95: 189
    repeated use in difficult second
      operations on head and neck,
      95: 156
  nasolabial, 93: 183
  omental, for tracheal
    autotransplantation (in pig),
    93: 202
  pectoralis major, for intraoral and
    pharyngeal reconstruction, 93: 176
  pharyngeal, effect on upper airway in
    children with velopharyngeal
    inadequacy, 95: 184
  radial forearm, sensate, bilobed design,
    to preserve tongue mobility after
    significant glossectomy, 95: 181
  sail, for coverage of opposite forehead
    defect, 95: 188
  skin, undermining in wound tension in
    rhytidectomy, 94: 202
  in skull base tumors, 93: 244

temporalis myofascial
    discussion of, 93: 161
    for maxillofacial reconstruction,
      93: 161
  temporoparietal fascial, in head and
    neck reconstruction, 94: 187
  thigh paddle, in mandibular
    reconstruction, 93: 163
  tissue expanders, rectangular,
    maximizing gain from, 93: 179
  trapezius, superiorly based, for
    emergency carotid artery coverage,
    94: 239
  V-Y, extended, 93: 175
Flow
  resistance, correlation with geometry in
    nose model, 95: 137
Fluid
  IV administration during radical neck
    surgery, 94: 242
  of middle ear, 93: 75
Flunarizine
  in tinnitus, 93: 30
Flunisolide
  intranasal spray as adjunct to oral
    antibiotics in sinusitis, 95: 172
Fluorescein
  IV, in perilymph at stapes surgery,
    negative observation, 94: 69
Fluoridation
  drinking water, effect on hearing in
    otosclerosis in low fluoride area,
    95: 65
Flying
  middle ear symptoms during, severe
    outcome prevention in, 95: 103
Footplate
  complication reduction in small fenestra
    microdrill stapedotomy, 94: 71
  in otosclerosis, obliterative, 93: 53
  stapedectomy, total, bone conduction
    threshold change by, and age,
    94: 72
  surgery, saccule and utricle in, 93: 51
Foramen
  cecum, core-out toward, in thyroglossal
    duct cyst operation, 93: 296
Forearm
  flap, sensate radial, bilobed design, to
    preserve tongue mobility after
    significant glossectomy, 95: 181
Forehead
  defect, coverage of opposite, expanded
    unilateral forehead flap for,
    95: 188
  flap
    expanded unilateral, for coverage of
      opposite forehead defect, 95: 188

in nasal reconstruction, anatomic
basis for design, 93: 167
Foreign body
of ear, removal, case review, 94: 99
in esophagus, causative factors, 93: 288
Formaldehyde
occupational exposure, and sinonasal
cancer, 94: 158
Foundry
workers, dust level reduction for,
93: 148
Fracture
facial
association with skull base fracture,
94: 185
extended access/internal approaches
for, 94: 178
microplates for repair, 93: 171
reconstruction, fate of plates of
screws after, 94: 170
mandible
in angular region, rigid internal
fixation of, complications, 94: 181
medical and economic considerations,
94: 185
patterns in children, 94: 180
plating vs. traditional techniques,
93: 170
vestibular and lingual wire splints in,
93: 164
midfacial, repair, sinusitis after, 94: 169
oblique, in children, 93: 45
orbital floor
repair, causing diplopia, Vicryl mesh
implant for, 95: 183
titanium implant in, 93: 166
otitis media and, 93: 83
petrous bone, in children, management,
95: 50
rhinoplasty making more susceptible to,
95: 205
serpiginous track, 93: 46
skull base, association with facial
fracture, 94: 185
temporal bone
in children, 93: 44
longitudinal or oblique, 93: 45
Frozen section
intraoperative, for diagnosis in head and
neck surgery, accuracy of, 94: 259
in thyroid tumors, distinguishing benign
from malignant, 94: 266

G

Gallium

scans in postradiotherapy osteonecrosis
of jaw, 93: 172
Gas
blood, analysis in laryngeal microsurgery
with small-bore endotracheal tubes,
95: 226
Gastric
transposition in head and neck cancer,
93: 161
Gastro-esophagonasopharyngeal acid
reflux, 93: 286
Gastroesophageal
reflux
airway manifestations in children,
93: 218
in obstructive sleep apnea, CPAP
reducing, 93: 294
Gastropharyngeal
reflux, pharyngeal pH monitoring in, in
children, 94: 284
Gastrostomy
endoscopic
in head and neck cancer, 93: 241
in head and neck carcinoma, 93: 279
percutaneous, in head injury, 95: 228
Gelfilm
myringoplasty for residual perforation,
93: 83
Gender
differences in sleep disordered
breathing, 95: 276
in joint noises prevalence, 94: 289
Gene
capsule, sequences in pharyngeal isolates
of nontypeable *Hemophilus
influenzae*, 95: 150
somatic gene therapy, ex vivo, in thyroid
follicular cell transplant (in dog),
94: 146
General practitioners
sinus x ray film use by, 95: 173
Gentamicin
accumulating in outer hair cells, 93: 17
intratympanic, in bilateral Ménière's
disease, 95: 61
kinetics in cochlear hair cells after
chronic use, 93: 16
vs. ciprofloxacin in chronic otitis media,
93: 65
Geometry
correlation with flow resistance in nose
model, 95: 137
Gillies temporal muscle
transfer in lagophthalmos, 93: 163
Glomus
jugulare tumor, benign, radiotherapy
for, lethal fibrosarcoma
complicating, 94: 89

tympanicum
  in infant, 95: 73
  tumor, Nd:YAG laser for, 94: 88
Glossectomy
  significant, tongue mobility preservation
      after, bilobed design for sensate
      radial forearm flap for, 95: 181
  total, without total laryngectomy in
      advanced tongue carcinoma,
      94: 269
Glottic
  cancer, partial laryngectomy after
      radiotherapy, 93: 196
  carcinoma
    early, open laryngeal procedures for,
        95: 251
    T1, radiotherapy of, 95: 244
    T1 and T2, surgery and radiotherapy
        of, 93: 229
  configuration, in laryngeal paralysis,
      95: 220
  insufficiency
    injectable collagen in, 93: 206
    Silastic medialization and arytenoid
        adduction in, 94: 231
    T1 lesions, microlaryngoscopic surgery
        for, as cost effective option,
        95: 232
Gloves
  surgical
    blood contact risk through, in
        aesthetic procedures, 95: 203
    perforations, prevention with
        cut-resistant gloves, 94: 290
Goblet cells
  of eustachian tube, distribution in
      children in otitis media, 93: 74
Gold
  weight implant, and MRI, 94: 82
Goode's tympanostomy tubes
  long-term results in children, 94: 113
Graft
  alar spreader, for pinched nasal tip
      correction, 94: 199
  auricular cartilage, in laryngotracheal
      reconstruction, 94: 222
  autograft (*see* Autoograft)
  baton, for short nose, 94: 206
  biologic, in facial plastic and
      reconstructive surgery, 94: 208
  bone
    craniofacial onlay, revascularization
        and resorption in endurance of (in
        rabbit), 95: 157
    reconstruction of orbital floor with
        iliac graft and titanium mesh plate
        (in monkey), 94: 149
  calvarial

bone, harvest, techniques,
    considerations and morbidity,
    94: 172
  split, for nasal reconstruction,
      94: 190
cartilage, irradiated, in nose, 94: 196
composite
  of bovine bone, demineralized, in
      growing cricoid reconstruction (in
      rabbit), 94: 147
  survival, pharmacologic and surgical
      enhancement (in rabbit), 94: 141
flap (*see* Flap)
iliac, for bone-graft reconstruction of
    orbital floor (in monkey), 94: 149
nerve, interposition, for facial nerve
    repair, results, 94: 174
nose tip, 20-year retrospective, 94: 207
olecranon bone, for nasal augmentation,
    93: 190
polytetrafluoroethylene, for permanent
    lip augmentation, 94: 204
of respiratory epithelia, cell
    differentiation after, 93: 132
rib cartilage, in laryngotracheal
    reconstruction in children, 93: 201
survival, increased, with elevated IGF-II
    and TGF-beta concentrations in
    calvarial bone and, 95: 138
temporalis fascia, in open secondary
    rhinoplasty, 95: 204
Granuloma
  excision in long-term tracheotomy, in
      children, 94: 228
  reparative, update on, American
      Otological Society and American
      Neurotology Society survey, 95: 70
  Teflon, as therapeutic challenge,
      95: 221
Granulomatosis
  Wegener's
    otologic manifestations of, 95: 42
    subglottic stenosis and, 94: 220
Graves' ophthalmopathy
  vision preservation with orbital
      decompression in, 94: 183
Grommet
  Mini-Shah, and tympanosclerosis,
      results, 94: 112
  swimming and, survey, 95: 107
Growth
  of cells on collagen, 93: 132
  craniofacial bone, pressure in regulation
      of, 95: 139
  facial, after tonsillar obstruction and
      tonsillectomy, 93: 289
  factor

angiogenic, in soft tissue wound
healing, 93: 131
epidermal, for chronic tympanic
membrane perforation repair,
95: 115
fibroblast, in healing of traumatic
tympanic membrane perforation,
94: 115
insulin-like, II, elevated
concentrations in calvarial bone,
95: 138
nerve, in Silastic tubes and facial nerve
regeneration (in rabbit), 94: 77
transforming beta, elevated
concentrations in calvarial bone,
95: 138
transforming beta, neutralizing
antibody to, to control scarring in
adult wounds, 93: 130
of squamous cell carcinoma cell line,
and hyperbaric oxygen therapy,
94: 143

H

Hair
cell
chronic use, gentamicin kinetics after,
93: 16
outer, gentamicin accumulating in,
93: 17
regeneration, after kanamycin
ototoxicity, 93: 15
regeneration, in basal turn, 93: 16
regeneration, in inner ear,
ultrastructural evidence (in
mammals), 94: 32
Hay fever
cost in U.S. in 1990, 95: 282
Head
dressings in middle ear surgery, 94: 129
injury, tracheostomy and endoscopic
gastrostomy in, 95: 228
and neck (*see below*)
Head and neck
cancer
advanced, chemoradiation in,
simultaneous, 93: 265
advanced, cisplatin in, 93: 278
cervical node evaluation in, 93: 230
defect repair, free flap for, 95: 195
enteral feeding in, 93: 241
evaluation, symptom-directed
selective endoscopy and cost
containment for, 95: 239
gastric transposition for, 93: 161
gastrostomy in, endoscopic, 93: 241

histologic grading DNA ploidy and
nodal status in, 93: 236
hyperalimentation in, 93: 241
intra-arterial infusions in, of cisplatin
and adriamycin, 93: 279
irradiated, bone-anchored
reconstruction of, 94: 186
pain in, types and causes, 93: 269
postoperative wound infection as
poor prognosis in, 94: 236
proliferation pattern, 93: 125
quality of life assessment in, 95: 240
radiotherapy, smoking in efficacy of,
94: 263
radiotherapy, thyroid dysfunction
after, 94: 262
surgery, quality of life after, 93: 246
trials, surgical reporting instrument to
improve outcome data of, 95: 245
carcinoma
basaloid squamous cell,
clinicopathology and
immunohistochemistry, 94: 247
fibronectin like substance secretion
from, 95: 145
gastrostomy in, endoscopic, 93: 279
MRI vs. CT in, 93: 254
radiotherapy, postoperative, 93: 267
recurrence, transfusion in, 93: 274
squamous cell, distant metastases of,
94: 238
squamous cell, hyperbaric oxygen
therapy in, 94: 144
squamous cell, locally advanced,
surgical resection leaving positive
margins in, 95: 242
suprafractionated radiotherapy in,
93: 237
complications in mucopolysaccharidoses
in children, 93: 307
endoscopy, open tube vs. flexible
esophagoscopy in, 93: 290
extracranial, interventional radiology of,
93: 244
hemangioma
MRI of, 94: 246
treatment, 94: 257
histiocytosis X, in children, 93: 276
injuries from physical abuse of children,
93: 291
masses, fine needle aspiration biopsy of,
cytopathology in, 94: 244
melanoma
lentigo maligna, 94: 260
mucosal, local control in survival,
95: 237
oncology, 93: 227, 94: 235, 95: 231

radiotherapy, oral sequelae of, protocol
    for prevention and treatment,
    94: 250
reconstruction
  arm free flap in, lateral, *94:* 176
  infrahyoid musculocutaneous flap in,
    93: 159
  temporoparietal fascial flap in,
    94: 187
rhabdomyosarcoma
  in children, *93:* 250
  surgery in, *93:* 231
surgeons, professional burnout among,
    survey results, *95:* 231
surgery, *94:* 137, *95:* 127
  intraoperative frozen section diagnosis
    in, accuracy of, *94:* 259
  research, advances in, *93:* 121,
    94: 141, *95:* 131
  second operations, difficult, repeated
    use of same myocutaneous flap in,
    95: 156
tumors, with AIDS, *94:* 235
vascular lesions, interventional radiology
    in, *93:* 245
vascular malformations, MRI of,
    94: 246
Healing
  mechanical evaluation by skin wound
    explants in tissue culture, *93:* 137
  of tympanic membrane perforation after
    fibroblast growth factor, *94:* 115
  wound
    early developmental, model for,
      monodelphis domesticus, *93:* 124
    in fetus, *93:* 124
    in ischemic skin tissue, hyperbaric
      oxygen improving, *95:* 147
    soft tissue, angiogenic growth factors
      in, *93:* 131
Health
  care
    cost of, *93:* 4
    professionals identifying dimensions
      of quality of life after laryngectomy,
      94: 265
  environmental, *95:* 275
Hearing, *94:* 23, *95:* 25
  after stapedotomy, long-term results,
    95: 67
  aid
    air conduction, *93:* 26
    for hearing loss at 65 and over,
      prevalence, *95:* 38
    infrared cross, *93:* 25
    irritation with, *93:* 26
    programmable, *93:* 3

programmable, as new technology,
    93: 28
programmable, cost, *93:* 28
super-base bone-anchored, *93:* 25
tissue breakdown and infection with,
    93: 26
traditional bone conduction,
    modification of, *94:* 42
bone conduction device, implant, in
    sensorineural hearing loss, *93:* 24
conservation acoustic tumor surgery,
    endoscopy of internal auditory
    canal during, *94:* 94
impaired children, otoacoustic
    emissions in, *93:* 14
levels in otosclerosis 10 years after
    stapedectomy, *94:* 72
loss
  500-Hz description of, *93:* 21
  after neurosurgery, low CSF pressure
    in, *95:* 34
  aged 65 and over, prevalence,
    screening and hearing aid provision,
    95: 38
  in automobile company, follow-up,
    94: 36
  conductive, tympanic membrane and
    middle war in, *93:* 43
  congenital, early acquired, *93:* 13
  in diabetes, *94:* 34
  high frequency, otitis media and,
    secretory, *93:* 42
  low-frequency, after spinal anesthesia,
    as perilymphatic hypotonia, *93:* 21
  music and, *93:* 20
  noise-induced, cassette players
    causing, personal, *93:* 18
  noise-induced, in children, *93:* 18
  noise-induced, "Walkman" causing,
    93: 18
  sensorineural, as more than meets the
    eye, *94:* 29
  sensorineural, bone conduction
    hearing device for, implant, *93:* 24
  sensorineural, from trumpets in
    symphony orchestra, *93:* 20
  sensorineural, idiopathic bilateral,
    clinical features, *95:* 33
  sensorineural, middle ear device for,
    contactless electromagnetic
    implant, *95:* 52
  sensorineural, otitis media with
    effusion and, *93:* 40
  sensorineural, sudden, vascular
    compression causing, *94:* 29
  sensorineural, tinnitus in, *93:* 31
  sensorineural, transient, with otitis
    media, acute, *94:* 53

sensorineural, with middle ear disease
in children, 94: 65
step-wise, and absent round window
reflex, 95: 58
sudden, acoustic neuroma causing,
small tumors in, 94: 95
sudden, as monosymptom of multiple
sclerosis, 95: 31
sudden, dextran for, 93: 23
sudden, idiopathic, and iron
metabolism disturbance, 93: 22
sudden, plasma expander in, 93: 23
sudden, procaine for, 93: 23
sudden, vasoactive therapy for, 93: 23
sudden, vasodilator in, 93: 23
transient, after spinal anesthesia,
94: 25
in Treacher Collins syndrome, 94: 30
tuning fork tests validity in, 95: 25
unchanged unilateral, in acoustic
neuroma ipsilateral growth, 94: 93
pathology resource registry, 94: 23
preservation
after meningioma affecting temporal
bone surgical removal, 94: 86
with early surgery in intracanalicular
acoustic neuroma, 95: 88
with modified translabyrinthine
approach, 94: 95
protection program for musicians,
93: 20
recovery, after fenestra stapes surgery
for otosclerosis, 94: 70
restoration
with type V tympanoplasty, 93: 95
of useful, after microvascular
decompression of cochlear nerve,
94: 28
tests, 94: 23, 95: 25
Heart
rate variability during sleep in snoring
with obstructive sleep apnea,
94: 285
Hemangioma
of head and neck
MRI of, 94: 246
treatment, 94: 257
nasal, early excision, L-approach,
95: 209
soft tissue, distinguishing from vascular
malformations, 93: 186
Hemifacial
spasm, microvascular decompression in,
93: 56
Hemithyroidectomy
in hyperthyroidism, surgery,
complications and results, 93: 307
Hemophilus influenzae

nasopharyngeal, and treatment failure in
otitis-prone children, 93: 81
nontypeable, capsule gene sequences in
pharyngeal isolates of, 95: 150
type B
invasive disease, retreat of,
immunization program in, 95: 283
large-scale vaccination of children,
epiglottitis disappearance during,
95: 280
Hemotympanum
spontaneous, and chronic middle ear
effusion, 93: 76
HEPP
in allergic rhinitis, 93: 147
Herniation, brain (*see* Brain herniation)
Herpes
simplex with pharyngitis in college
students, 94: 295
zoster oticus
acyclovir in, 93: 55
steroids in, 93: 55
Hiccups
case presentation and etiologic review,
94: 278
treatment methods, 94: 281
Histamine
challenge in allergy, nasal response to,
and rhinovirus 39 infection,
95: 178
H_1 receptors in nasal turbinates,
autoradiographic localization,
93: 151
induced nasal provocation, topical
steroids in, 93: 143
in middle ear effusion, 93: 77
release, antigen-mediated, from blood
in allergic rhinitis, astemizole in,
94: 156
topical application, effect on cochlear
electrophysiology, 94: 67
Histiocytosis X
classification system, 93: 277
of head and neck, in children, 93: 276
HIV
cervical node biopsy in, open,
indications for, 94: 288
parotid lesions in, benign cystic vs. solid,
93: 284
(*See also* AIDS)
HLA
A2 antigen, protective association with
nasopharyngeal carcinoma, 95: 284
Home care
after tracheostomy in children, 93: 207
Hormone
parathyroid

assay, in parathyroid enlargement
localization, 93: 232
"quick" test, 93: 239
Hunter's syndrome
tracheobronchomalacia in, 94: 225
Hurthle cell
tumors of thyroid, 93: 235
Hydralazine
topical application, effect on cochlear
electrophysiology, 94: 67
Hydrops
endolymphatic
in Ménière's disease, 93: 6
in Ménière's disease, vestibular,
94: 16
and otosclerosis, extensive, temporal
bone histopathology, 95: 43
symptomatic vs. asymptomatic,
histopathology, 94: 12
tympanic electrocochleography in,
93: 6
perilymphatic, perilymph fistula and,
93: 38
Hydroxyapatite
cement
for calvarial defect reconstruction,
93: 135
cranioplasty (in cat), 93: 134
laryngeal implant, for medialization,
95: 222
prosthesis, 93: 87
for incus long process defects,
94: 117
in ossiculoplasty, 93: 90
Hyperalimentation
in head and neck cancer, 93: 241
Hyperbaric oxygen (*see* Oxygen,
hyperbaric)
Hyperkeratosis
obturans differentiated from ear canal
cholesteatoma, 93: 64
Hyperparathyroidism
association with nonmedullary thyroid
carcinoma, 94: 271
normocalcemic, biochemical and
symptom profiles before and after
surgery, 94: 268
primary, cervical exploration for,
94: 245
Hyperplasia
pulmonary, in Potter's syndrome in
infant, 94: 58
Hypertension
perilymphatic, 93: 35
pseudoephedrine in, cardiovascular
effects, 93: 312
sympathomimetics and, 93: 313
Hyperthermia

malignant, in otology patient, UCLA
experience, 95: 48
Hyperthyroidism
surgery for, complications and results,
93: 307
Hypertrophy
adenoids, assessment, 93: 321
tonsil
in sleep apnea, obstructive, in
children, 93: 305
upper airway obstruction and,
93: 289
Hypnosis
for tinnitus, 95: 37
Hypoglossal
facial nerve anastomosis for facial nerve
palsy after cerebellopontine angle
tumor surgery, 94: 83
lingual nerve transfer, for tongue
reinnervation, 95: 151
Hypopharynx
carcinoma, hypothyroidism after
treatment, 93: 234
reconstruction, total, 94: 237
Hypopnea
sleep apnea syndrome
inheritance of, 95: 262
posture and upper airway dimensions,
93: 197
Hyposmia
in rhinitis, allergic, 94: 164
Hypothyroidism
after hypopharyngeal and laryngeal
carcinoma treatment, 93: 234
after radiotherapy, 94: 262
Hypotonia
perilymphatic, and low-frequency
hearing loss after spinal anesthesia,
93: 21

I

Iliac
graft for bone-graft reconstruction of
orbital floor (in monkey), 94: 149
Imaging
bone and gallium, in postradiography
osteonecrosis of jaw, 93: 172
bone and gallium, in postradiotherapy
osteonecrosis of jaw, 93: 172
DentaScan, of mandible and maxilla,
94: 270
magnetic resonance (*see* Magnetic
resonance imaging)
surface contour three-dimensional, in
congenital aural atresia, 94: 100
Imbalance

after vestibular rehabilitation, 93: 9
Immune
  inhibition of repair of skull trephine
    defects (in dog), 93: 126
  inner ear disease, laboratory diagnosis,
    95: 26
  regulation in rhinopathy, 93: 142
  vestibular injury after immune reaction
    of endolymphatic sac, 95: 19
Immunization
  program, and *Hemophilus influenzae*
    type B invasive disease retreat,
    95: 283
Immunoglobulin
  concentration in nasal secretions differ
    with IgE-mediated rhinopathy and
    non-IgE-mediated rhinopathy,
    93: 142
  distribution patterns in tonsils, 93: 318
  E
    mediated allergy, from vegetable
      allergens, 95: 269
    in tonsillitis, chronic, in children,
      93: 318
  secreting cells in adenoids, 93: 317
Immunologic
  abnormality in Ménière's disease, 93: 5
    bilateral disease, 93: 5
  approach to Ménière's disease, 95: 19
  aspects of allergic reactions, 94: 301
Immunotherapy
  subcutaneous, oral and nasal, humoral
    response to, for allergic rhinitis due
    to *Dermatophagoides*
    pteryonyssinus, 95: 167
Implant
  alloplastic
    in facial plastic and reconstructive
      surgery, 94: 208
    qualities of, 93: 87
  Audiant XA-II, experiences with,
    95: 124
  bone conduction
    hearing device in sensorineural
      hearing loss, 93: 24
    transcutaneous vs. percutaneous,
      93: 66
  Branemark, in cleft palate, 93: 160
  cochlea (*see* Cochlea implant)
  Dacron mesh tube in tracheal
    replacement with jejunal autograft
    (in dog), 94: 143
  facial silicone, safety of, 95: 214
  gold weight, and MRI, 94: 82
  of human keloid in athymic mice, effects
    of pharmacologic agents on,
    93: 121

hydroxylapatite laryngeal, for
    medialization, 95: 222
middle ear device, contactless
    electromagnetic, for sensorineural
    hearing loss, 95: 52
osseointegrated
  in ear abnormalities in children,
    94: 43
  into free vascularized radius, in
    mandibular reconstruction, 95: 192
of ossicular replacement device,
    electromagnetic, 95: 54
rigid internal fixation, in midfacial
    trauma, postoperative infection
    rates in, 94: 169
spring, and MRI, 94: 82
in temporal bone, percutaneous, results,
    95: 125
titanium, in orbital floor fracture,
    93: 166
trephine defects of skull with bovine
    morphogenetic protein (in dog),
    93: 126
Vicryl mesh, for orbital floor fracture
    repair, causing diplopia, 95: 183
Incus
  long process defects, hydroxylapatite
    prosthesis for, 94: 117
  transposition
    first stage tympanoplasty technique
      and, 93: 86
    mastoidectomy and, cortical, 93: 86
Infant
  glomus tympanicum in, 95: 73
  tracheostomy
    communicative development after,
      93: 205
    medical and social factors predicting
      outcome, 93: 204
  vomiting, protracted, with minimal
    middle ear effusion indicating
    ventilation tubes, 94: 111
  x-ray therapy for enlarged thymus,
    thyroid cancer later, 95: 288
Infection
  after face lift surgery, hospital
    readmission for, incidence,
    treatment and sequelae, 95: 212
  disease team approach for infections in
    children requiring parenteral
    antibiotics, 94: 124
  of ear, chronic, with tympanic
    membrane perforation, temporal
    bone histopathology in, 94: 125
  postoperative rates in midfacial trauma,
    intermaxillary fixation, wire fixation
    and rigid internal fixation implant
    in, 94: 169

postoperative wound, and poor
prognosis in head and neck cancer,
94: 236
Staphylococcus aureus,
methicillin-resistant
community-acquired, 94: 302
streptococcal throat, group A
beta-hemolytic, cephalexin and
penicillin in, 94: 302
Infectious mononucleosis
tonsillectomy in, acute, 94: 294
Inflammatory
mechanisms of allergic reactions,
94: 301
Influenza A virus
in ciliary activity and dye transport
function in eustachian tube (in
chinchilla), 94: 105
Infrahyoid
musculocutaneous flap in head and neck
reconstruction, 93: 159
Infrared
cross hearing aid, 93: 25
Ingestion
caustic cosmetic products, 95: 285
fishbone, possible, radiography in,
95: 268
Insulin
like growth factor II, elevated
concentrations in calvarial bone,
95: 138
Intelligibility
of tracheoesophageal speech among
naive listeners, 95: 225
Interdental
immobilization, new device for, 93: 177
Interleukin
1 and DNA synthesis after ozone
exposure, 93: 157
Intracranial
complications of vestibular nerve
section, 93: 11
extension of middle ear meningioma,
94: 86
Intranasal
cocaine in benzoylecgonine screening,
93: 144
Intraoral
flap
facial artery flap, 93: 180
free muscle flap, skin in, 94: 173
reconstruction, pectoralis major flap for,
93: 176
Intubation
lidocaine before, to prevent
postoperative stridor and
laryngospasm, 93: 197

Iodine-123
scintigraphy in thyroid disorder
evaluation in children, 93: 311
Iodine-131
imaging for diagnosis and assessment of
metastatic differentiated thyroid
carcinoma, 95: 234
Iodine, radioactive
to evaluate thyroidectomy in thyroid
carcinoma, 93: 280
in thyroid carcinoma, well
differentiated, 93: 275
Iron
metabolism disturbance and sudden
hearing loss, 93: 22
Irradiated
cartilage graft in nose, 94: 196
ear, in nasopharyngeal carcinoma,
tympanomastoidectomy for chronic
suppurative otitis media of, 95: 120
mandible, distraction osteogenesis in (in
dog), 95: 131
Irradiation
as risk factor for carotid atherosclerosis,
93: 231
Ischemia
acute, for preconditioning in latissimus
dorsi model for skeletal muscle
survival augmentation (in pig),
94: 144
skin tissue, hyperbaric oxygen improving
wound healing in, 95: 147
Isopropanol
production workers, mortality study,
93: 152
Isshiki
thyroplasty type I, vocal quality
long-term changes after, 95: 227

J

Jaw
osteonecrosis after radiotherapy, bone
and gallium scans in, 93: 172
Jejunal
autograft, revascularized, for tracheal
replacement (in dog), 94: 143
flap, free, recurrence, complications and
functional results with, 95: 250
transfer, microvascular free, for
hypopharynx and esophagus
reconstruction, 94: 237
Joint
noises, prevalence, age and gender in,
94: 289

K

Kanamycin
  ototoxicity, hair cell regeneration after, 93: 15
Kaposi's sarcoma
  in AIDS, 94: 235
Kawasaki disease
  cervical node enlargement in, 93: 310
  early presentation, 94: 297
  five-year experience in children, 93: 309
Keloids
  human, implants, effects of pharmacologic agents on (in athymic mice), 93: 121
Keratinocyte
  proliferated and differentiated on collagen sponge containing fibroblasts, as new skin equivalent, 95: 152
Keratosis
  laryngeal, laryngoscopy in, 93: 202
Kerr flap
  in myringoplasty for anterior perforation, 93: 84
Kidney
  agenesis in Potter's syndrome in infant, 94: 58
  transplant, skin cancer after, 95: 287
Kikuchi-Fujimoto disease
  of neck, update, 94: 287
Killer cell
  activity, natural, in laryngeal carcinoma, 94: 263
KTP laser
  in revision stapedectomy, 95: 68

L

Labyrinth
  membranous
    inner ear, injury after cytomegalic inclusion disease, 94: 28
    particulate matter within, pathology vs. normality, 95: 17
  MRI of, 94: 30
  vestibular, middle ear effusion and, 93: 43
Labyrinthectomy
  with cochlear implant, 94: 47
  transmastoid, for vertigo, 95: 23
Lacrimal
  drainage system injury in functional endoscopic sinus surgery, 94: 167
Lagophthalmos
  Gillies temporal muscle transfer for, 93: 163

temporal muscle transposition in, 93: 164
Language
  development in children with recurrent acute otitis media, follow-up for seven years, 94: 108
Laryngectomy
  partial, for glottic cancer after radiotherapy, 93: 196
  pharyngeal contraction pressures after, cricopharyngeus myotomy in, 94: 252
  quality of life after, dimensions identified by patients and health care professionals, 94: 265
  supraglottic, bilateral neck dissection in recovery after, 94: 261
  thyroid during, intraoperative management, 93: 255
Laryngobronchoscopy
  rigid, complications in children, 94: 227
Laryngocele
  in children, 93: 208
Laryngopharyngeal
  cancer, advanced, radiotherapy failure, surgery after, 95: 252
Laryngopharyngectomy
  thyroid function tests after, 93: 235
Laryngoscope
  microbial adherence to, and disinfection of, in office practice, 94: 233
Laryngoscopy
  fiberoptic
    in laryngeal keratosis, 93: 202
    in vocal cord paralysis, 93: 223
Laryngospasm
  after tonsillectomy and adenotonsillectomy, 93: 197
  postoperative
    lidocaine before intubation, 93: 197
    prevention with topical lidocaine, 93: 196
Laryngotracheal
  reconstruction
    auricular cartilage graft in, 94: 222
    cricoid cartilage division in, four-quadrant, 94: 217
    perioperative management, 93: 200
    rib cartilage graft in, in children, 93: 201
  stenosis
    classification, 94: 229
    stenting in children, 93: 213
Laryngotracheobronchitis
  complicating measles epidemic, 94: 218
Larynx, 93: 195, 94: 211, 95: 217
  cancer

occupational exposure to sulfuric acid
and, 94: 216
severity staging system, five-year
survival rates, 95: 235
carcinoma
cells, living, during invasion of healthy
cell formation, 93: 133
hypothyroidism after treatment,
93: 234
natural killer cell activity in, 94: 263
squamous cell, thyroidectomy in,
93: 255
verrucous, papillomavirus, radiation
and surgery in, 94: 211
collagen injections in, 93: 207
edema after tracheal extubation,
dexamethasone to prevent, 93: 212
hydroxylapatite implant, for
medialization, 95: 222
keratosis, laryngoscopy in, 93: 202
microsurgery under general anesthesia
with small-bore endotracheal tubes,
blood gas analysis in, 95: 226
model, in posterior cricoarytenoid
muscle function in phonation,
95: 218
motoneurons modulated by respiratory
cycle, 94: 142
movements, coordinated with oral cavity
movements during swallowing,
95: 146
muscles
coordinated with oral muscle during
swallowing, 95: 155
intrinsic, during respiration, single
motor unit activity of, 94: 142
muscular tenotomy, for bilateral midline
vocal cord fixation, 95: 223
nerve, superior, surgical anatomy of
external branch, 93: 217
open procedures, for early glottic
carcinoma, 95: 251
paralysis
bilateral, airway management with
endoscopic laser medial
arytenoidectomy, 94: 214
glottis configuration in, 95: 220
stroboscopy of, 93: 223
pharyngolaryngeal carcinoma with
palpable nodes, 93: 239
phrenic nerve reinnervation in, new
technique (in cat), 95: 143
precancer, vs. oral leukoplakia, 93: 201
reconstruction, vascularized fascia as
transferable bed for (in rabbit),
95: 160
tuberculosis, case review, 94: 212
Laser

carbon dioxide, microspot microslad
for, 93: 284
dacryocystorhinostomy, endoscopic,
95: 186
endoscopic, for medial arytenoidectomy
for airway management in laryngeal
paralysis, 94: 214
in head and neck hemangioma, 94: 258
KTP, in revision stapedectomy, 95: 68
Nd:YAG, for glomus tympanicum
tumor, 94: 88
tunable pulsed-dye, in capillary vascular
malformations, 95: 202
Latissimus dorsi
model, acute ischemic preconditioning
for skeletal muscle survival
augmentation (in pig), 94: 144
Lentigo
maligna melanoma of head and neck,
94: 260
Leukoplakia
oral, vs. laryngeal precancer, 93: 201
Lidocaine
before intubation in postoperative
stridor and laryngospasm, 93: 197
in tinnitus, 32, 93: 30
topical, to prevent postoperative stridor
and laryngospasm, 93: 196
vs. cocaine with oxymetazoline for nasal
procedures, 95: 165
xylometazoline solution,
vasoconstrictive and anesthetics
effects, vs. intranasal cocaine,
94: 164
Lightning
injury of tympanic membrane, 95: 46
strike, unusual otolaryngologic
manifestation of, 95: 45
Lignocaine
in tinnitus, 93: 32
Lingual
hypoglossal nerve transfer, for tongue
reinnervation, 95: 151
Lining
cells, incomplete coverage of bone
matrix (in mammals), 94: 24
Lip
augmentation, permanent, with
polytetrafluoroethylene graft,
94: 204
cleft (see /iunder/I Cleft)
flap, cross-lip bipedicled axial, to
correct major vermilion deficiency
after cleft lip repair, 95: 206
Lobectomy
vs. total thyroidectomy for thyroid
differentiated carcinoma, 95: 253
Lung

disease, children set home with
tracheostomy, 93: 208
Lymph node
cervical (*see* Cervical nodes)
extracapsular, extension of head and
neck carcinoma, 93: 267
Lymphadenitis
cervical, mycobacterial, curettage of,
93: 308
Lymphadenopathy
cervical, in AIDS, 93: 285
Lymphangioma
cystic, bleomycin in, 93: 262
Lymphocyte
migration to middle ear mucosa,
95: 111
Lymphoma
malignant, in AIDS, 94: 235
Lymphoproliferative disease
of salivary gland, 93: 234

M

Magnetic resonance angiography
of tinnitus, pulsatile, 95: 49
Magnetic resonance arteriography
to distinguish soft tissue hemangioma
from vascular malformation,
93: 187
Magnetic resonance imaging
of acoustic neuroma, and histology,
94: 92
of acoustic tumor growth, 94: 94
of cervical nodes, necrosis and
neoplastic spread in, 93: 254
of endolymphatic sac tumors, 94: 19
gold weight implant and, 94: 82
of head and neck carcinoma, squamous
cell, vs. CT, 93: 254
of head and neck hemangioma and
vascular malformations, 94: 246
high-resolution, of temporal bone,
93: 47
of paranasal sinus disease, inflammatory,
in Bell's palsy, 94: 80
of parotid tumors, malignant, 94: 254
of perilymphatic fistula (in cat), 94: 59
in sensorineural hearing loss, 94: 29
spring implant and, 94: 82
in stridor in children, 93: 209
of tinnitus, pulsatile, 95: 49
Malformations
ear, congenital, cochlear implant in,
94: 45
vascular
capillary, tunable pulsed-dye laser for,
95: 202

of head and neck, MRI of, 94: 246
Malignancy (*see* Cancer)
Malocclusion
dental, after tonsillar obstruction,
93: 289
Mandible
contouring, intraoperative custom,
95: 210
DentaScan imaging of, 94: 270
fracture (*see* Fracture, mandible)
irradiated, distraction osteogenesis in (in
dog), 95: 131
lengthening by gradual distraction,
93: 164
maxillofacial fixation, system for,
93: 179
nerve localization during neck
dissection, 93: 256
reconstruction
AO plate with myocutaneous flap
instead of revascularized tissue
transfer for, 95: 185
cost and complications, 94: 175
with femoral condyle flap, 93: 162
with osseointegrated implant into free
vascularized radius, 95: 192
with recombinant bone-inducing
factor, 93: 122
thigh paddle flap for, 93: 163
Marrow transplant
nasal mucociliary clearance impairment
during, 95: 174
Mastoid, 93: 59, 94: 99, 95: 95
cavities grafted with epithelium from
epidermal cells to prevent chronic
otorrhea, 95: 119
pressure dressing not necessary after
middle ear surgery, 94: 130
Mastoidectomy
cortical, and incus transposition, 93: 86
radical
modified, and single-stage
management of cholesteatoma,
93: 108
reconstruction by obliteration
technique, 93: 111
with tympanoplasty in chronic otitis
media in children, 94: 128
Mastoiditis
chronic, in Southern Israel, 93: 111
latent, no room for complacency,
93: 97
with otitis media, medical therapy failure
in, 93: 110
otomastoiditis, tuberculous, 93: 96
Maxilla
DentaScan imaging of, 94: 270

intermaxillary fixation in midfacial
  trauma and postoperative infection
  rates, 94: 169
removal and reinsertion in cranial base
  tumors, 93: 169
Maxillary
continuity defects, stabilized with plates
  and screws, motion across, 95: 154
craniomaxillofacial internal fixation
  devices, CT imaging artifacts from,
  95: 132
and ethmoidal arterial occlusion in
  epistaxis, 93: 155
sinusitis, chronic, antrum bacteriology
  in, 95: 179
Maxillofacial
reconstruction, temporalis myofascial
  flap for, 93: 161
skeleton, rigidly fixated, impact
  tolerances of, 94: 148
trauma, blunt, blindness after, optic
  nerve decompression surgery in,
  95: 190
Maxillomandibular
fixation, system for, 93: 179
Measles
epidemic, laryngotracheobronchitis
  complicating, 94: 218
Meatal
fibrosis, medial, experience with,
  94: 122
Medications (*see* Drugs)
Melanoma
cervical node dissection in, 93: 253
cutaneous malignant, neck dissection
  for, 93: 252
of head and neck, lentigo maligna,
  94: 260
mucosal, of head and neck, local control
  in survival, 95: 237
Ménière's disease
bilateral, intratympanic gentamicin for,
  95: 61
classification, 94: 17
diet effect on, committee evaluation,
  95: 20
diuretic effect on, committee evaluation,
  95: 20
endolymphatic sac ballooning surgery
  for, 95: 22
hydrops and, endolymphatic, 93: 6
immunologic abnormality in, 93: 5
  bilateral disease, 93: 5
immunologic approach to, 95: 19
suspected, temporal bone in, 94: 18
systemic disease process in, 93: 6
vertigo in
  benign paroxysmal postural, 94: 7
endolymphatic sac surgery efficacy in,
  94: 14
vestibular diagnosis with
  electrocochleography, 94: 16
Meningioma
temporal, presenting as chronic otitis
  media, 94: 85
temporal bone affected, surgical
  removal, hearing preservation after,
  94: 86
Meningitis
sensorineural damage and tympanogenic
  labyrinthitis, 93: 33
Mesh
Dacron tube, implantable, for tracheal
  replacement, with jejunal autograft
  (in dog), 94: 143
titanium, plate with iliac graft for
  bone-graft reconstruction of orbital
  floor (in monkey), 94: 149
Vicryl implant, for orbital floor fracture
  repair, causing diplopia, 95: 183
Mesotympanic
cholesteatoma, posterior, management,
  93: 102
Metal
industry, cancer of nose and paranasal
  sinuses in, 93: 147
Metastases
cervical node, CT and palpation in,
  93: 245
distant, in head and neck squamous cell
  carcinoma, 94: 238
in neck adenocarcinoma, 93: 227
of thyroid carcinoma, thyroglobulin and
  iodine-131 imaging for diagnosis
  and treatment assessment in,
  95: 234
Methicillin
resistant *Staphylococcus aureus*
  infections, community-acquired,
  94: 302
Metoclopramide
reducing vomiting after tonsillectomy in
  children, 93: 316
Metoprolol
in sleep apnea, 93: 199
Microbial
adherence to laryngoscope in office
  practice, 94: 233
Microdrill
stapedotomy, small fenestra, footplate
  complication reduction in, 94: 71
Microlaryngoscopic
surgery, for T1 glottic lesions, as cost
  effective option, 95: 232
Micromanipulator
for laser, carbon dioxide, 93: 285

Microplate
  repair of facial fracture, 93: 171
Microscopically
  controlled excision of medial canthus
    basal cell carcinoma, limits in,
    94: 195
Microscopy
  electron, brush biopsies of nasal mucosa
    for, 93: 152
Microslad
  microspot, for carbon dioxide laser,
    93: 284
Microspot
  microslad, for carbon dioxide laser,
    93: 284
Microsurgery
  of ear, high-definition television for,
    93: 60
  laryngeal, under general anesthesia with
    small-bore endotracheal tubes,
    blood gas analysis in, 95: 226
  for repair of parotid duct, 94: 176
Microvascular
  decompression
    of cochlear nerve, restoration of
      useful hearing after, 94: 28
    in hemifacial spasm, 93: 56
  free jejunal transfer for hypopharynx
    and esophagus reconstruction,
    94: 237
Midfacial
  trauma, postoperative infection rates in,
    and intermaxillary fixation, wire
    fixation and rigid internal fixation
    implant, 94: 169
Mini-Grommet
  tympanosclerosis and, results, 94: 112
Mini-Shah grommet
  tympanosclerosis and, results, 94: 112
Model
  animal, for tinnitus research, 93: 29
  for cholesteatoma (in animal), 94: 130
  laryngeal, in posterior cricoarytenoid
    muscle function in phonation,
    95: 218
  latissimus dorsi, acute ischemic
    preconditioning for skeletal muscle
    survival augmentation (in pig),
    94: 144
  of middle ear contamination by
    amniotic fluid in newborn, 94: 101
  nose, correlations between flow
    resistance and geometry in, 95: 137
  sinusitis, natural ostiotomy vs. inferior
    antrostomy in (in rabbit), 95: 136
  skin substitute, living, production and
    transplantation (in rat), 93: 135

  of subperiosteal tissue expansion (in
    dog), 95: 140
  for wound healing, early developmental,
    monodelphis domesticus, 93: 124
Molecular
  bioengineering of biomaterials, 93: 128
  biology and polymers, 93: 128
Mondini dysplasia
  bilateral, with normal hearing, 94: 30
Monitoring
  airway pressure, in airway collapse site in
    obstructive sleep apnea, 95: 217
  cranial nerve, during otologic and
    neurotologic surgery, 95: 91
  of facial nerve
    intraoperative, electrophysiological, is
      it standard of practice, 95: 92
    intraoperative, in parotid gland
      pleomorphic adenoma, 95: 247
  global, of positive surgical outcome,
    95: 279
  nasal packing with pulse oximetry,
    93: 314
  of parathyroid hyperfunction, operative,
    93: 238
  pH
    nasopharyngeal, in rhinopharyngitis in
      children, 93: 286
    pharyngeal, in gastropharyngeal reflux
      in children, 94: 284
Monodelphis
  domesticus, model for early
    developmental wound healing,
    93: 124
Mononucleosis
  infectious, acute tonsillectomy in,
    94: 294
Morbidity
  in brain abscess, 93: 115
  in calvarial bone graft harvest, 94: 172
  of facial nerve, after parotid surgery for
    benign disease, 94: 294
  in facial plastic surgery with coronal
    approach, 94: 193
  in head and neck cancer radiotherapy,
    thyroid dysfunction after, 94: 262
Mortality
  in brain abscess, 93: 115
  in ethanol production workers, 93: 152
  in isopropanol production workers,
    93: 152
  in tracheobronchial disruption in
    children, 93: 203
Motion
  across maxillary continuity defects
    stabilized with plates and screws,
    95: 154

sickness, in children, experimental,
    95: 8
Motoneurons
  laryngeal, modulated by respiratory
    cycle, 94: 142
Motor
  unit activity, single, of intrinsic laryngeal
    muscles during respiration, 94: 142
Movement
  of oral cavity and larynx, coordinated
    during swallowing, 95: 146
Mucin
  in effusions in otitis media, 93: 75
Mucociliary
  transport
    disorders, brush biopsies in, 93: 152
    nasal, of chronic sinusitis in children,
      94: 162
Mucopolysaccharidoses
  head and neck complications in
    children, 93: 307
  otolaryngologic manifestations of,
    93: 305
Mucosa
  early changes in sinusitis (in rabbit),
    94: 151
  of middle ear, lymphocyte migration to,
    95: 111
Multiple sclerosis
  sudden hearing loss as monosymptom
    of, 95: 31
Muscle
  cricoarytenoid, posterior, function in
    phonation, laryngeal model,
    95: 218
  intraoral, flap, skin in, 94: 173
  laryngeal
    coordinated with oral muscle during
      swallowing, 95: 155
    during respiration, single motor unit
      activity of, 94: 142
    tenotomy for bilateral midline vocal
      cord fixation, 95: 223
  oral, coordinated with laryngeal muscle
    during swallowing, 95: 155
  pectoralis major flap for intraoral and
    pharyngeal reconstruction, 93: 176
  skeletal, survival augmentation in
    latissimus dorsi model with acute
    ischemic preconditioning (in pig),
    94: 144
  temporal (see Temporal muscle)
Musculoaponeurotic
  system suspension in wound tension in
    rhytidectomy, 94: 202
Music
  hearing loss and, 93: 20
Musicians

hearing protection program for, 93: 20
rock, auditory temporary threshold shift
    after heavy metal concert, 94: 37
Mycobacterial
  cervical
    adenitis in children, management,
      95: 272
    lymphadenitis, curettage of, 93: 308
Myocutaneous flap (see Flap,
    myocutaneous)
Myotomy
  cricopharyngeus, in postlaryngectomy
    pharyngeal contraction pressures,
    94: 252
Myringoplasty
  for anterior perforation, and Kerr flap,
    93: 84
  Gelfilm, for residual perforation, 93: 83
  success and pitfalls, follow-up case
    review, 94: 116
Myringostomy
  in vomiting infant with minimal middle
    ear effusion, 94: 111

N

Nasal
  airway resistance and middle ear
    pressure in upper respiratory tract
    infection, 94: 153
  augmentation with olecranon bone
    graft, 93: 190
  cancer
    formaldehyde occupational exposure
      and, 94: 158
    in metal industry, 93: 147
    occupational exposures and, 94: 157
    sinonasal cancer, occupational risk
      factors for, 93: 148
  cartilage graft in, irradiated, 94: 196
  cavity, fiberoptic exam, in children,
    93: 320
  challenge, unilateral, with allergen,
    terfenadine in, 95: 171
  cilia, ultrastructural changes due to
    common cold, 94: 154
  corticosteroids, topical, long-term
    effects, 94: 166
  disorders, and lower respiratory tract
    symptoms and illness in children,
    94: 159
  endonasal (see Endonasal)
  epithelium, endotoxin or cytokines
    attenuating ozone-induced DNA
    synthesis in (in rat), 93: 156
  hemangioma, early excision,
    L-approach, 95: 209

model, correlations between flow
resistance and geometry in, 95: 137
mucociliary clearance impairment during
marrow transplant, 95: 174
mucociliary transport of chronic sinusitis
in children, 94: 162
mucosa
brush biopsies for electron
microscopy, 93: 152
histamine H_1 receptors in, Scatchard
analysis, 93: 151
vasoconstriction, epinephrine for,
93: 320
packing
after nasal surgery, routine, 95: 166
in epistaxis, 93: 156
materials used in nasal surgery,
95: 175
pulse oximetry monitoring of,
93: 314
papilloma, inverting, treatment options,
93: 150
provocation, ragweed and histamine,
topical steroids in, 93: 143
reconstruction
forehead flaps in, anatomic basis for
design, 93: 167
platyrrhine nose, 93: 188
refinements, 93: 173
reconstruction with split calvarial grafts,
94: 190
response to exercise in rhinitis and
asthma, 95: 163
response to histamine and cold air
challenges in allergy, and rhinovirus
39 infection, 95: 178
rhinoplasty making more susceptible to
fracture, 95: 205
secretion, immunoglobulin
concentrations in, differing in
IgE-mediated and
non-IgE-mediated rhinopathy,
93: 142
structure reconstruction at donor site,
93: 174
surgery
adrenaline for, catecholamine levels
after, 93: 319
cocaine and epinephrine for,
ventricular fibrillation after, 93: 315
cocaine vs. lidocaine with
oxymetazoline for, 95: 165
intranasal, dental sensation alteration
after, 95: 257
nasal packing materials used in,
95: 175
routine, nasal packing after, 95: 166

tip
graft, 20-year retrospective, 94: 207
pinched, correction with alar spreader
grafts, 94: 199
turbinates, histamine H_1 receptors in,
autoradiographic localization,
93: 151
(*See also* Nose)
Nasolabial
flap, 93: 183
fold, and rhytidectomy, 94: 200
Nasopharyngeal
angiofibroma, treatment, in children,
93: 249
carcinoma
irradiated ears of,
tympanomastoidectomy for chronic
suppurative otitis media of, 95: 120
protective association with HLA-A2
antigen, 95: 284
radiotherapy results, 93: 273
recurrence, 93: 274
fiberoptic exam in children, 93: 320
Hemophilus influenzae and treatment
failure in otitis-prone children,
93: 81
pH monitoring in rhinopharyngitis in
children, 93: 286
Nasopharyngoscopy
fiberoptic flexible, of upper airway
narrowing in obstructive sleep
apnea, 94: 284
in obstructive sleep apnea, 93: 198
Natural
killer cell activity in laryngeal carcinoma,
94: 263
Nausea
postoperative, in ear surgery,
transdermal scopolamine for,
95: 11
Nd:YAG laser
for glomus tympanicum tumor, 94: 88
Neck
adenocarcinoma, metastatic, 93: 227
dissection
bilateral, in recovery after supraglottic
laryngectomy, 94: 261
mandibular nerve localization during,
93: 256
in melanoma, cutaneous malignant,
93: 252
supraomohyoid, in oral cavity
carcinoma, 93: 230, 247
and head (*see* Head and neck)
Kikuchi-Fujimoto disease, update,
94: 287
mass, evaluation by surgeon, 93: 228

nodes, uncontrolled, in head and neck
squamous cell carcinoma distant
metastases, *94:* 239
surgery, radical, IV fluid administration
and urine output during, *94:* 242
treatment in salivary cancer, *93:* 248
whiplash injury, cerebral symptoms
after, *94:* 277
Necrosis
cervical nodes, MRI vs. CT in, *93:* 254
Needle
aspiration of peritonsillar abscess in
children, *94:* 275
Neoglottis
functional, creation methods, *94:* 223
Neolarynx
functionally adequate, creation
methods, *94:* 223
Neomycin, *93:* 66
Neoplasia (*see* Tumors)
Nerve
cochlear, microvascular decompression,
restoration of useful hearing after,
94: 28
cranial, monitoring during otologic and
neurotologic surgery, *95:* 91
facial, *93:* 55, *94:* 75, *95:* 73
anomalous, avulsion at stapedectomy,
93: 51
degenerating, electroneurography and
histology (in cat), *94:* 76
how to find it, *95:* 82
with hypoglossal anastomosis for
facial nerve palsy after
cerebellopontine angle tumor
surgery, *94:* 83
injury during cochlear implant, *94:* 49
management in cranial base surgery,
94: 267
monitoring, intraoperative,
electrophysiological, is it standard
of practice, *95:* 92
monitoring, intraoperative, in parotid
pleomorphic adenoma, *95:* 247
morbidity after parotid surgery for
benign disease, *94:* 294
neuroma, presenting as acoustic
tumor, *95:* 86
palsy, after cerebellopontine angle
tumor surgery, hypoglossal-facial
nerve anastomosis for, *94:* 83
paralysis, after epidural blood patch,
94: 80
paralysis, idiopathic, prednisone for,
95: 84
paralysis, in chronic otitis media,
93: 57
paralysis, surgery of, *93:* 58

reconstruction, results, *95:* 87
regeneration, in nerve growth factor
containing Silastic tubes (in rabbit),
94: 77
repair by interposition nerve graft,
results, *94:* 174
graft, interposition, for facial nerve
repair, results, *94:* 174
growth factor containing Silastic tubes
for facial nerve regeneration (in
rabbit), *94:* 77
hypoglossal lingual nerve transfer, for
tongue reinnervation, *95:* 151
laryngeal, superior, surgical anatomy of
external branch, *93:* 217
mandibular, localization during neck
dissection, *93:* 256
optic, decompression surgery, for
maxillofacial blunt trauma, with
blindness after, *95:* 190
peripheral, repair, silicone cuffs for (in
rat), *94:* 77
phrenic, reinnervation, of larynx, new
technique (in cat), *95:* 143
vestibular, section
caloric function return in ear after,
93: 10
intracranial complications, *93:* 11
translabyrinthine, for vertigo, *95:* 23
vestibular function patterns after,
93: 10
Neuralgia, trigeminal (*see* Trigeminal
neuralgia)
Neurectomy
vestibular, for inner ear vertigo, *93:* 11
Neuroblastoma
olfactory, modern treatment approaches
results, *94:* 258
Neuroimaging
of acoustic neuroma, cystic, *94:* 90
Neuroma
acoustic
cystic, neuroimaging and histology of,
94: 90
hearing loss due to, sudden, and small
tumors, *94:* 95
intracanalicular, early surgery for
hearing preservation, *95:* 88
ipsilateral growth, unchanged
unilateral hearing loss in, *94:* 93
recurrent disappearing, in aged
woman, *94:* 92
translabyrinthine removal, technique
to avoid cerebrospinal fluid
otorhinorrhea, *95:* 88
facial, of cerebellopontine angle and
internal auditory canal, *94:* 84

facial nerve, presenting as acoustic
tumor, 95: 86
Neuronitis
vestibular
epidemiological survey by
questionnaire in Japan, 94: 8
respiratory infection before, viral
upper, 94: 8
vertigo after, benign paroxysmal
positional, 94: 6
vestibular compensation in, long-term
follow-up, 94: 9
Neuropsychological study
of cerebral symptoms after whiplash
injury of neck, 94: 277
Neurosurgery
hearing loss, low CSF pressure in,
95: 34
Neurotologic
surgery, cranial nerve monitoring during,
95: 91
Neutralization
biochemistry of, 95: 168
Neutralizing
antibody to transforming growth factor
β to control scarring in adult
wounds, 93: 130
Neutrophil
constituents, autoantibodies against, in
subglottic stenosis diagnosis,
94: 219
Newborn
ear abnormalities in, 94: 101
otitis media, diagnosis, 93: 71
with Potter's syndrome, temporal bone
histopathology in, 94: 57
Nicotine
replacement therapy, effective in
smoking cessation, 95: 278
Nicotinic acid
topical application, effect on cochlear
electrophysiology, 94: 67
Nitroprusside
topical application, effect on cochlear
electrophysiology after, 94: 67
Noise
attenuation of foam earplugs, earphone
vs. sound field methods for
estimating, 94: 36
drill-generated noise levels during ear
surgery, 93: 36
exposure in rural setting, 94: 38
inducing hearing loss in children, 93: 18
Nortriptyline
for tinnitus, 93: 31
Nose
short, lengthening, 94: 204
(See also Nasal)

O

Occupational
exposure
in nose and paranasal sinus cancer,
94: 157
to sulfuric acid and laryngeal cancer,
94: 216
risk factors for sinonasal cancer,
93: 148
Oculinum
in facial dyskinesia, 93: 192
Olecranon
bone graft for nasal augmentation,
93: 190
Olfactory
neuroblastoma, modern treatment
approaches results, 94: 258
Omental
flap for tracheal autotransplant (in pig),
93: 202
Oncology
head and neck, 93: 227, 94: 235,
95: 231
Operating room
fire safety of patient in, 95: 196
Ophthalmopathy
Graves', vision preservation with orbital
decompression in, 94: 183
Optic
nerve decompression surgery in
maxillofacial blunt trauma, with
blindness after, 95: 190
Oral
cancer
changing trends in U.S., 93: 241
recurrences, due to discontinuous
periosteal involvement, 93: 228
rising in females, 93: 242
second cancer after, tobacco and
alcohol in, 95: 281
vitamin supplement to reduce risk of,
93: 302
carcinogenesis and vitamin E, 93: 303
carcinoma, squamous cell, multiple
tumor risk after, 95: 275
cavity
cancer, resection, frozen section at,
93: 252
cancer, stage I and II squamous cell,
recurrence, 93: 251
carcinoma, neck dissection and frozen
section biopsy in, 93: 230
carcinoma, squamous cell,
supraomohyoid neck dissection in,
93: 247

movements coordinated with
  laryngeal movements during
  swallowing, 95: 146
 reconstruction, pectoralis major flap
  for, 93: 177
 intraoral (*see* Intraoral)
 leukoplakia vs. laryngeal precancer,
  93: 201
 muscle, coordinated with laryngeal
  muscle during swallowing, 95: 155
 sequelae of head and neck radiotherapy,
  protocol for prevention and
  treatment, 94: 250
Orbit
 calvarial bone graft for, 94: 191
 complications in functional endoscopic
  sinus surgery, 95: 176
 decompression for vision preservation in
  Graves' ophthalmopathy, 94: 183
 floor bone-graft reconstruction with
  iliac graft and titanium mesh plate
  (in monkey), 94: 149
 floor fracture
  repair, Vicryl mesh implant for,
   causing diplopia, 95: 183
  titanium implant in, 93: 166
Oromandibular
 reconstruction, vascularized bone flaps
  in, 95: 132
Oscillopsia
 with vestibular function loss, 94: 10
Osseointegrated
 implant
  in ear abnormalities in children,
   94: 43
  in mandibular reconstruction, into
   free vascularized radius, 95: 192
Ossicular
 chain defects, hydroxylapatite prosthesis
  for, 93: 89
 replacement
  device, electromagnetic, implant of,
   95: 54
  prosthesis, 93: 91
  prosthesis, total and partial, in
   children, 95: 123
Ossiculoplasty
 auditory brain stem response in, 93: 91
 hydroxylapatite prosthesis in, 93: 90
Ossification
 of tympanic membrane, clinical records,
  94: 118
Osteogenesis
 distraction, 93: 165
  in irradiated mandible (in dog),
   95: 131
Osteonecrosis

 of jaw, postradiotherapy, bone and
  gallium scans in, 93: 172
Osteoporosis
 resistance, and elevated IGF-II and
  TGF-beta concentrations in
  calvarial bone and, 95: 138
Ostiomeatal unit
 development in children, radiography
  of, 94: 156
Ostiotomy
 natural, vs. inferior antrostomy in
  sinusitis (in rabbit model), 95: 136
Otic
 topical preparation, ciprofloxacin as,
  93: 66
Oticus
 herpes zoster
  acyclovir in, 93: 55
  steroids in, 93: 55
Otitis externa
 malignant, nondiabetic, 95: 47
 management of recalcitrant case, 95: 95
Otitis media
 acute
  antibiotics for, outcome in children,
   94: 105
  middle ear susceptibility to
   Pseudomonas infection during,
   94: 106
  recurrent, language development in
   children with, follow-up for seven
   years, 94: 108
  risk factors for, temporal aspect
   control in, in children, 94: 103
  with transient sensorineural hearing
   loss, 94: 53
 in adult trauma, 93: 82
 with cholesteatoma, ceftazidime in,
  93: 109
 chronic, 93: 3
  in children, conservative surgical
   approach for, 94: 128
  ciprofloxacin vs. gentamicin for,
   93: 65
  facial nerve paralysis secondary to,
   93: 57
  with mastoiditis, medical therapy
   failure in, 93: 110
  noncholesteatomatous, in children,
   surgery results, 94: 128
  suppurative, incidence and risk factors
   in children, 93: 110
  suppurative, of irradiated ears in
   nasopharyngeal carcinoma,
   tympanomastoidectomy for,
   95: 120
  suppurative, therapy effective against
   anaerobic bacteria in, 95: 118

suppurative, with cholesteatoma in
children, outpatient management,
93: 108
suppurative, without cholesteatoma,
medical treatment in children,
94: 123
temporal meningioma presenting as,
94: 85
with tympanic membrane perforation,
94: 125
tympanomastoidectomy in, 93: 109
clinical profile of, 94: 104
with effusion, 93: 3
adult onset, 95: 108
chronic, quality of life issues in,
93: 70
components contributing to viscous
properties, 93: 75
middle ear effusion causing (in
chinchilla), 93: 77
mucin in, 93: 75
pars tensa micropathologic changes in
children, 95: 112
sensorineural hearing loss and, 93: 40
ventilation tube surgery in, 93: 70
eustachian tube goblet cell and gland
distributions in children in, 93: 74
induced cochlear damage, cochlear
polyamines marking, 95: 62
in newborn, diagnosis, 93: 71
perforation in (*see* Perforation in otitis
media with effusion)
prevention, continuous vs. intermittent
amoxicillin in, 93: 78
prone children, treatment failure with
tympanotomy tube and *Hemophilus
influenzae*, 93: 81
Pseudomonas species causing, 93: 65
secretory
adenotonsillectomy in, 95: 104
hearing loss and, high-frequency,
93: 42
serous and purulent, round window
membrane structure in (in rat),
94: 64
suppurative, extracranial and intracranial
complications of, 95: 51
temporal bone fracture and, 93: 83
Otoacoustic
emissions in hearing-impaired children,
93: 14
Otogenic
brain abscess, 93: 114
Otolaryngologic
manifestation
of child abuse, 94: 288
of mucopolysaccharidoses, 93: 305
unusual, of lightning strike, 95: 45

surgery
eye protection in, 95: 272
robotics in, image-directed, 95: 158
Otolaryngologist
survey of ototoxicity of ototopical drugs,
94: 109
Otolaryngology
comprehensive, 95: 257
general, 94: 275
journals, biostatistics in, 93: 123
Otologic
manifestations of Wegener's
granulomatosis, 95: 42
surgery, cranial nerve monitoring during,
95: 91
Otology
general, 93: 283
Otomastoiditis
tuberculous, 93: 96
Otopathology, 94: 3
with cochlear implant, multichannel,
95: 28
studies of temporal bone, 93: 53
Otorhinolaryngologic
conditions, teleconsultation in, 95: 266
Otorhinorrhea
cerebrospinal fluid, technique to avoid,
with translabyrinthine removal of
acoustic neuroma, 95: 88
Otorrhea
after tympanostomy, topical
prophylaxis, 93: 80
after ventilation tube, 93: 79
chronic, prevention with mastoid cavity
graft with epithelium from
epidermal cells, 95: 119
postoperative, antibiotic/steroid ear
drops to reduce, 94: 111
ventilation tubes and swimming,
94: 113
Otosclerosis, 93: 49, 94: 69, 95: 65
extensive, and endolymphatic hydrops,
temporal bone histopathology,
95: 43
far-advanced, 94: 73, 95: 66
hearing in, effect of drinking water
fluoridation on, in low fluoride
area, 95: 65
obliterative, 93: 53
footplate, 93: 53
regrowth in, 95: 69
stapedectomy for, hearing levels 10
years after, 94: 72
U. of Minnesota temporal bone
collection, 93: 52
Otoscopy
in children, clinical and histologic
correlation, 93: 71

of ear abnormalities in newborn,
94: 101
Otosurgery
endoscopy guiding, to prevent residual
cholesteatoma, 94: 134
Otosyphilis
diagnostic and therapeutic update,
95: 32
Ototopical drugs
ototoxicity of, otolaryngologists survey,
94: 109
Ototoxicity
kanamycin, hair cell regeneration after,
93: 15
of ototopical drugs, otolaryngologists
survey, 94: 109
"Outcome studies," 93: 4
Oxazepam
in tinnitus, 93: 30
Oximetry
pulse, monitoring nasal packing,
93: 314
Oxygen
hyperbaric
improving wound healing in ischemic
skin tissue, 95: 147
therapy, and squamous cell carcinoma
cell line growth, 94: 143
Oxymetazoline
with cocaine vs. lidocaine for nasal
procedures, 95: 165
Ozone
induced DNA synthesis, in nasal
epithelium, endotoxin or cytokines
attenuating (in rat), 93: 156

P

Packing (*see* Nasal packing)
Pain
in head and neck cancer, types and
causes, 93: 269
of tonsillectomy and adenoidectomy,
reduction by bupivacaine in
children, 94: 282
Palate
adhesion, unilateral, for paralysis after
high vagal injury, 95: 133
cleft (*see under* Cleft)
impalement injuries in children, case
review, 94: 189
Palatoplasty
for cleft palate, long-term speech results
with, 94: 179
Palsy
Bell's, 93: 56
infection in, 93: 57

inflammatory paranasal sinus disease
in, MRI of, 94: 80
cerebral, drooling in, treatment, 93: 287
facial
acute idiopathic peripheral,
corticosteroids and findings in,
94: 81
and infection, unfolding story, 93: 56
nerve, after cerebellopontine angle
tumor surgery, hypoglossal-facial
nerve anastomosis for, 94: 83
Panendoscopy
justifications and controversies, 93: 278
Papilloma
inverting
of nose and paranasal sinuses,
treatment options, 93: 150
recurrence after through removal,
93: 150
Papillomatosis
respiratory
epidemiologic origins, 93: 210
risk factors in, 93: 209
Papillomavirus
in laryngeal carcinoma, verrucous,
94: 211
Paralysis
after vagal injury, high, unilateral palatal
adhesion for, 95: 133
facial nerve
after epidural blood patch, 94: 80
idiopathic, prednisone for, 95: 84
in otitis media, chronic, 93: 57
surgery of, 93: 58
laryngeal
bilateral, airway management with
endoscopic laser medial
arytenoidectomy for, 94: 214
glottis configuration in, 95: 220
stroboscopy, 93: 223
vocal cord
laryngoscopy of, fiberoptic, 93: 223
videostroboscopy of, 93: 221
Paranasal sinus (*see* Sinus, paranasal)
Parathyroid
autotransplantation, 93: 270
enlargement localization with fine
needle aspiration for parathyroid
hormone assay, 93: 232
hormone "quick" test, 93: 239
hyperfunction, operative monitoring,
93: 238
Parotid
adenoma, recurrent pleomorphic, facial
nerve intraoperative monitoring in,
95: 247
duct
ligation in drooling, 93: 287

microsurgical repair, 94: 176
lesions, cystic vs. solid in HIV, 93: 284
surgery for benign disease, facial nerve
    morbidity after, 94: 294
tumors
    adenoid cystic, 93: 240
    advanced, subtotal petrosectomy in,
        94: 254
    malignant, MRI and histology of,
        94: 254
Parotidectomy
face lift incision for, modified, 95: 208
outpatient, 93: 283
Pars tensa
micropathologic changes in otitis media
    with effusion in children, 95: 112
Pectoralis
major flap for intraoral and pharyngeal
    reconstruction, 93: 176
Pediatric (*see* Children)
Penicillin
in streptococcal throat infections, group
    A beta-hemolytic, 94: 302
V, for streptococcal pharyngitis during
    childhood and adolescence,
    94: 282
Percussion
instruments and temporary threshold
    shift, 93: 19
Perforation in otitis media with effusion
anterior perforation, myringoplasty for,
    Kerr flap in, 93: 84
residual, Gelfilm myringoplasty in,
    93: 83
Perichondrium
autogenous, in growing cricoid
    reconstruction (in rabbit), 94: 147
free and vascularized, in airway,
    chondrogenic potential of, 95: 157
in tympanomastoid reconstruction,
    93: 93
Perilymph
fistula (*see* Fistula, perilymph)
fluorescein in, IV, at stapes surgery,
    negative observation, 94: 69
hydrops, perilymph fistula and, 93: 38
hypertension, 93: 35
hypertonia, and low-frequency hearing
    loss after spinal anesthesia, 93: 21
Periosteal
discontinuous periosteal involvement
    causing oral cancer recurrence,
    93: 228
Peripheral nerve
repair, silicone cuffs for (in rat), 94: 77
Peritonsillar
abscess, needle aspiration of, in
    children, 94: 275

Peritubal
adenoidectomy, 95: 261
Petrosectomy
subtotal, in advanced parotid tumors,
    94: 254
Petrous
apex cholesteatoma, diagnostic and
    treatment dilemmas, 94: 133
bone, fracture, in children,
    management, 95: 50
pH
monitoring
    nasopharyngeal, in rhinopharyngitis in
        children, 93: 286
    pharyngeal, in gastropharyngeal reflux
        in children, 94: 284
Pharmacologic
agents, effect on human keloid implant
    (in athymic mice), 93: 121
treatment of tinnitus, review, 93: 30
Pharmacotherapy
topical, in allergic rhinitis, 93: 146
Pharyngitis
with herpes simplex in college students,
    94: 295
streptococcal, cefixime and penicillin V
    for, during childhood and
    adolescence, 94: 282
Pharyngolaryngeal
carcinoma with palpable nodes, 93: 239
Pharyngoplasty
transpalatal advancement, in obstructive
    sleep apnea, 94: 292
Pharyngoscopy
nasopharyngoscopy in obstructive sleep
    apnea, 93: 198
Pharynx
cancer
    second cancer after, tobacco and
        alcohol in, 95: 281
    vitamin supplement to reduce risk of,
        93: 302
contraction pressures after
    laryngectomy, cricopharyngeus
    myotomy in, 94: 252
flap, effect on upper airway in children
    with velopharyngeal inadequacy,
    95: 184
isolated of nontypeable *Hemophilus
    influenzae, capsule gene sequences
    in,* 95: 150
narrowing predicting outcome of
    obstructive sleep apnea surgery,
    94: 283
nasopharyngeal (*see* Nasopharyngeal)
pH monitoring in gastropharyngeal
    reflux in children, 94: 284

reconstruction, pectoralis major flap for,
93: 176
Phenotype
neoplastic-like, induction of, and
cholesteatoma fibroblast alteration,
94: 132
Phenytoin
in trigeminal neuralgia, 93: 303
Phonation
posterior cricoarytenoid muscle function
in, posterior, laryngeal model in,
95: 218
Phonosurgical
procedures, Silastic medialization and
arytenoid adduction in, 94: 231
Phrenic
nerve reinnervation of larynx, new
technique (in cat), 95: 143
Physical abuse
of children, otolaryngology perspective,
93: 291
Pimozide
in trigeminal neuralgia, 93: 303
Plasma
expander in sudden hearing loss, 93: 23
Plastic surgery
facial, 93: 185, 95: 199
biologic grafts and alloplastic implants
in, 94: 208
coronal approach, anatomic and
technical considerations and
morbidity, 94: 193
speech pathology interaction in
velopharyngeal insufficiency,
95: 191
Plate
AO, with myocutaneous flap, instead of
revascularized tissue transfer, for
mandibular reconstruction, 95: 185
fate of, after facial fracture
reconstruction, 94: 170
microplate repair of facial fracture,
93: 171
neutral reconstruction, in mandibular
fracture at angular region, 94: 182
to stabilize maxillary continuity defects,
motion across, 95: 154
titanium mesh, with iliac graft for
bone-graft reconstruction of orbital
floor (in monkey), 94: 149
Plating
systems for mandibular fractures,
94: 186
vs. traditional techniques in mandibular
fracture, 93: 170
Platysma
myocutaneous flap, indications and
caveats, 95: 189

Polyamines
cochlear, marking otitis media induced
cochlear damage, 95: 62
Polyglactin-910
mesh implant for orbital floor fracture
repair, causing diplopia, 95: 183
Polymers
molecular biology and, 93: 128
synthetic, seeded with chondrocytes
provide template for new cartilage
formation, 93: 127
Polysomnography
findings in obstructive sleep apnea in
children, 93: 304
Polysomnographyy
one negative, not excluding obstructive
sleep apnea, 94: 296
Polytetrafluoroethylene
graft, for permanent lip augmentation,
94: 204
Posture
upper airway dimensions and sleep
apnea/hypopnea syndrome,
93: 197
Potter's syndrome
temporal bone histopathology in,
94: 57
Pott's puffy tumor
with mastoiditis, 93: 99
Precancer
laryngeal, vs. oral leukoplakia, 93: 201
Preconditioning
acute ischemic, in latissimus dorsi model
for skeletal muscle survival
augmentation (in pig), 94: 144
Prednisone
for facial nerve paralysis, idiopathic,
95: 84
Prematurity
history of, in adenotonsillectomy for
upper airway obstruction, 93: 299
Presbycusis
cochlear pathology in, 94: 35
Procaine
for sudden hearing loss, 93: 23
Programmable hearing aid
cost, 93: 28
as new technology, 93: 28
Prostaglandin
E$_2$ in middle ear effusion, 93: 77
Prosthesis
hydroxylapatite, 93: 87
for incus long process defects,
94: 117
in ossiculoplasty, 93: 90
ossicular replacement, 93: 91
total and partial, for children, 95: 123

positioning guidance with intraoperative auditory brain stem responses, 93: 90

Protein
bovine morphogenetic, for implant of skull trephine defects (in dog), 93: 126

Pseudoephedrine
in hypertension, cardiovascular effects, 93: 312

Pseudomonas
infection, middle ear susceptibility to, during acute otitis media, 94: 106
species causing otitis media, 93: 65

Psychological
limits in excision of basal cell carcinoma of medial canthus, 94: 195

Pulmonary
bronchopulmonary suction, 93: 195
hyperplasia in Potter's syndrome in infant, 94: 58

Pulse oximetry
monitoring nasal packing, 93: 314

Q

Quality of life
after laryngectomy, dimensions identified by patients and health care professionals, 94: 265
in chronic otitis media with effusion, 93: 70
in head and neck cancer, 95: 240
after surgery, 93: 246

R

Radial
forearm flap, sensate, bilobed design, to preserve tongue mobility after significant glossectomy, 95: 181

Radiation
exposure and CT development, 93: 142
as risk for carotid atherosclerosis, 93: 231

Radiography
of adenoids, assessment methods, 93: 300
autoradiographic localization of histamine H_1 receptors in nasal turbinates, 93: 151
of endolymphatic sac tumors, 94: 19
in fishbone ingestion, possible, 95: 268
of ostiomeatal unit development in children, 94: 156

Radiology

interventional, of extracranial head and neck, 93: 244

Radiotherapy
CT-based 3-dimensional, in paranasal sinus cancer, 95: 241
failure, in laryngopharyngeal cancer, advanced, surgery after, 95: 252
of glomus jugulare tumor, benign, lethal fibrosarcoma complicating, 94: 89
of glottic cancer, partial laryngectomy after, 93: 196
of glottic carcinoma
T1, 95: 244
T1 and T2, 93: 229
of head and neck, oral sequelae of, protocol for prevention and treatment, 94: 250
of head and neck cancer
bone-anchored reconstruction after, 94: 186
smoking in efficacy of, 94: 263
thyroid dysfunction after, 94: 262
of head and neck carcinoma, 95: 242
postoperative, 93: 267
hypothyroidism after, 94: 262
jaw osteonecrosis after, bone and gallium scans in, 93: 172
in laryngeal carcinoma, verrucous, 94: 211
in nasopharyngeal carcinoma, results, 93: 273
superfractionated, in head and neck carcinoma, 93: 237

Radiotherapy
chemoradiation of head and neck cancer, 93: 265

Radius
vascularized, free, in mandibular reconstruction with osseointegrated implant, 95: 192

Ragweed
induced nasal provocation, topical steroids in, 93: 143

Ramsay Hunt syndrome, 93: 56

Reconstruction, 93: 159, 94: 169, 95: 181
airway, upper, in obstructive sleep apnea syndrome, 95: 258
bone-anchored, of irradiated head and neck cancer, 94: 186
bone-graft, of orbital floor with iliac graft and titanium mesh plate (in monkey), 94: 149
calvarial defects, hydroxyapatite cement for, 93: 135
computer, in facial canal dehiscence, 94: 75

of cricoid, growing, with bovine bone
  graft and perichondrium (in rabbit),
  94: 147
esophagus, cervical total, 94: 237
face, biologic grafts and alloplastic
  implants in, 94: 208
facial fracture, fate of plates and screws
  after, 94: 170
facial nerve, results, 95: 87
head and neck
  arm free flap in, lateral, 94: 176
  infrahyoid musculocutaneous flap in,
    93: 159
  temporoparietal fascial flap in,
    94: 187
hypopharynx, total, 94: 237
intraoral, pectoralis major flap for,
    93: 176
laryngotracheal
  auricular cartilage grafts in, 94: 222
  cricoid cartilage division in,
    four-quadrant, 94: 217
  perioperative management, 93: 200
larynx, vascularized fascia as transferable
  bed for (in rabbit), 95: 160
mandible (*see* Mandible, reconstruction)
of mastoidectomy, radical, by
  obliteration technique, 93: 111
maxillofacial, temporalis myofascial flap
  for, 93: 161
middle ear, alloplastic, problems with,
    93: 87
nasal
  forehead flaps in, anatomic basis for
    design, 93: 167
  platyrrhine nose, 93: 188
  refinements, 93: 173
  with split calvarial grafts, 94: 190
oromandibular, vascularized bone flaps
  in, 95: 132
pharyngeal, pectoralis major flap for,
    93: 176
rib cartilage graft in children, 93: 201
trachea
  epithelial equivalent for, 95: 141
  and respiratory epithelium free
    grafting, 93: 133
of tympanic membrane by "crown-cork"
  technique, 93: 92
tympanomastoid, tragal and conchal
  palisade cartilage and
  perichondrium, 93: 93
Recontouring
  cervical, submentoplasty to enhance, in
    face lift, 94: 203
Red blood cell

scintigraphy to distinguish soft tissue
  hemangioma from vascular
  malformations, 93: 186
Reflex
  round window, absent, possible relation
    to step-wise hearing loss, 95: 58
Reflux
  gastro-esophagonasopharyngeal acid,
    93: 286
  gastroesophageal (*see* Gastroesophageal
    reflux)
  gastropharyngeal, pharyngeal pH
    monitoring in, in children, 94: 284
Regrowth
  in otosclerosis, 95: 69
Rehabilitation
  balance therapy, 94: 20
  vestibule, 94: 20
    dizziness and imbalance after, 93: 9
    peripheral vestibular disorders and,
      93: 9
Reinnervation
  phrenic nerve, of larynx, new technique
    (in cat), 95: 143
  tongue, by hypoglossal lingual nerve
    transfer, 95: 151
Research
  head and neck surgery, advances in,
    93: 121, 95: 131
  in tinnitus, animal model for, 93: 29
Respiration
  laryngeal muscles during, intrinsic, single
    motor unit activity of, 94: 142
Respiratory
  allergy, upper, in chronic or recurrent
    sinusitis, 93: 146
  compromise after adenotonsillectomy in
    children with obstructive sleep
    apnea, 93: 313
  cycle, modulating laryngeal
    motoneurons, 94: 142
  epithelia grafting, cell differentiation
    after, 93: 132
  infection, viral upper, before vestibular
    neuronitis, 94: 8
  papillomatosis
    epidemiologic origins, 93: 210
    recurrent, risk factors in, 93: 209
  tract
    lower, symptoms and illness of, and
      nasal disorders in children, 94: 159
    upper, acute infection, nasal airway
      resistance and middle ear pressure
      in, 94: 153
Retraction
  pockets, surgery of, 93: 91
Revascularization

in endurance of craniofacial onlay bone grafts (in rabbit), 95: 157
jejunal autograft for tracheal replacement (in dog), 94: 143
synchronous, for composite thyrotracheal transplant (in dog), 94: 145
tissue transfer, for mandibular reconstruction, AO plate with myocutaneous flap instead of, 95: 185
Rhabdomyosarcoma
of head and neck
in children, 93: 250
surgery in, 93: 231
Rheumatic fever
prevention in Costa Rica, 94: 286
Rhinitis
allergic
ascorbic acid in, 93: 147
astemizole in antigen-mediated histamine release from blood in, 94: 156
corticosteroids in, intranasal, in mild asthma, 94: 155
HEPP in, 93: 147
hyposmia in, 94: 164
immunotherapy for, subcutaneous, oral and nasal, humoral response to, due to *Dermatophagoides pteronyssinus*, 95: 167
topical pharmacotherapy, 93: 146
nose response to exercise in, 95: 163
Rhinology, 93: 141, 94: 153, 95: 163
Rhinopathy
immune regulation in, 93: 142
immunoglobulin concentration in nasal secretions differing in IgE-mediated and non-IgE-mediated, 93: 142
Rhinopharyngitis
chronic, in children, nasopharyngeal pH monitoring in, 93: 286
Rhinoplasty
external approach in children, 93: 187
making nose more susceptible to fracture, 95: 205
open
secondary, temporal fascia grafts in, 95: 204
vertical dome division in, indications, techniques and results, 95: 200
revision
with esthetic deformity analysis, 93: 191
of skin excision, 94: 206
Rhinosinusitis

chronic, endoscopic sinus surgery in, 93: 143
Rhinovirus
39 infection in nasal response to histamine and cold air challenges in allergy, 95: 178
Rhytidectomy
nasolabial fold and, 94: 200
wound tension in, skin flap undermining and musculoaponeurotic system suspension in, 94: 202
Rib
cartilage graft in laryngotracheal reconstruction, 93: 201
Robotics
image-directed, in otolaryngologic surgery, 95: 158
Rock musicians
auditory temporary threshold shift after heavy metal concert, 94: 37
Round window
membrane
bacteria and, 93: 33
fistula, and auditory threshold (in guinea pig), 93: 40
under pathologic and normal conditions, 93: 34
semipermeable, 93: 34
in serous and purulent otitis media, structure of (in rat), 94: 64
perilymph fistula (in guinea pig), 93: 38
reflex, absent, possible relation to step-wise hearing loss, 95: 58

S

Saccule
cyst in children, 93: 208
footplate surgery and, 93: 51
stapedotomy and, 93: 50
Sail
flap, for coverage of opposite forehead defect, 95: 188
Saline
sterile, vs. tap water for cleaning acute traumatic soft tissue wounds, 94: 181
Salivary
cancer, elective treatment of neck in, 93: 248
gland lesions, fine needle aspiration cytology of, 95: 254
lymphoepithelial lesions and AIDS, 93: 233
lymphoproliferative disease, 93: 234
Sarcoma
Kaposi's, in AIDS, 94: 235

Scala vestibuli
  of cochlea, air intrusion to, causing
      inner ear injury, 95: 59
Scanning (*see* Imaging)
Scarring
  control in adults' wounds by neutralizing
      antibody to transforming growth
      factor β, 93: 130
Scatchard analysis
  of histamine H_1 receptors in nasal
      mucosa, 93: 151
Scintigraphy
  to distinguish soft tissue hemangioma
      from vascular malformations,
      93: 186
  iodine-123, in thyroid disorder
      evaluation in children, 93: 311
  thallium-201, for thyroid cancer
      postoperative follow-up, 93: 242
Sclerosis
  multiple, sudden hearing loss as
      monosymptom of, 95: 31
Scopolamine
  transdermal
      effect on vestibular system, 94: 13
      to reduce postoperative nausea in ear
          surgery, 95: 11
Screw
  fate of, after facial fracture
      reconstruction, 94: 170
  to stabilize maxillary continuity defects,
      motion across, 95: 154
Scuba divers
  inner ear barotrauma, long-term
      follow-up with continued diving,
      94: 55
SCUD missile explosion
  tympanic membrane perforation in
      survivors of, 95: 113
Semicircular canal
  lateral, streptomycin applied to, acute
      and chronic effects, 94: 15
Sensorineural
  damage, tympanogenic labyrinthitis and
      meningitis, 93: 33
  deafness, tinnitus suppression by
      electrical promontory stimulation
      in, 94: 40
  hearing loss (*see* Hearing loss,
      sensorineural)
Sentence
  scores, postoperative, in postlinguistic
      deafness with cochlear implant,
      93: 27
Septal
  perforation, management, 94: 161
Serax
  in tinnitus, 93: 31

Shah Perma-Vent, 94: 114
Short nose
  lengthening, 94: 204
Silastic
  medialization and arytenoid adduction,
      94: 231
  sheet, Swiss roll, in laryngotracheal
      stenosis in children, 93: 213
  tubes, nerve growth factor containing, in
      facial nerve regeneration (in rabbit),
      94: 77
Silicone
  cuffs for peripheral nerve repair (in rat),
      94: 77
  facial implant, safety of, 95: 214
Sinonasal
  cancer, occupational risk factors for,
      93: 148
Sinus
  cancer, and formaldehyde occupational
      exposure, 94: 158
  CT of, screening, technique
      optimization, 93: 141
  disease, interface of allergy in sinus
      disease, 93: 145
  endonasal sinus surgery in children,
      93: 149
  paranasal, 93: 141, 94: 153, 95: 163
      cancer, and occupational exposures,
          94: 157
      cancer, CT-based 3-dimensional
          radiotherapy of, 95: 241
      cancer, in metal industry, 93: 147
      inflammatory disease in Bell's palsy,
          MRI of, 94: 80
      papilloma of, inverting, treatment
          options, 93: 150
  surgery, complications of, major,
      95: 170
  surgery, endoscopic
      in chronic rhinosinusitis, 93: 143
      functional, local vs. general anesthesia
          for, 94: 165
      functional, orbital complications in,
          95: 176
      and intranasal, anatomic
          considerations in complications of,
          95: 169
      lacrimal draining system injury in,
          94: 167
      revision functional, review of, 95: 164
  x-ray films, use by general practitioners,
      95: 173
Sinusitis
  antibiotics for, oral, intranasal
      flunisolide spray as adjunct to,
      95: 172

chronic, nasal mucociliary transport of,
    in children, 94: 162
chronic and recurrent
  in children, endonasal sinus surgery
      for, 93: 150
  upper respiratory allergy in, 93: 146
diagnosis by history and physical
    examination, 94: 160
maxillary, chronic, antrum bacteriology
    in, 95: 179
in midfacial fracture repair, 94: 169
mucosal changes in, early (in rabbit),
    94: 151
ostiotomy for, natural, vs. inferior
    antrostomy (in rabbit model),
    95: 136
rhinosinusitis, chronic, endoscopic sinus
    surgery in, 93: 143
Sistruck procedure, 93: 297
Skeletal
  muscle survival augmentation in
      latissimus dorsi model with acute
      ischemic preconditioning (in pig),
      94: 144
Skin
  cancer
    non-melanoma, after kidney
        transplant, 95: 287
    skin carcinoma risk after, 94: 253
  carcinoma, risk after skin cancer,
      94: 253
  excision revision rhinoplasty, 94: 206
  expanded, long-term histopathologic
      evaluation, 94: 182
  flap undermining in wound tension in
      rhytidectomy, 94: 202
  in intraoral free muscle flap, 94: 173
  ischemic tissue, hyperbaric oxygen
      improving wound healing in,
      95: 147
  melanoma, malignant, neck dissection
      for, 93: 252
  new skin equivalent, keratinocytes
      proliferated and differentiated on
      collagen sponge containing
      fibroblasts, 95: 152
  substitute, living, production and
      transplantation in model (in rat),
      93: 135
  wound explants in tissue culture,
      93: 137
Skull
  base
    fracture association with facial
        fracture, 94: 185
    surgery, anterior, 93: 277
    tumors, extended frontal approach,
        93: 243

trephine defects, immune inhibition of
    repair (in dog), 93: 126
Sleep
  apnea
    antihypertensives and, 93: 198
    cilazapril in, 93: 199
    hypopnea syndrome, inheritance of,
        95: 262
    hypopnea syndrome, posture and
        upper airway dimensions in,
        93: 197
    metoprolol in, 93: 199
    obstructive, adenotonsillectomy in,
        respiratory compromise after, in
        children, 93: 313
    obstructive, airway collapse site in,
        airway pressure monitoring in,
        95: 217
    obstructive, CPAP vs. surgery in,
        93: 199
    obstructive, nasopharyngoscopy in,
        93: 198
    obstructive, one negative
        polysomnogram not excluding,
        94: 296
    obstructive, pharyngeal narrowing
        predicting outcome of surgery for,
        94: 283
    obstructive, pharyngoplasty for,
        transpalatal advancement, 94: 292
    obstructive, polysomnographic and
        clinical findings in children,
        93: 304
    obstructive, snoring in, heart rate
        variability during sleep in, 94: 285
    obstructive, syndrome, CPAP
        reducing, gastroesophageal reflux
        in, 93: 294
    obstructive, syndrome, in children
        with habitual snoring, early tonsil
        surgery in, 94: 299
    obstructive, syndrome, surgical
        protocol for upper airway
        reconstruction in, 95: 258
  disordered breathing, gender differences
      in, 95: 276
  pattern and antihypertensives, 93: 198
Smoking
  cessation
    nicotine replacement therapy
        effectiveness in, 95: 278
    predictors of, Framingham Study,
        93: 298
  in radiotherapy efficacy in head and
      neck cancer, 94: 263
  in second cancers after oral and
      pharyngeal cancers, 95: 281
Snoring

cardiovascular risk factors in, 94: 292
habitual, in obstructive sleep apnea
    syndrome in children, early tonsil
    surgery in, 94: 299
in obstructive sleep apnea, heart rate
    variability during sleep in, 94: 285
Sodium
  amylobarbitone in tinnitus, 93: 30
  nitroprusside, topical application,
    cochlear electrophysiology after,
    94: 67
Soft tissue
  hemangioma, distinguishing from
    vascular malformation, 93: 186
  wound healing, angiogenic growth
    factors in, 93: 131
  wounds, acute traumatic, sterile saline
    vs. tap water for cleaning, 94: 181
Somatic
  gene therapy, ex vivo, in thyroid
    follicular cell transplant (in dog),
    94: 146
Sound field
  vs. earphone methods for estimating
    noise attenuation of foam earplugs,
    94: 36
Spasm
  esophageal, and foreign bodies, 93: 288
  hemifacial, microvascular
    decompression in, 93: 56
Spasmodic dysphonia (*see* Dysphonia,
  spasmodic)
Speech
  long-term results of cleft palate with
    palatoplasty, 94: 179
  outcome in cleft palate repair, 93: 171
  pathology plastic surgery interaction in
    velopharyngeal insufficiency,
    95: 191
  tonsils' functional role in, 95: 265
  tracheoesophageal, intelligibility among
    naive listeners, 95: 225
Spine
  anesthesia
    auditory function after, 94: 25
    low-frequency hearing loss after, as
      perilymphatic hypotonia, 93: 21
Splint
  wire, vestibular and lingual, in
    mandibular fracture, 93: 164
Spring
  implant, and MRI, 94: 82
Stapedectomy
  air-borne gap improved by, 93: 49
  facial nerve avulsion at, 93: 51
  fallopian canal and, 93: 51

footplate, total, bone conduction
    threshold change by, and age,
    94: 72
for otosclerosis, hearing levels 10 years
    after, 94: 72
results, influence of age on, 93: 49
revision, KTP laser in, 95: 68
Stapedial
  persistent stapedial artery in middle ear,
    95: 79
Stapedotomy
  fenestra microdrill, small, footplate
    complication reduction in, 94: 71
  hearing long-term results after, 95: 67
  utricle, saccule and cochlear duct in
    relation to, 93: 50
Stapes
  malformation of superstructure, in
    congenital perilymphatic fistula,
    94: 63
  mobilization, 93: 3
  surgery, 93: 49, 94: 69
    fenestra, large and small, for
      otosclerosis, hearing recovery after,
      94: 70
    fluorescein, IV, in perilymph at,
      negative observation, 94: 69
Staphylococcus aureus
  infections, methicillin-resistant
    community-acquired, 94: 302
Stenosis
  laryngotracheal
    classification, 94: 229
    stenting in children, 93: 213
  subglottic
    cannulation in, long-term, 94: 212
    in children, auricular cartilage graft
      for laryngotracheal reconstruction
      in, 94: 223
    congenital, early expansion surgery in,
      94: 212
    implant/replacement tissue
      composite in, 94: 148
    inducing anesthesia and gaining
      airway in, 93: 201
    isolated, autoantibodies against
      neutrophil constituents in diagnosis
      of, 94: 219
    tracheotomy in, 94: 212
    Wegener's granulomatosis and,
      94: 220
Stent
  Aboulker, for laryngotracheal stenosis in
    children, 93: 213
Stenting
  for laryngotracheal stenosis in children,
    93: 213
Stereolithography

CT guided, new in craniofacial surgery,
95: 148
Steroids
with antibiotics for ear drops to reduce
postoperative otorrhea and
ventilation tube blockage, 94: 111
in herpes zoster oticus, 93: 55
in inner ear disorders, 93: 21
in stomatitis, aphthous, 93: 312
topical, in ragweed and
histamine-induced nasal
provocation, 93: 143
Stomatitis, aphthous
features of, and steroids in, 93: 312
triamcinolone in, 93: 312
Streptococcal
pharyngitis, cefixime and penicillin V
for, during childhood and
adolescence, 94: 282
throat infections, group A
beta-hemolytic, cephalexin and
penicillin in, 94: 302
Streptomycin
applied to lateral semicircular canal,
acute and chronic effects of, 94: 15
Stridor
in children, CT and MRI in, 93: 209
postoperative
lidocaine before intubation, 93: 197
prevention with topical lidocaine,
93: 196
with thyroid mass, 94: 225
Stroboscopy
of laryngeal paralysis, 93: 223
Subglottic stenosis (see Stenosis,
subglottic)
Submandibular
duct diversion in drooling, 93: 287
Submentoplasty
to enhance cervical recontouring in face
lift surgery, 94: 203
Subperiosteal
tissue expansion, model (in dog),
95: 140
Suction
bronchopulmonary, 93: 195
continuous vs. intermittent, effect on
tracheal tissue, 93: 195
damaging tracheal epithelium, 93: 195
Sulfuric acid
occupational exposure to, and laryngeal
cancer, 94: 216
Super-base
bone anchored hearing aid, 93: 25
Surface contour
three-dimensional imaging in congenital
aural atresia, 94: 100
Surgeon

head and neck, professional burnout in,
survey results, 95: 231
Surgery, plastic (see Plastic surgery)
Surgical
glove perforations, prevention with
cut-resistant gloves, 94: 290
positive surgical outcome, global
monitoring of, 95: 279
Swallowing
oral and laryngeal muscle coordination
during, 95: 155
oral cavity movements and laryngeal
movements coordinated during,
95: 146
Swimming
grommets and, survey, 95: 107
otorrhea and ventilation tubes, 94: 113
Sympathomimetics
hypertension and, 93: 313

T

T tubes
insertion retrospective review, 94: 114
tympanic membrane perforation after,
94: 115
Taste
effect of unilateral chorda tympani
damage on, 95: 90
Team
assessment and management of
drooling, 93: 294
Technetium
erythrocyte scintigraphy to distinguish
soft tissue hemangioma from
vascular malformations, 93: 186
Technology
modern, vs. biopsy, 95: 3
Teeth
interdental immobilization, new device
for, 93: 177
Teflon
granuloma and overinjection, as
therapeutic challenge, 95: 221
for vocal cord augmentation, 93: 212
Teleconsultation
in otorhinolaryngologic conditions,
95: 266
Telendoscopic
study, 95: 266
Television
high-definition, for ear microsurgery,
93: 60
high-resolution, 93: 62
Temporal aspect
control in risk factors for acute otitis
media in children, 94: 103

Temporal bone
    carcinoma, squamous cell, surgery
        efficacy, 95: 41
    in carotid canal dehiscence, prevalence
        in middle ear, 95: 98
    endolymphatic hydrops in, 94: 13
    in facial canal dehiscence prevalence,
        95: 79
    fracture (*see* Fracture, temporal bone)
    histopathology
        14 years after cytomegalic inclusion
            disease, 94: 25
        in chronic ear infections with
            tympanic membrane perforation,
            94: 125
        in endolymphatic hydrops and
            extensive otosclerosis, 95: 43
        in Potter's syndrome, 94: 57
    implant, percutaneous, results, 95: 125
    in Ménière's disease, suspected, 94: 18
    meningioma affecting, surgical removal,
        hearing preservation after, 94: 86
    MRI of, high-resolution, 93: 47
    otopathologic studies, 93: 53
    pathology resource registry, 94: 23
    in persistent stapedial artery, 95: 79
    study in stapedectomy, 93: 50
    U. of Minnesota collection, and
        otosclerosis, 93: 52
Temporal meningioma
    presenting as chronic otitis media,
        94: 85
Temporal muscle
    transfer of Gillies for lagophthalmos,
        93: 163
    transposition in lagophthalmos, 93: 164
Temporalis
    fascia grafts, in open secondary
        rhinoplasty, 95: 204
    myofascial flap
        discussion of, 93: 161
        for maxillofacial reconstruction,
            93: 161
Temporomandibular
    disorder
        tinnitus in, 93: 8
        vertigo in, 93: 8
    joint
        noises, in aged, 94: 290
        in resection of regional tumors,
            95: 248
Temporoparietal
    fascial flap in head and neck
        reconstruction, 94: 187
Tenotomy
    laryngeal muscular, for bilateral midline
        vocal cord fixation, 95: 223
Terfenadine

interactions with, possible, 95: 169
    in unilateral nasal challenge with
        allergen, 95: 171
Textile
    workers, dust level reduction for,
        93: 148
Thallium-201
    scintigraphy for thyroid cancer
        postoperative follow-up, 93: 242
Thermal
    continuous change in air caloric test,
        95: 6
Thigh
    paddle flap in mandibular
        reconstruction, 93: 163
Threshold shift
    temporary, and percussion instruments,
        93: 19
Throat
    streptococcal infections, group A
        beta-hemolytic, cephalexin and
        penicillin in, 94: 302
Thymus
    enlarged, x-ray treatment in infancy for,
        thyroid cancer after, 95: 288
Thyroglobulin
    for diagnosis and assessment of
        metastatic differentiated thyroid
        carcinoma, 95: 234
    measurement for thyroid cancer
        postoperative follow-up, 93: 242
Thyroglossal
    duct cyst operation, core-out toward the
        foramen cecum in, 93: 296
Thyroid
    artery, anatomical variations, 93: 218
    cancer
        after radiotherapy in infancy for
            thymus enlargement, 95: 288
        medullary, in multiple endocrine
            neoplasia IIb, 93: 260
        papillary, determinants of, 95: 277
        postoperative follow-up, with
            scintigraphy and thyroglobulin
            measurement, 93: 242
        resection of airway in, 93: 256
        in young patient, 93: 265
    carcinoma
        airway invaded by resection, 93: 255
        differentiated, completion
            thyroidectomy for, necessity and
            safety of, 94: 249
        differentiated, in children, 93: 263
        differentiated, lobectomy vs. total
            thyroidectomy in, 95: 253
        follicular, diagnosis, treatment and
            outcome, 95: 233

metastatic differentiated,
thyroglobulin and iodine-131
imaging in diagnosis and treatment
assessment, 95: 234
nonmedullary, association with
hyperparathyroidism, 94: 271
papillary, locally invasive, 1940-1990,
95: 246
papillary, management method and
outcome, 95: 243
thyroidectomy in, total, radioactive
iodine to evaluate, 93: 280
well differentiated, radioactive iodine
in, 93: 275
well differentiated, treatment results,
93: 275
disorders in children, evaluation with
iodine-123 scintigraphy, 93: 311
dysfunction after radiotherapy of head
and neck cancer, 94: 262
follicular cell transplant, and ex vivo
somatic gene therapy (in dog),
94: 146
function tests after
laryngopharyngectomy, 93: 235
Hurthle cell tumors of, 93: 235
during laryngectomy, intraoperative
management, 93: 255
mass, with stridor, 94: 225
nodules
ectopic, management, 95: 238
fine-needle aspiration cytology of,
93: 271
surgery, airway complications in,
94: 224
tumors, follicular, distinguishing benign
from malignant, frozen section and
clinical parameters in, 94: 266
vascular proliferation of, complicating
fine needle aspiration, 94: 248
Thyroidectomy
completion, for differentiated thyroid
carcinoma, necessity and safety of,
94: 249
total
in thyroid carcinoma, radioactive
iodine evaluation, 93: 280
vs. lobectomy for differentiated
thyroid carcinoma, 95: 253
Thyroplasty
Isshiki, type I, vocal quality long-term
changes after, 95: 227
Thyrotracheal
transplant, composite, synchronous
revascularization of (in dog),
94: 145
Tinnitus
antidepressants for, 93: 31

chronic, biofeedback for, 94: 39
clonazepam in, 93: 30
eperisone hydrochloride in, 93: 30
flunarizine in, 93: 30
high blood pressure and, 93: 8
hypnosis for, 95: 37
lidocaine in, 32, 93: 30
lignocaine in, 93: 32
nortriptyline for, 93: 31
oxazepam in, 93: 30
pharmacologic treatment, review,
93: 30
pulsatile, MRI and magnetic resonance
angiography of, 95: 49
research, animal model for, 93: 29
sensorineural hearing loss and, 93: 31
Serax in, 93: 31
severe, vascular decompression surgery
for, selection criteria and results,
94: 41
sodium amylobarbitone in, 93: 30
suppression
by cochlear implant, 95: 63
by electrical promontory stimulation
in sensorineural deafness, 94: 40
in temporomandibular disorder, 93: 8
Valium in, 93: 31
weight loss due to (in rat), 93: 29
xylocaine in, 93: 32
Tip, nose (*see* Nose, tip)
Tissue
engineering with scaffolds containing
extracellular matrix, 93: 132
expanders, rectangular, maximizing gain
from, 93: 179
expansion, subperiosteal, model of (in
dog), 95: 140
soft (*see* Soft tissue)
transfer, revascularized, for mandibular
reconstruction, AO plate with
myocutaneous flap instead of,
95: 185
transformation in vivo, potential
practical application, 93: 126
Titanium
implant in orbital floor fracture, 93: 166
mesh plate with iliac graft for bone-graft
reconstruction of orbital floor (in
monkey), 94: 149
Tobacco
in second cancers after oral and
pharyngeal cancers, 95: 281
Tomography, computed (*see* Computed
tomography)
Tongue
cancer, oral, under 40 years, aggressive
therapy, 95: 251

carcinoma, advanced, total glossectomy
without total laryngectomy in,
94: 269
mobility preservation after significant
glossectomy, bilobed design of
sensate radial forearm flap for,
95: 181
reinnervation by hypoglossal lingual
nerve transfer, 95: 151
Tonsil
bacteriology of, 95: 263
functional role in speech, 95: 265
hypertrophy
in sleep apnea, obstructive, in
children, 93: 305
upper airway obstruction and,
93: 289
immunoglobulin distribution patterns in,
93: 318
obstruction in facial growth and dental
arch morphology, 93: 289
surgery, early, in habitual snoring and
obstructive sleep apnea syndrome
in children, 94: 299
Tonsillectomy
acute, in infectious mononucleosis,
94: 294
adenotonsillectomy (*see*
Adenotonsillectomy)
in children, ambulatory, and high-risk
subgroup identification, 95: 270
facial growth and dental arch
morphology after, 93: 289
laryngospasm after, 93: 197
outpatient
for children, 93: 292
complications and recommendations,
95: 264
pain reduction with bupivacaine in
children, 94: 282
two methods, comparison of, 94: 298
vomiting after, metoclopramide
reducing in children, 93: 316
Tonsillitis
chronic, immunoglobulin E in, in
children, 93: 318
Toxin, botulinum (*see* Botulinum toxin)
Trachea
epithelium damage from suction,
93: 195
extubation, laryngeal edema after,
dexamethasone to prevent, 93: 212
laryngotracheal (*see* Laryngotracheal)
reconstruction
epithelial equivalent for, 95: 141
respiratory epithelium free grafting
and, 93: 133
replacement

allograft for (in dog), 94: 145
with revascularized jejunal autograft
and implantable Dacron mesh tube
(in dog), 94: 143
tissue, effects of continuous vs.
intermittent suction on, 93: 195
transplant with omental flap (in pig),
93: 202
Tracheitis
bacterial, in children, airway endoscopy
in, 95: 229
Tracheobronchial
disruption, mortality in, in children,
93: 203
injuries in children, 93: 203
tree replacement with vascularized,
semisynthetic composite implant (in
dog), 94: 143
Tracheobronchomalacia
in children, and airway collapse, 93: 215
classification system for, 93: 216
in Hunter's syndrome, 94: 225
Tracheoesophageal
speech, intelligibility among naive
listeners, 95: 225
Tracheostomy
Carden anesthetic tube for surgery
around, 95: 224
in children, and home care, 93: 207
in head injury, 95: 228
in infant
communicative development after,
93: 205
medical and social factors predicting
outcome, 93: 204
tubes, airway resistance and work of
breathing in, 95: 221
Tracheotomy
long-term, granuloma excision in, in
children, 94: 228
in subglottic stenosis, 94: 212
Tragal
palisade cartilage in tympanomastoid
reconstruction, 93: 93
Transfusion
in head and neck carcinoma recurrence,
93: 274
Translabyrinthine
approach, modified, for hearing
preservation, 94: 95
Transplantation
airway, upper, 93: 203
kidney, skin cancer after, 95: 287
marrow, nasal mucociliary clearance
impairment during, 95: 174
parathyroid, autotransplantation,
93: 270

of skin substitute, living, in model (in
   rat), 93: 135
thyroid follicular cell, and ex vivo
   somatic gene therapy (in dog),
   94: 146
thyrotracheal, composite, synchronous
   revascularization of (in dog),
   94: 145
trachea, with omental flap (in pig),
   93: 202
Trapezius
flap, superiorly based, for emergency
   carotid artery coverage, 94: 239
Trauma, 93: 159, 94: 169, 95: 181
adult, and otitis media, 93: 82
face, management, extended
   access/internal approaches for,
   94: 177
maxillofacial, blunt, blindness after,
   optic nerve decompression surgery
   in, 95: 190
midfacial, postoperative infection rates
   in, and intermaxillary fixation, wire
   fixation and rigid internal fixation
   implant, 94: 169
Traumatic
soft tissue wounds, acute, sterile saline
   vs. top water for cleaning of,
   94: 181
Treacher Collins syndrome
ear malformation and hearing loss in,
   94: 30
Trephine
defects, skull, immune inhibition of
   repair (in dog), 93: 126
Triamcinolone
in aphthous stomatitis, 93: 312
Trigeminal neuralgia
baclofen in, 93: 303
carbamazepine in, 93: 303
clonazepam in, 93: 303
medical management, 93: 303
phenytoin in, 93: 303
pimozide in, 93: 303
valproic acid in, 93: 303
Trumpets
in symphony orchestra causing
   sensorineural hearing loss, 93: 20
Tube
Dacron mesh, implantable, for tracheal
   replacement, with jejunal autograft
   (in dog), 94: 143
endotracheal, small-bore, for laryngeal
   microsurgery under general
   anesthesia, blood gas analysis in,
   95: 226
Goode's tympanostomy, long-term
   results in children, 94: 113

T tubes (see T tubes)
tracheostomy, airway resistance and
   work of breathing in, 95: 221
tympanostomy (see Tympanostomy
   tube)
ventilation (see Ventilation tubes)
Tuberculosis
cervical, contemporary management,
   93: 292
laryngeal, case review, 94: 212
Tuberculous
otomastoiditis, 93: 96
Tumors
acoustic
   facial nerve neuroma presenting as,
      95: 86
   hearing conservation surgery,
      endoscopy of internal auditory
      canal during, 94: 94
aerodigestive tract, upper, neck staging
   procedure for, 93: 248
cell kinetics, higher proliferative rate,
   discussion of, 93: 125
cerebellopontine angle, surgery of, facial
   nerve palsy after, hypoglossal-facial
   nerve anastomosis for, 94: 83
cranial base, maxillary removal and
   reinsertion in, 93: 169
craniofacial, devascularization by
   puncture, 95: 246
endolymphatic sac, radiographic
   appearance, 94: 19
facial, 93: 55, 94: 75, 95: 73
glomus jugulare, benign, radiotherapy
   for, lethal fibrosarcoma
   complicating, 94: 89
glomus tympanicum, Nd:YAG laser for,
   94: 88
head and neck, in AIDS, 94: 235
Hurthle cell, of thyroid, 93: 235
multiple endocrine neoplasia type IIb,
   natural course of, 93: 260
multiple tumors risk after oral squamous
   cell carcinoma, 95: 275
necrosis factor, and DNA synthesis after
   ozone exposure, 93: 157
parotid (see Parotid tumors)
Pott's puffy, with latent mastoiditis,
   93: 99
regional, resection, temporomandibular
   joint surgical management in,
   95: 248
skull base, extended frontal approach,
   93: 243
thyroid, follicular, distinguishing benign
   from malignant, frozen section and
   clinical parameters in, 94: 266
Tuning fork

tests, validity in hearing loss diagnosis,
    95: 25
Tympanic
  electrocochleography in endolymphatic
      hydrops, 93: 6
  membrane
    conductive hearing loss and, 93: 43
    lightning injury of, 95: 46
    ossification, clinical records, 94: 118
    perforation, after ventilation tube
        removal in children, 94: 115
    perforation, chronic, repair with
        epidermal growth factor, 95: 115
    perforation, ear infection with,
        chronic, temporal bone
        histopathology in, 94: 125
    perforation, in survivors of SCUD
        missile explosion, 95: 113
    perforation, traumatic, healing after
        fibroblast growth factor, 94: 115
    reconstruction with "crown-cork"
        technique, 93: 92
  mesotympanic cholesteatoma, posterior
      management, 93: 102
Tympanogenic
  labyrinthitis, bacterial, meningitis and
      sensorineural hearing loss, 93: 33
Tympanomastoid
  reconstruction, tragal and conchal
      palisade cartilage and
      perichondrium in, 93: 93
Tympanomastoidectomy
  in otitis media, chronic, 93: 109
    suppurative, of irradiated ears in
        nasopharyngeal carcinoma, 95: 120
Tympanoplasty
  first stage technique and incus
      transposition, 93: 86
  in intact canal wall, for cholesteatoma
      recurrence prevention, 95: 121
  with mastoidectomy in chronic otitis
      media in children, 94: 128
  obliteration, in radical mastoidectomy
      reconstruction, 93: 112
  transcanal, in cholesteatoma, 93: 105
  type 1, in children, 95: 116
  type V
    hearing restoration with, 93: 95
    usefulness and risks with, 93: 96
  xenograft vs. autograft for, 95: 117
Tympanosclerosis
  Mini-Shah grommet and, results,
      94: 112
  tympanic membrane ossification
      secondary to, 94: 119
Tympanostomy
  Goode's tubes, long-term results in
      children, 94: 113

otorrhea after, topical prophylaxis,
    93: 80
tube
  insertion, effect of water exposure
      after, 95: 106
  medical appropriateness for children
      under 16, 95: 105
  treatment failure in otitis-prone
      children, and *Hemophilus
      influenzae*, 93: 81

U

Ultrasound
  guided fine needle aspiration in
      parathyroid enlargement
      localization, 93: 232
Ultrastructure
  changes in nasal cilia by common cold,
      94: 154
  of cochlea in AIDS, 95: 35
  of endolymphatic sac, absorption
      activity and barrier properties,
      95: 15
  of hair cell regeneration in inner ear (in
      mammals), 94: 32
Urine
  output during radical neck surgery,
      94: 242
Utricle
  footplate surgery and, 93: 51
  hair cell regeneration in (in animal
      model), 94: 34
  stapedotomy and, 93: 50

V

V-Y flap
  extended, 93: 175
Vaccination
  Hemophilus influenzae type B
      conjugate, in children, epiglottitis
      disappearance during, 95: 280
Vagal
  injury, high, paralysis after, unilateral
      palatal adhesion for, 95: 133
Valium
  in tinnitus, 93: 31
Valproic acid
  in trigeminal neuralgia, 93: 303
Vascularized
  bone flaps in oromandibular
      reconstruction, 95: 132
  fascia, as transferable bed for laryngeal
      reconstruction (in rabbit), 95: 160
  perichondrium in airway, chondrogenic
      potential of, 95: 157

radius, free, in mandibular
  reconstruction with osseointegrated
  implant, 95: 192
Vasoactive
  therapy in sudden hearing loss, 93: 23
Vasoconstriction
  of nasal mucosa, epinephrine for,
    93: 320
Vasoconstrictive
  effects of intranasal cocaine vs.
    xylometazoline/lidocaine solution,
    94: 164
Vasoconstrictors
  potentiating cilia loss during common
    cold, 94: 154
Vasodilating
  agent topical application, effect on
    cochlear electrophysiology, 94: 66
Vasodilator
  in sudden hearing loss, 93: 23
Velopharyngeal
  inadequacy, in children, pharyngeal flap
    for upper airway in, 95: 184
  insufficiency, plastic surgery speech
    pathology interaction in, 95: 191
Velopharyngoplasty
  self-lined superiorly based pull-through,
    plastic surgery and speech
    pathology interaction in
    velopharyngeal insufficiency,
    95: 191
Ventilation tube
  with antibiotic eardrops, prophylactic,
    93: 79
  in atelectasis surgery, 93: 92
  blockage, antibiotic/steroid ear drops
    for, 94: 111
  for lignocaine in tinnitus, 93: 32
  middle ear effusion, minimal, indicating,
    in vomiting infant, 94: 111
  otorrhea after, 93: 79
  removal, tympanic membrane
    perforation after, in children,
    94: 115
  surgery in chronic otitis media with
    effusion, 93: 70
  swimming and otorrhea, 94: 113
Ventricle
  fibrillation after cocaine and
    epinephrine for nasal surgery,
    93: 315
Vermilion
  deficiency, major, after cleft lip repair,
    bipedicled axial cross-lip flap to
    correct, 95: 206
Vertigo
  benign paroxysmal positional, after
    vestibular neuronitis, 94: 6

inner ear, vestibular neurectomy for,
  93: 11
in Ménière's disease, endolymphatic sac
  surgery efficacy in, 94: 14
sudden deafness and, outcome, 95: 12
surgery, in nonserviceable hearing ear,
  95: 23
in temporomandibular disorder, 93: 8
Vessels
  decompression surgery for severe
    tinnitus, selection criteria and
    results, 94: 41
  head and neck lesions, interventional
    radiology in, 93: 245
  malformations
    capillary, tunable pulsed-dye laser for,
      95: 202
    distinguishing soft tissue hemangioma
      from, 93: 186
    of head and neck, MRI of, 94: 246
  proliferation of thyroid, complicating
    fine needle aspiration, 94: 248
Vestibule
  autorotation in dizziness, 95: 7
  compensation in vestibular neuronitis,
    long-term follow-up, 94: 9
  consequences of ear blast injury, 95: 44
  disturbances in middle ear effusion in
    children, 93: 44
  enlarged vestibular aqueduct syndrome,
    95: 5
  function, 94: 5, 95: 5
    loss, with oscillopsia, 94: 10
    patterns after vestibular nerve section,
      93: 10
  immune injury after immune reaction of
    endolymphatic sac, 95: 19
  labyrinth, middle ear effusion and,
    93: 43
  Ménière's disease, diagnosis with
    electrocochleography, 94: 16
  nerve (see Nerve, vestibular)
  neurectomy, for inner ear vertigo,
    93: 11
  neuronitis (see Neuronitis, vestibular)
  peripheral, disorders
    electronystagmography in, 93: 7
    exercise in, conditioning, 93: 9
    vestibular rehabilitation and, 93: 9
  rehabilitation, 94: 20
    dizziness and imbalance after, 93: 9
    vestibular disorders and, peripheral,
      93: 9
  symptoms, and central disorders, 93: 9
  system
    effect of transdermal scopolamine on,
      94: 13
    recovery after injury, 93: 10

test battery, standardization of, 93: 7
testing equipment, 93: 3
Vestibulopathy
   high impact aerobics inducing, 95: 10
Vicryl
   mesh implant for orbital floor fracture
      repair, causing diplopia, 95: 183
Videostroboscopy
   in vocal fold paralysis, 93: 221
Violence
   family, and physical abuse of children,
      93: 291
Viruses
   influenza A, effect on ciliary activity and
      dye transport function in eustachian
      tube (in chinchilla), 94: 105
   rhinovirus 39 infection in nasal response
      to histamine and cold air challenges
      in allergy, 95: 178
   in upper respiratory infection before
      vestibular neuronitis, 94: 8
Vision
   preservation in Graves' ophthalmopathy,
      orbital decompression for, 94: 183
Vitamin
   E and oral carcinogenesis, 93: 303
   supplement to reduce risk of oral and
      pharyngeal cancer, 93: 302
Vocal
   cord augmentation
      collagen for, 93: 212
      with fat, autologous, 93: 210
      Teflon for, 93: 212
   cord fixation, bilateral midline, laryngeal
      muscular tenotomy for, 95: 223
   cord paralysis, fiberoptic laryngoscopy
      of, 93: 223
   fold
      paralysis, videostroboscopy of,
         93: 221
      problems, injectable collagen in,
         93: 207
   quality
      in aged, 93: 206
      long-term changes after Isshiki
         thyroplasty type I, 95: 227
Vomiting
   after tonsillectomy in children,
      metoclopramide reducing, 93: 316
   protracted, in infant, with minimal
      middle ear effusion indicating
      ventilation tubes, 94: 111

W

Walkman

causing noise-induced hearing loss,
   93: 18
Wardill-Kilner technique
   for cleft palate, experience with,
      95: 194
Water
   exposure, effect after tympanostomy
      tube insertion, 95: 106
   fluoridation, drinking, effect on hearing
      in otosclerosis in low fluoride area,
      95: 65
   tap, vs. sterile saline for cleaning acute
      trauma soft tissue wounds, 94: 181
Wegener's granulomatosis (*see*
      Granulomatosis, Wegener's)
Weight
   loss, tinnitus causing (in rat), 93: 29
Whiplash
   injury of neck, cerebral symptoms after,
      94: 277
Wire
   fixation in midfacial trauma, and
      postoperative infection rates,
      94: 169
   splints, vestibular and lingual, in
      mandibular fracture, 93: 164
Wood dust exposure
   increasing risk of adenocarcinoma of
      sinonasal cavities, 94: 159
Work
   of breathing in tracheostomy tubes,
      95: 221
Wound
   adults, scarring control by neutralizing
      antibody to transforming growth
      factor β, 93: 130
   contraction, living skin substitute for,
      93: 137
   healing (*see* Healing, wound)
   infection, postoperative, for poor
      prognosis in head and neck cancer,
      94: 236
   skin, explants in tissue culture, 93: 137
   soft tissue, acute traumatic, sterile saline
      vs. tap water for cleaning, 94: 181
   tension in rhytidectomy, skin flap
      undermining and
      musculoaponeurotic system
      suspension in, 94: 202

X

X-ray
   films, sinus, use by general practitioners,
      95: 173
   therapy for sinus enlargement in infancy,
      thyroid cancer after, 95: 288

Xenograft
  vs. autograft for tympanoplasty, 95: 117
Xylocaine
  in tinnitus, 93: 32
Xylometazoline
  lidocaine solution, vasoconstrictive and
      anesthetic effects, vs. intranasal
      cocaine, 94: 164

Z

Zoster
  oticus
      acyclovir in, 93: 55
      steroids in, 93: 55
Zygoma
  calvarial bone graft for, 94: 191

Author Index

A

Aalto H, 61
Achauer BM, 202
Adamson PA, 200
Ahmad K, 245
Aitchison FA, 173
Al-Sarraf M, 242, 245
Altissimi G, 226
Amble FR, 76
Anderl H, 148
Anderson JR, 174
Andresen E, 288
Aoki H, 101
Applebaum EL, 141
Arcamone D, 226
Ariyan S, 156
Aslan T, 179
Austin DF, 104, 281
Austin JR, 84
Austin SG, 84
Avraham A, 234
Axelson O, 277

B

Backhaus JW, 172
Bagger-Sjöbäck D, 13
Bailey HAT Jr, 67
Baker TM, 204
Ballester E, 163
Barna BP, 26
Baroody FM, 171
Bartels J, 113
Bartlett SP, 139
Bartoshuk LM, 90
Basch C, 172
Bass JW, 283
Battista RA, 66
Beck RA, 283
Becker CJ, 5
Belenky WM, 5
Belser R, 52
Ben-David J, 57
Benninger MS, 136, 239
Berg Rvd, 124
Berger SI, 57
Bergstralh EJ, 246
Berke GS, 218
Berman S, 37
Berti C, 269
Berwick M, 284
Besteiro JM, 87
Biller HF, 132, 181, 270
Bizzaro N, 167
Blackwell KE, 48
Blank C, 244
Blatter DD, 49
Blot WJ, 281
Bonding P, 54
Borum P, 34
Boyd JB, 192

Bradford CR, 189, 250
Briant D, 252
Brightwell AP, 175
Brokx JPL, 30
Brook I, 118
Brook RH, 105
Brown TP, 103
Browner I, 276
Buchbinder D, 132
Buchman SR, 139
Bucky LP, 157
Bumsted R, 176
Bundo J, 111
Burgess BJ, 28
Burkey BB, 189
Burnett A, 268
Burrow GN, 233
Burt RD, 284
Busse WW, 172

C

Cafferkey MT, 263
Calcaterra TC, 237
Caldarelli DD, 164
Calhoun KH, 225
Callanan VP, 117
Campbell BH, 242
Cannito MP, 191
Cannoni M, 170
Canonico D, 244
Carroll WR, 189, 250
Casasco A, 246
Casiano RR, 245
Caslin AW, 254
Castro F, 170
Catalano P, 270
Catton P, 131
Chang BW, 196
Chang HK, 137
Chen NT, 157
Chepeha DB, 143
Choi H-S, 218
Clark OH, 233
Cohen O, 47
Constantinides MS, 200
Corey JP, 176
Courtiss EH, 204, 213
Crabtree JA, 96
Cremers CWRJ, 125
Cummings CW, 222
Curran AJ, 117

D

D'Amelio LF, 228
Damm M, 229
Daube JR, 247
Davidson J, 252
Davis WE, 221
Davis WL, 49
Day GL, 281

Deffresne D, 246
DeGroot LJ, 243
Delaere PR, 160
DeSanto LW, 251
Dessi P, 170
De Vries N, 275
Dharker D, 253
Diamond JS, 174
Diaz-Ordaz EA, 68
Dietz RR, 49
Disher MJ, 185
Dobie RA, 20
Dodd KT, 113
Donaldson I, 38
Dornhoffer JL, 67
Douglas NJ, 262
Doweck I, 44
Doyle PJ, 143
Doyle WJ, 178
Drago P, 52
Drake AF, 184, 261
Dreschler WA, 124
Druce HM, 172
Drulović B, 31
Dubois RW, 105
Duff BE, 141
Duh Q-Y, 233
Dvoretsky P, 288
Dyer WK II, 199

E

Eason AL, 138
East CA, 279
Eckel HE, 229
Eiselt-Proteau D, 169
Elander A, 194
Ellis H, 267
Emerick GT, 233
Enrique RR, 239
Erkan M, 179
Ervin TJ, 242
Esclamado RM, 157, 185, 189, 250
Esko E, 150
Eskola J, 280
Evans PJ, 151

F

Fabre JW, 119
Facer GW, 76
Falk T, 52
Falkow S, 150
Farioli L, 269
Fee WE Jr, 208
Feenstra L, 160
Feiglin H, 57
Feinmesser R, 47, 234
Feinstein AR, 235
Fenton JE, 42
Ferreira MC, 87

Ferrette V, 276
Fiala TGS, 132
Finkelman RD, 138
Finkelstein Y, 108, 265
Fireman P, 178
Fisch U, 50
Fischer ND, 261
Fleming DM, 38
Flint PW, 222
Flynn SD, 238
Fooanant S, 51
Fradis M, 57
Fraumeni JF Jr, 281
Freeman DF, 263
Frenz W, 52
Friedberg J, 100
Friede H, 194
Funk GF, 154
Furuta H, 15

G

Gaffney RJ, 263
Gahbauer RA, 242
Gallati V, 50
Gallucci L, 226
Gantous A, 131
Garth RJN, 175
Gay T, 146, 155
Geelhoed GW, 238
Genden E, 132
George B, 246
Gilbert JG, 107
Gilbert PM, 209
Glarner H, 50
Glasgold AI, 210, 214
Glasgold MJ, 210
Glasscock ME III, 86
Gleich LL, 32
Glover MT, 287
Glowacki J, 157
Goepfert H, 195, 231
Goldwyn RM, 213
Golledge J, 267
Gordon CR, 44
Gormley PK, 117
Gotoh Y, 19
Goycoolea MV, 79, 98
Grace ARG, 224
Graham SS, 67
Greco RJ, 203
Greenberg RS, 281
Gruber B, 285
Guilleminault C, 258
Gullane P, 252
Guyuron B, 205
Gwaltney JM, 178
Gyo K, 121

H

Haapaniemi T, 147

Haga D, 266
Haines SJ, 88
Hall RA, 20
Hammond JS, 228
Hannenberg AA, 213
Harada T, 33
Harari PM, 251
Hardesty RA, 138
Harner SG, 76
Harnsberger HR, 49
Hartig GK, 157
Hartviksen G, 266
Haruna S-I, 110
Harvey SA, 58
Haselow RE, 242
Hassan SJ, 240
Hatschek T, 277
Havlik R, 156
Hawkins DB, 272
Haxby D, 169
Hay ID, 246
Hazuka MB, 241
Hedges JR, 169
Henley CM, 62
Herbreteau D, 246
Hildreth N, 288
Hillman DE, 35
Hinderink JB, 30
Hinohira Y, 121
Hinson J Jr, 221
Ho CM, 137
Hof E, 50
Holinger LD, 141
Holmberg D, 131
Hong H-Z, 157
Hoshikawa H, 15
Hotaling AJ, 5
Houdart E, 246
Houghton DJ, 173
Houlden D, 151
Huang T-S, 22, 78
Hughes GB, 26, 70
Hughes LF, 20
Hunter RE, 62
Hyrkäs T, 190

I

Iizuka T, 190
Ikezono T, 19
Incorvaia C, 269
Innes DJ, 271
Ishizaki H, 61
Ispano M, 269
Isshiki N, 152
Itaya T, 6
Ito J, 63
Iwahira Y, 188

J

Jackler RK, 91, 115

Jackson CG, 86
Jackson IJB, 224
Jacobs IN, 73
Jacobs JM, 49
Jacobs JR, 242, 245
Janecka IP, 41
Joffe JM, 213
Johns DF, 191
Johnson JT, 231, 232
Jones AS, 254
Jovanovic A, 275
Juillard G, 237

K

Kaasinen S, 60
Kaczor J, 136
Kagey-Sobotka A, 171
Kahlstrom EJ, 272
Kallela I, 190
Kambiss S, 283
Kamide Y, 112
Kangsanarak J, 51
Kanzaki J, 8
Kaplan EL, 243
Karjalainen S, 65
Kartush JM, 68
Kashgarian M, 17
Kasperbauer JL, 221
Kato BM, 115
Kato H, 111
Katsantonis GP, 217
Kavanagh KT, 158
Kaye JM, 37
Keane T, 252
Keller J, 132
Kessler A, 116, 123
Ketten DR, 28
Kikuchi S, 33
Kim W-K, 157
Kinder B, 238
King JM, 164
Kitahara M, 6
Klein KW, 11
Kleinman LC, 105
Knapp R, 148
Ko WH, 52
Kobayashi T, 59
Koç N, 179
Kokatsu T, 145
Kong J, 221
Kosecoff J, 105
Kostense PJ, 275
Kostić VS, 31
Kozol RA, 238
Kraut R, 183
Kreiman J, 218
Kreutziger KL, 248
Kroll SS, 195
Kuga Y, 140
Kump K, 276
Kveton JF, 17, 90
Kwan JTC, 287

L

Langman AW, 23
Laramore G, 245
Laramore GE, 242
Law M, 278
Leder SB, 227
Lee AJ, 115
Lee FP, 78
Lee SP, 237
Leider JS, 5
Leigh IM, 287
LeRoy JL Jr, 212
Levine SC, 88
Levy R, 47, 234
Li W, 43
Lichtenstein LM, 171
Lichter AS, 241
Liff JM, 281
Lilja J, 194
Lim J, 35
Lin C-C, 22
Lindeman RC, 23
Lindqvist C, 190
Linstrom CJ, 32
Lippy WH, 66
Lohmander-Agerskov A, 194
Loree TR, 253
Loscalzo G, 37
Lubin E, 234
Luke M, 262
Lurie AG, 146

M

McCabe BF, 46
McCaffrey TV, 246
McDonald TJ, 76
MacDougall G, 257
McGee TM, 68
McGraw-Wall BL, 200
McKellop HA, 154
McKenna P, 203
Mackinnon SE, 151
Macknin ML, 96
MacLaughlin EF, 272
McLaughlin JK, 281
McMenamin P, 282
McMenomey SO, 86
Maddox MR, 106
Madgy DN, 5
Maloney AP, 219
Maly PV, 268
Maniglia AJ, 52
Manson PN, 196
Maragos NE, 221
Marchi M, 195
Marlowe FI, 37
Marsh RR, 116, 123
Martel MK, 241
Maruguchi T, 152
Maruguchi Y, 152
Maruyama Y, 188

Mathur R, 262
Matsuda K, 152
Matsune S, 101
Matsuo T, 140
Mauriello JA Jr, 183
Mechlis-Frish S, 234
Meltzer EO, 172
Mens LHM, 30
Merland JJ, 246
Metson R, 186
Metzger WJ, 172
Meuli M, 50
Meyerhoff WL, 92
Meyers A, 45
Millen SJ, 58
Miller MJ, 195
Miltenburg DM, 25
Milton CM, 119
Minor LB, 86
Mitchell DQ, 172
Miyazaki S, 217
Mizuno A, 140
Mochimatsu I, 145
Mogi G, 111
Monacelli C, 226
Montgomery PQ, 272
Montserrat JM, 163
Moreano EH, 79, 98
Mori N, 15
Morris MR, 244
Morrison MD, 219
Morrow TA, 200
Moscicki R, 26
Moscoso JF, 132
Moseson M, 288
Mosier K, 146
Moss K, 217
Mounsey RA, 192
Mühlbauer W, 148
Mullins JB, 221
Mullol J, 163
Murphy TP, 7
Myers EN, 232
Mylanus EAM, 125

N

Nachmani A, 265
Nachtigal D, 44
Naclerio RM, 171
Nadal D, 50
Nadol JB Jr, 28
Naguib MB, 62
Nakashima T, 12
Namon A, 176
Navacharoen N, 51
Neel HB III, 251
Netterville JL, 133
Newman MH, 206
Nichols RD, 239
Nielsen OA, 34
Nilsson G, 147
Niranjan N, 287
Nisperos B, 284

Nolan WB III, 212
Nonaka M, 19
Noorily AD, 165
Novelline RA, 132
Nuutinen J, 65
Nylander G, 147

O

Ogren FP, 174
Ohyama K, 59
Olsen KD, 247, 251
Ophir D, 108, 265
Orgel HA, 172
Ortolani C, 269
O'Sullivan TJ, 42
Otto RA, 169
Özcan M, 179

P

Padilla JF III, 202
Panarese A, 254
Panje W, 176
Paparella MM, 43, 79, 98,
   110, 112
Pappas DG, 35
Parker GS, 106
Pasternack B, 288
Pastorello EA, 269
Patow CA, 113
Paukku P, 190
Pedersen S, 266
Pellinen P, 65
Peltola H, 280
Perkins SW, 199
Persson E-C, 194
Peskind SP, 84
Petty P, 196
Phillips JH, 131
Piazza I, 167
Picado C, 163
Piccirillo JF, 235
Pigato JB, 164
Podoshin L, 57
Potsic WP, 73, 116, 123
Powell NB, 258
Prasad S, 41
Prattichizzo L, 226
Pravettoni V, 269
Premachandra DJ, 119
Preston-Martin S, 281
Prior AJ, 272
Pulec JL, 82, 88
Puliafito CA, 186
Purcell LL, 222
Pyykkö I, 61

R

Rakijian DR, 138
Ramchandani D, 37

Rawlinson E, 252
Redleaf MI, 46
Redline S, 276
Reece GP, 195
Reed EC, 174
Rees TD, 212
Reinhart DJ, 11
Rendell JK, 146, 155
Rennard SI, 174
Ribarić-Jankes K, 31
Rice DH, 84
Richardson GL, 224
Riley RW, 258
Rizer FM, 66
Roa WHY, 241
Robbins RA, 174
Robinson M, 69
Robinson P, 166
Roddi R, 209
Rohrich RJ, 191
Roland NJ, 254
Roland PS, 92
Rontal E, 223
Rontal M, 223
Rosenbaum M, 52
Roth B, 229
Rothschild MA, 270
Ruckphaopunt K, 51
Rueger RM, 231
Ryan R, 166
Ryan RM, 279

S

Sahupak A, 44
St Geme JW III, 150
Sakai CS, 165, 169
Sakai S-I, 15
Sakakihara J, 63
Sakumoto M, 145
Sakurada T, 59
Salomon G, 54
Sanderson RJ, 257
Sandler HM, 241
Sando I, 101
San Martin JE, 26
Sano S, 112
Sano S-I, 110
Santos PM, 20
Sarkar S, 281
Sarkaria JN, 251
Sasaki CT, 227, 235
Sasaki Y, 121
Schachern PA, 43, 110, 112
Schindler B, 37
Schloss B, 264
Schloss MD, 264
Schoenberg JB, 281
Schreck S, 137
Schroff E, 11
Schuller D, 245
Schuller DE, 242
Schulten EAJM, 275

Schuring AG, 66
Schusterman MA, 195
Schwade JG, 242
Schwarz DWF, 143
Scott CB, 242, 245
Scott NM, 115
Segal K, 47, 234
Seicshnaydre MA, 70
Sekhar HKC, 35
Selesnick SH, 91, 95
Selner JC, 172
Senders CW, 142
Sergeant RJ, 119
Seroky JT, 178
Serra-Batlles J, 163
Shabtai A, 108
Shah JP, 253
Shapiro GG, 172
Shih L, 96
Shimizu KT, 237
Shimoni A, 234
Shindo ML, 272
Shore RE, 281, 288
Shpitzer T, 47
Shukla MS, 243
Silver FH, 214
Simo F, 199
Siperstein AE, 233
Sirsjö A, 147
Sismanis A, 70
Sisson JH, 174
Skoner DP, 178
Slavit DH, 221
Smith LF, 225
Smith PA, 254
Snik AFM, 30, 125
Snow GB, 275
Snyder JM, 20
Söderpalm E, 194
Spain DA, 228
Spiro J, 146, 155
Spitzer O, 44
Srinivasan V, 272
Stanley RB Jr, 154
Stauffer UG, 50
Stenson K, 285
Stern Y, 47
Šternić N, 31
Stone C, 136
Strachan DR, 224
Strasnick B, 86
Straus FH, 243
Strauss M, 108
Streitmann MJ, 169
Strong EW, 253
Sullivan KJ, 137
Sullivan MJ, 185, 250
Suman VJ, 251
Sundgren PC, 268
Suntioinen S, 65
Sutyak JP, 228
Suzuki S, 152
Swanson M, 284

T

Takahashi H, 101
Takahashi M, 8
Takala A, 150
Takala AK, 280
Takasaka T, 59
Takei Y, 8
Talmi YP, 108
Talo H, 96
Tami TA, 106
Tan AKW, 264
Tang JL, 278
Tange RA, 124
Tarver CP, 165
Tebbetts JB, 191
Telian SA, 157
Templer JW, 221
Teotrakul S, 51
Terris DJ, 208
Tewfik TL, 264
Thomas JV, 251
Thornton AF, 241
Timon CI, 263
Tinling SP, 142
Tishler PV, 276
Toda K-I, 152
Todd DH, 45
Tominaga K, 140
Tomiyama S, 19
Toriyabe I, 8
Tos M, 54
Tran LM, 237
Tran Ba Huy P, 246
Trevino RJ, 168
Triglia JM, 170
Tsukuda M, 145
Tuffo KM, 208
Tuma P Jr, 87
Turnbull LS, 254
Turrisi AT, 241
Tutundzhyan Y, 138
Twerdy K, 148

U

Uhl E, 147
Urba S, 241
Urken ML, 132, 181

V

Van Bavel JH, 172
Van Damme B, 160
van den Berge NW, 125
van den Broek P, 30
VanderBrug Medendorp S, 96
Vander Kam VM, 202
van der Meulen JC, 209
Van Der Tol IGH, 275
Van Der Waal I, 275
Vartiainen E, 65

Vaughan TL, 284
Von Schoenberg M, 166
Vrabec JT, 133

W

Wackym PA, 48
Wagenmann M, 171
Wagner JD, 206
Wagner RL, 231, 232
Wald N, 278
Walsh J, 217
Walsh MA, 263
Walsted A, 34
Warren DW, 184
Wasserman B, 183
Watanabe N, 111
Wei WI, 120
Weiland LH, 76
Weinberg H, 132
Weinberger JM, 151
Weintraub MI, 10
Wells CK, 235
Wenig BL, 141
Wenig BM, 141
Werning J, 52

Westerberg BD, 143
Weymuller EA Jr, 240, 245
Wheatley M, 203
Wheeler R, 242
Whitaker LA, 139
White C, 279
Wicke K, 148
Widemann B, 229
Wilkinson L, 173
Wilson JA, 173
Wilson JF, 106
Wilson PS, 38
Wingren G, 277
Winther B, 271
Witsell DL, 184
Wolf GT, 241
Woodson GE, 220
Woodward B, 119
Woog JJ, 186
Wornom IL III, 139

X

Xaubet A, 163

Y

Yagi M, 33
Yagi T, 19
Yago T, 145
Yamasoba T, 33
Yanagihara N, 121
Yanagita N, 12
Yaremchuk MJ, 132, 157
Ye M, 218
Yeates DB, 141
Yuen PW, 120

Z

Zanaret M, 170
Zanon E, 148
Zanussi C, 269
Zarandy S, 205
Zatz S, 234
Zechnich AD, 169
Zelterman D, 79, 98
Zhu W-L, 52
Zohar Y, 108
Zuidema T, 124
Zur Nedden D, 148